Oxford Handbook of
Clinical Dentistry

Fourth edition

**David A. Mitchell and
Laura Mitchell**

with contributions from

Paul Brunton

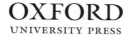
OXFORD
UNIVERSITY PRESS

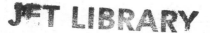

OXFORD

UNIVERSITY PRESS

Great Clarendon Street, Oxford OX2 6DP

Oxford New York

Auckland Bangkok Buenos Aires Cape Town Chennai
Dar es Salaam Delhi Hong Kong Istanbul Karachi Kolkata
Kuala Lumpur Madrid Melbourne Mexico City Mumbai
Nairobi São Paulo Shanghai Taipei Tokyo Toronto

Oxford is a trade mark of Oxford University Press

Published in the United States
by Oxford University Press, Inc., New York

First published 1991
Second edition 1995
Reprinted 1996, 1997
Third edition 1999
Reprinted 2000, 2001, 2003
Fourth edition 2005

The moral rights of the author have been asserted

British Library Cataloguing in Publication Data

Data available

Library of Congress Cataloging in Publication Data
ISBN 0-19-852920-1

1 3 5 7 9 10 8 6 4 2

Typeset by Newgen Imaging Systems (P) Ltd., Chennai, India
Printed in Italy
on by acid-free paper by Lego Print s.r.l.

Preface to the first edition

Dental students are introduced to real live patients at an early stage of their undergraduate course in order to fulfil the requirements for clinical training, with the result that they are expected to absorb a large quantity of information in a relatively short time. This is often compounded by clinical allocations to different specialities on different days, or even the same day. Given the obvious success of the Oxford handbooks of clinical medicine and clinical specialties, evidenced by their position in the white coat pockets of the nation's medical students, the extension of the same format to dentistry seems logical. However, it is hoped that the usefulness of this idea will not cease on graduation, particularly with the introduction of Vocational Training. While providing a handy reference for the recently qualified graduate, it is envisaged that trainers will also welcome an aide mémoire to help cope with the enthusiastic young trainee who may be more familiar with recent innovations and obscure facts. We also hope that there will be much of value for the hospital trainee struggling towards FDS.

The *Oxford Handbook of Clinical Dentistry* contains those useful facts and practical tips that were stored in our white coat pockets as students and then postgraduates; initially on scraps of paper, but as the collection grew, transferred into notebooks to give a readily available reference source.

The dental literature already contains a great number of erudite books which, for the most part deal exclusively, in some depth, with a particular branch or aspect of dentistry. The aim of this handbook is not to replace these specialist dental texts, but rather to complement them by distilling together theory and practical information into a more accessible format. In fact, reference is made to sources of further reading where necessary.

Although the authors of this handbook are not the specialized authorities usually associated with dental textbooks, we are still near enough to the coal-face to provide, we hope, some useful practical tips based on sound theory. We were fortunate whilst compiling this handbook in being able to draw on the expertise of many colleagues; the contents, however, remain our sole responsibility. The format of a blank page opposite each page of text has been plagiarized from the other Oxford handbooks. This gives space for the reader to add his own comments and updates. Please let us know of any that should be made available to a wider audience.

We hope that the reader will find this book to be a useful addition to their white coat pocket or a companion to the BNF in the surgery.

Preface to the second edition

It would appear that our 'baby' is now a toddler and rapidly outgrowing his previous milieu. Caring for such a precocious child is hard work and therefore we have again relied on the help of understanding friends and colleagues who have contributed their knowledge and expertise.

The pace of change in dentistry, both scientifically and politically, is so fast that although the first edition was only published in 1991, this second edition has involved extensive revision of all chapters. Advances in dental materials and restorative techniques have necessitated major revision of these sections and we are indebted to Mr Andrew Hall, who has helped update the chapter on restorative dentistry.

Since the first edition was published, political changes in the UK have resulted in a shift towards private dentistry. This changing emphasis is reflected in the practice management chapter, which now includes a new page on independent and private practice. In addition recent developments in cross-infection control and UK health and safety law have been included.

That old favourite, temporomandibular pain dysfunction syndrome, has also been given the treatment and is now situated on a newly devised page in the chapter on oral medicine. Non-accidental injury, guided tissue regeneration, AIDS, ATLS, and numerous other topical issues have been expanded in this edition.

One aspect of this developing infant remains, however, unchanged. The sole purpose of this book is to enable you, the reader, to gain easy access to the sometimes confusing conglomerate of facts, ideas, opinions, dogma, anecdote, and truth that constitutes clinical dentistry. To this framework you should add, on the blank pages provided, the additional information which will help you treat the next patient or pass the next exam, or more importantly the practical hints and tips which you will glean with experience. It is the potential for that interaction which makes this book distinctive in clinical dentistry. It is participating in that interaction which makes your book unique.

Preface to the third edition

Like any proud parents we are surprised and delighted with the continued development of our 'baby', and we are grateful to all those who have helped or provided positive feedback. We are also grateful to our colleagues who have helped with the 'baby-care'.

Of course, now being of school age, peer group rivalry has arrived, but ours is a robust child and despite being the first kid on the block welcomes both competition and change.

Some of this change is reflected by bringing in a new contributor who has overseen a complete overhaul of the restorative dentistry chapters and a large number of new contributions to reflect dentistry in the late 1990s.

Our own areas of (increasingly erudite) specialist expertise have grown apace but we think we have curbed the temptation to dwell on these in what is, after all, a generalist text for the earlier years; we trust the odd excursion will be forgiven.

We hope that the new sections, which include: evidence-based medicine/dentistry; the new NHS complaints procedure, objective structured clinical examinations, the 1997 Advanced Life Support Guidelines, and the completely revised restorative chapters will prove helpful and informative. We would, however, like to remind you that the blank pages are there for your additional notes—and it is this that makes your copy of this Handbook unique. Please do not hesitate to share these annotations with us, we would be happy to include the best we receive in the next edition and to acknowledge the contributor.

As always while we are grateful for the contributions of our colleagues the contents and the brickbats remain our sole responsibility.

Preface to the fourth edition

A new millennium means new technology and new challenges.

So the time has come to update the *Oxford Handbook of Clinical Dentistry*. In fact the pace of change is such that all chapters in this new edition have been completely revised. To continue the analogy of earlier prefaces: our teenager is keen on exploring new avenues, so we are going to indulge this by expanding our horizons into new attitudes and technology with a section on Dentistry and the World Wide Web, and also a section on web-based learning. This new, twenty-first century edition has the added bonus of colour plates and more diagrams to aid understanding.

We are, as ever, indebted to contributors past and present. The new recruits bring both knowledge and enthusiasm to their areas of expertise as well as to the book as a whole, and build on the work of previous contributors. To all we are greatly indebted. The ultimate responsibility for errors or oversights remains, as always, ours.

Please keep sending us feedback—this is the best way for us to improve future editions.

Let's just hope the teenager doesn't rebel!!

Acknowledgements

In addition to those readers whose comments and suggestions have been incorporated into the fourth edition, we would like to thank the following for their time and expertise: Mr N. Barnard, Mr P. Chambers, Dr Abdul Dalghous, Dr I. D. Grime, Mr S. Fayle, Dr H. Gorton, Mr W. Jones, Ms E. McDerra and Dr J. E. Paul. Thanks also to Dr R. Dookun for his helpful comments.

In addition, this book is the sum and distillate of its previous incarnations, which would not have been possible without Mr B. S. Avery, Ms F. Carmichael, Mr N. E. Carter, Mr M. Chan, Mrs J. J. Davison, Ms S. Dowsett, Dr C. Flynn, Ms V. Hind, Mr A. Hall, Mr H. Harvie, Dr J. Hunton, Mr D. Jacobs, Ms K. Laidler, Mr C. Lloyd, Mr P. J. Knibbs, Mr M. Manogue, Professor J. F. McCabe, Dr B. Nattress, Mr R. A. Ord, Professor A. Rugg-Gunn, Professor R. A. Seymour, Professor J. V. Soames, Ms A. Tugnait, Dr D. Wood, and Professor R. Yemm.

We are grateful to the editor of the *BMJ*, the *BDJ* and Professor M. Harris, the Royal National Institute of the Deaf, Laerdal, and the Resuscitation Council UK for granting permission to use their diagrams, and VUMAN for allowing us to include the Index of Orthodontic Treatment Need.

Once again the staff of OUP deserve thanks for their help and encouragement.

Note Although this is an equal opportunity publication, the constraints of space have meant that in some places we have had to use 'he' or 'their' to indicate 'he/she', 'his/hers', etc.

Contents

List of colour plates

Symbols and abbreviations

Some of these are included because they are in common usage, others because they are big words and we were trying to save space.

▶	this is important
Δ	diagnosis
$	supernumerary
−ve	negative
+ve	positive
&/or	and/or
↑	increased
↓	decreased
<	lesser than
>	greater than
~	approximately
#	fracture
μ	micro (e.g. μg, μm)
?	question/ask about (when ? appears alone)
∴	therefore
1°	primary
2°	secondary
3°	tertiary
5̅; i̅n̅c̅	lower second premolar, lower incisor
2̲; i̲n̲c̲	upper lateral incisor, upper incisor
ACS	American College of Surgeons
ACTH	adrenocorticotrophic hormone
ADH	antidiuretic hormone
ADJ	amelo-dentinal junction
Ag	antigen
AIDS	acquired immune deficiency syndrome
ALS	advanced life support
AP	antero-posterior
APPT	activated partial thromboplastin time
ARF	acute renal failure
ASAP	as soon as possible
ATLS	advanced trauma life support
AZT	3'-azido-3'-deoxythimidine
BCC	basal cell carcinoma
bd	twice daily
BDA	British Dental Association
BDJ	*British Dental Journal*
BIPP	bismuth iodoform paraffin paste
BLS	basic life support
b/w	bitewing radiograph
BMA	British Medical Association
BNF	British National Formulary
BP	blood pressure

BSS	black silk suture
Ca^{2+}	calcium
CAP	chronic adult periodontitis
C&S	culture and sensitivity
CDS	Community Dental Service
CEJ	cemento-enamel junction
C/I	contraindication
Class I	Class I relationship
Class II/1	Class II division 1 relationship
Class II/2	Class II division 2 relationship
Class III	Class III relationship
CLP	cleft lip and palate
cm	centimetre
CMV	cytomegalovirus
CNS	central nervous system
C/O	complaining of
COPD	chronic obstructive pulmonary disease
CPR	cardiopulmonary resuscitation
CSF	cerebrospinal fluid
CSM	Committee on Safety of Medicines
CT	computed tomography
CVA	cerebro-vascular accident
CVS	cardiovascular system
CXR	chest X-ray
dl	decilitre
DMARD	disease modifying antirheumatic drug
DMF	Decayed, Missing, Filled
DN	dental nurse
DNA	did not attend
DOH/DH	Department of Health
DPB	Dental Practice Board
DPF	Dental Practitioner's Formulary
DPT	dental panoramic tomogram (politically correct: OPT/OPG)
DVT	deep venous thrombosis
EBM/D	evidence-based medicine/dentistry
EBV	Epstein–Barr virus
ECG	electrocardiograph
EDTA	ethylene diamine tetraacetic acid
e.g.	for example
EMD	enamel matrix derivative
EMLA	eutectic mix of lignocaine and prilocaine
ENT	ear, nose, and throat
EO	extra-oral
ESR	erythrocyte sedimentation rate
EUA	examination under anaesthesia
F	female
F/-	full upper denture (and -/F for lower)
FA	fixed appliance
FABP	flat anterior bite plane
FB	foreign body
FBC	full blood count

Fe	iron
FESS	functional endoscopic sinus surgery
fl	femtolitre
FNAC	fine-needle aspiration cytology
f/s	flssure sealant
FWS	freeway space
g	gram
GA	general anaesthesia
GAP	generalized aggressive periodontitis
GDC	General Dental Council
GDP	general dental practitioner
GDS	General Dental Services
GI	glass ionomer
GKI	glucose, potassium, insulin
GMP	general medical practitioner
GP	gutta-percha
GTR	guided-tissue regeneration
h	hour
H2	histamine 2 receptor antagonist
HA	Health Authority
Hb	haemoglobin
HBeAg	hepatitis B e antigen (high-risk marker)
HBsAg	hepatitis B surface antigen
HDU	high dependency unit
Hep B/C	hepatitis B/C
Hg	mercury
HIV	human immunodeficiency virus
HLA	human leucocyte antigen
HPV	human papilloma virus
HRT	hormone replacement therapy
HSV	herpes simplex virus
i.e.	that is
ICP	intercuspal position
ICU	intensive care unit
ID	inferior dental
IDB	inferior dental block
IDN	inferior dental nerve
IE	infective endocarditis
Ig	immunoglobulin (e.g. IgA, IgG, etc.)
IM	intramuscular
IMF	intermaxillary fixation
inc	incisor
INR	International Normalized Ratio
IO	intra-oral
ITP	idiopathic thrombocytopenic purpura
IU	international units
IV	intravenous
JP	juvenile periodontitis
K$^+$	potassium
KCT	kaolin–cephalin clotting time
kg	kilogram

kV	kilovolt
l	litre
LA	local anaesthesia
LAP	localized aggressive periodontitis
LFH	lower face height
LFT	liver function test
LLS	lower labial segment
LMA	laryngeal mask airway
m	metre
M	male
mand	mandible/mandibular
MAOI	monoamine oxidase inhibitor
max	maxilla/maxillary
MCV	mean corpuscular volume
MEN	multiple endocrine neoplasia
mg	milligram
MHz	megahertz
MI	myocardial infarction
micromol	micromoles
min	minute
ml	millilitre
mm	millimetre
mmHg	millimetres of mercury
mmol	millimole
MMPA	maxillary mandibular planes angle
MRI	magnetic resonance imaging
MST	slow release morphine
MSU	mid-stream urine
MTA	mineral trioxide aggregate
NAD	nothing abnormal detected
NAI	non-accidental injury
NGT	naso-gastric tube
NHS	National Health Service
nm	nanometre
nocte	at night
NUG	necrotising ulcerative gingivitis
O_2	oxygen
NSAID	non-steroidal anti-inflammatory drug
o/b	overbite
od	once daily
OD	overdenture
O/E	on examination
OH	oral hygiene
OHCM	*Oxford Handbook of Clinical Medicine*
OHI	oral hygiene instruction
o/j	overjet
OP	out patient
ORIF	open reduction and internal fixation
OTC	over the counter
OVD	occlusal vertical dimension
P/-	partial upper denture (and -/P for lower)

PA	posteroanterior
PCA	patient-controlled analgesia
PCD	professional complementary to dentistry
PCT	Primary Care Trust
PDH	past dental history
PDL	periodontal ligament
PEA	pulseless electrical activity
PEG	percutaneous endoscopic gastrostomy
PFM	porcelain fused to metal (crown)
PJC	porcelain jacket crown
PM	premolar
PMH	past medical history
PMMA	polymethylmethacrylate
PO	per orum (by mouth)
ppm	parts per million
PR	per rectum
prn	as required
PRR	preventive resin restoration
PTFE	(poly)tetrafluoroethene
PU	pass urine
qds	four times daily
RA	relative analgesia
RAS	recurrent aphthous stomatitis
RBC	red blood cell count
RCCT	randomized controlled clinical trial
RCP	retruded contact position
RCT	root canal treatment/therapy
RIG	radiologically inserted gastrostomy
RMGIC	resin-modified glass ionomer composite
Rx	treatment
SC	subcutaneous
SCC	squamous cell carcinoma
sec	second
SF	sugar free
SLE	systemic lupus erythematosus
SS	stainless steel
STD	sexually transmitted diseases
TANI	target average net income
TB	tuberculosis
TC	tungsten carbide
tds	thrice daily
TENS	transcutaneous electrical nerve stimulation
TIBC	total iron binding capacity
TMA	titanium molybdenum alloy
TMJ	temporomandibular joint
TMPDS	temporomandibular pain dysfunction syndrome
TNF	tissue necrosis factor
TTP	tender to percussion
ULS	upper labial segment
URA	upper removable appliance

URTI	upper respiratory tract infection
US (S)	ultrasound (scan)
UTI	urinary tract infection
U&Es	urea and electrolytes
VF	ventricular fibrillation
Xbite	crossbite
X-rays	either X-rays or radiographs
yr	year
ZOE	zinc oxide eugenol

History and examination

Relevant pages in other chapters   It could, of course, be said that all pages are relevant to this section, because history and examination are the first steps in the care of any patient. However, as that is hardly helpful, the reader is referred specifically to the following: dental charting, p. 764; medical conditions, Chapter 11; the child with toothache, p. 66; pre-operative management of the dental patient, p. 584; the cranial nerves, p. 548; orthodontic assessment, p. 140; pulpal pain, p. 260.

Principal sources: Experience.

Listen, look, and learn

Much of what you need to know about any individual patient can be obtained by watching them enter the surgery and sit in the chair, their body language during the interview, and a few well-chosen questions. One of the great secrets of health care is to develop the ability to actually listen to what your patients tell you and to use that information. Doctors and dentists are often concerned that if they allow patients to speak rather than answer questions, history-taking will prove inefficient and prolonged. In fact, most patients will give the information necessary to make a provisional diagnosis, and further useful personal information, if allowed to speak uninterrupted. Most will lapse into silence after 2–3 minutes of monologue. History-taking should be conducted with the patient sitting comfortably; this rarely equates with supine! In order to produce an all-round history it is, however, customary and frequently necessary to resort to directed questioning, here are a few hints:

- Always introduce yourself to the patient and any accompanying person, and explain, if it is not immediately obvious, what your role is in helping them.
- Remember that patients are (usually) neither medically nor dentally trained, so use plain speech without speaking down to them.
- Questions are a key part of history-taking and the manner in which they are asked can lead to a quick diagnosis and a trusting patient, or abject confusion with a potential litigant. Leading questions should be, by and large, be avoided as they impose a preconceived idea upon the patient. This is also a problem when the question suggests the answer, e.g. 'is the pain worse when you drink hot drinks?' To avoid this, phrase questions so that a descriptive reply rather than a straight yes or no is required. However, with the more reticent patient it may be necessary to ask leading questions to elicit relevant information.
- Notwithstanding earlier paragraphs, you will sometimes find it necessary to interrupt patients in full flight during a detailed monologue on their grandmother's sick parrot. Try to do this tactfully, e.g. 'but to come more up to date' or 'this is rather difficult—please slow down and let me understand how this affects the problem you have come about today'.

Specifics of a medical or dental history are described on p. 8 and p. 6. The object is to elicit sufficient information to make a provisional diagnosis for the patient whilst establishing a mutual rapport, thus facilitating further investigations and/or treatment.

Presenting complaint

The aim of this part of the history is to have a provisional differential diagnosis even before examining the patient. The following is a suggested outline, which would require modifying according to the circumstances:

C/O (complaining of) In the patient's own words. Use a general introductory question, e.g., 'Why did you come to see us today? What is the problem?'

Avoid 'What brought you here today?', unless you want to give them the chance to make a joke.

If symptoms are present:

Onset and pattern When did the problem start? Is it getting better, worse or staying the same?

Frequency How often, how long does it last? Does it occur at any particular time of day or night.

Exacerbating and relieving factors What makes it better, what makes it worse? What started it?

If pain is the main symptom:

Origin and radiation Where is the pain and does it spread?

Character and intensity How would you describe the pain: sharp, shooting, dull, aching, etc. This can be difficult, but patients with specific 'organic' pain will often understand exactly what you mean whereas patients with symptoms with a high behavioural overlay will be vague and prevaricate.

Associations Is there anything, in your own mind, which you associate with the problem?

The majority of dental problems can quickly be narrowed down using a simple series of questions such as these to create a provisional diagnosis and judge the urgency of the problem.

The dental history

It is important to assess the patient's dental awareness and the likelihood of raising it. A dental history may also provide invaluable clues as to the nature of the presenting complaint and should not be ignored. This can be achieved by some simple general questions:

How often do you go to the dentist?
   (this gives information on motivation, likely attendance patterns, and may indicate patients who change their GDP frequently)
When did you last see a dentist and what did he do?
   (this may give clues as to the diagnosis of the presenting complaint, e.g. a recent RCT)
How often do you brush your teeth and how long for?
   (motivation and likely gingival condition)
Have you ever had any pain or clicking from your jaw joints?
   (TMJ pathology)
Do you grind your teeth or bite your nails?
   (TMPDS, personality)
How do you feel about dental treatment?
   (dental anxiety)
What do you think about the appearance of your teeth?
   (motivation, need for orthodontic treatment)
What is your job?
   (socio-economic status, education)
Where do you live?
   (fluoride intake, travelling time to surgery)
What types of dental treatment have you had previously?
   (previous extractions, problems with LA or GA, orthodontics, periodontal treatment)
What are your favourite drinks/foods?
   (caries rate, erosion)

The medical history

There is much to be said for asking patients to complete a medical history questionnaire, as this encourages more accurate responses to sensitive questions. However, it is important to use this as a starting point, and clarify the answers with the patient.

Example of a medical questionnaire

QUESTION   YES/NO

Are you fit and well?
Have you ever been admitted to hospital?
  If yes, please give brief details:

Have you ever had an operation?
  If so, were there any problems?

Have you ever had any heart trouble or high blood pressure?
Have you ever had any chest trouble?
Have you ever had any problems with bleeding?
Have you ever had asthma, eczema, hayfever?
Are you allergic to penicillin?
Are you allergic to any other drug or substance?
Have you ever had:
– rheumatic fever?
– diabetes?
– epilepsy?
– tuberculosis?
– jaundice?
– hepatitis?
– other infectious disease?

Are you pregnant?
Are you taking any drugs, medications, or pills?
  If yes, please give details:

Who is your doctor?

▶ Check the medical history at each recall.
▶ If in any doubt contact the patient's GMP, or the specialist they are attending, before proceeding.

NB A complete medical history (as required when clerking in- patients) would include details of the patient's family history (for familial disease) and social history (for factors associated with disease, e.g. smoking, drinking, and for home support on discharge). It would be completed by a systematic enquiry:

Cardiovascular chest pain, palpitations, breathlessness.

Respiratory breathlessness, wheeze, cough—productive or not.

Gastrointestinal appetite and eating, pain, distension, and bowel habit.

Genitourinary pain, frequency (day and night), incontinence, straining, or dribbling.

Central nervous system fits, faints, and headaches.

Medical examination

For the vast majority of dental patients attending as out-patients to a prac-tice, community centre, or hospital, simply recording a medical history should suffice to screen for any potential problems. The exceptions are patients who are to undergo general anaesthesia and anyone with a posi-tive medical history undergoing extensive treatment under LA or seda-tion. The aim in these cases is to detect any gross abnormality so that it can be dealt with (by investigation, by getting a more experienced or spe-cialist opinion, or by simple treatment if you are completely familiar with the problem).

General jaundice   look at sclera in good light, anaemia ditto. Cyanosis, peripheral: blue extremities, central: blue tongue. Dehydration, lift skin between thumb and forefinger.

Cardiovascular system   Feel and time the pulse. Measure blood pressure. Listen to the heart sounds along the left sternal edge and the apex (norm-ally 5th intercostal space midclavicular line on the left), murmurs are whooshing sounds between the 'lup dub' of the normal heart sounds. Palpate peripheral pulses and look at the neck for a prominent jugular venous pulse (this is difficult and takes much practice).

Respiratory system   Look at the respiratory rate (12–18/min) is expansion equal on both sides? Listen to the chest, is air entry equal on both sides, are there any crackles or wheezes indicating infection, fluid, or asthma? Percuss the back, comparing resonance.

Gastrointestinal system   With the patient lying supine and relaxed with hands by their sides, palpate with the edge of the hand for liver (upper right quadrant) and spleen (upper left quadrant). These should be just palpable on inspiration. Also palpate bimanually for both kidneys in the right and left flanks (healthy kidneys are not palpable) and note any masses, scars, or hernia. Listen for bowel sounds and palpate for a full bladder.

Genitourinary system   Mostly covered by abdominal examination above. Patients with genitourinary symptoms are more likely to go into post-operative urinary retention. Pelvic and rectal examinations are neither appropriate nor indicated and should not be conducted by the non-medically qualified.

Central nervous system   Is the patient alert and orientated in time, place, and person? Examination of the cranial nerves, p. 548. Ask the patient to move their limbs through a range of movements, then repeat passively and against resistance to assess tone, power, and mobility. Reflexes: bra-chioradialis, biceps, triceps, knee, ankle, and plantar are commonly elicited (stimulation of the sole normally causes plantar flexion of the great toe).

Musculoskeletal system   Note limitations in movement and arthritis, espe-cially affecting the cervical spine, which may need to be hyperextended in order to intubate for anaesthesia.

Examination of the head and neck

This is an aspect of examination that is both undertaught and overlooked in both medical and dental training. In the former, the tendency is to approach the area in a rather cursory manner, partly because it is not well understood. In the latter it is often forgotten, despite otherwise extensive knowledge of the head and neck, to look beyond the mouth. For this reason the examination below is given in some detail, but so thorough an inspection is only necessary in selected cases, e.g. suspected oral cancer, facial pain of unknown origin, trauma, etc.

Head and facial appearance   Look for specific deformities (p. 196), facial disharmony (p. 194), syndromes (p. 755), traumatic defects (p. 492–6), and facial palsy (p. 463).

Assessment of the cranial nerves is covered on p. 548.

Skin   lesions of the face should be examined for colour, scaling, bleeding, crusting, palpated for texture and consistency and whether or not they are fixed to, or arising from, surrounding tissues.

Eyes   Note obvious abnormalities such as proptosis and lid retraction (e.g. hyperthyroidism) and ptosis (drooping eyelid). Examine conjunctiva for chemosis (swelling), pallor, e.g. anaemia or jaundice. Look at the iris and pupil. Ophthalmoscopy is the examination of the disc and retina via the pupil. It is a specialized skill requiring an adequate ophthalmoscope and is acquired by watching and practising with a skilled supervisor. However, direct and consensual (contralateral eye) light responses of the pupils are straightforward and should always be assessed in suspect head injury (p. 490).

Ears   Gross abnormalities of the external ear are usually obvious. Further examination requires an auroscope. The secret is to have a good auroscope and straighten the external auditory meatus by pulling upwards, backwards, and outwards using the largest applicable speculum. Look for the pearly grey tympanic membrane; a plug of wax often intervenes.

The mouth,   p. 14

Oropharynx and tonsils   These can easily be seen by depressing the tongue with a spatula, **the hypopharynx and larynx** are seen by indirect laryngoscopy, using a head-light and mirror, and the **post-nasal space** is similarly viewed.

The neck   Inspect from in front and palpate from behind. Look for skin changes, scars, swellings, and arterial and venous pulsations. Palpate the neck systematically, starting at a fixed standard point, e.g. beneath the chin, working back to the angle of the mandible and then down the cervical chain, remembering the scalene and supraclavicular nodes. Swellings of the thyroid move with swallowing. Auscultation may reveal bruits over the carotids (usually due to atheroma).

TMJ   Palpate both joints simultaneously. Have the patient open and close and move laterally whilst feeling for clicking, locking, and crepitus. Palpate the muscles of mastication for spasm and tenderness. Auscultation is not usually used.

Examination of the mouth

Most dental textbooks, quite rightly, include a very detailed and comprehensive description of how to examine the mouth. These are based on the premise that the examining dentist has never before seen the patient, who has presented with some exotic disease. Given the constraints imposed by routine clinical practice, this approach needs to be modified to give a somewhat briefer format that is as equally applicable to the routine dental attender who is symptomless as to the new patient attending with pain of unknown origin.

The key to this is to develop a systematic approach, which becomes almost automatic, so that when you are under pressure there is less likelihood of missing any pathology. As any abnormal findings indicate that further investigation is required, the reader is referred to the page numbers in parenthesis, as necessary.

EO examination (p. 12). For routine clinical practice this can usually be limited to a visual appraisal, e.g. swellings, asymmetry, patient's colour, etc. More detailed examination can be carried out if indicated by the patient's symptoms.

IO examination
- Oral hygiene.
- Soft tissues. The entire oral mucosa should be carefully inspected. Any ulcer of >3 weeks' duration requires further investigation (p. 480).
- Periodontal condition. This can be assessed rapidly, using a periodontal probe. Pockets >5 mm indicate the need for a more thorough assessment (p. 220).
- Chart the teeth present (p. 764).
- Examine each tooth in turn for caries (p. 30) and examine the integrity of any restorations present.
- Occlusion. This should involve not only getting the patient to close together and examining the relationship between the arches (p. 136), but also looking at the path of closure for any obvious prematurities and displacements (p. 178). Check for evidence of tooth wear (p. 310).

For those patients complaining of pain, a more thorough examination of the area related to their symptoms should then be carried out, followed by any special investigations (p. 18).

Investigations—general

▶ Do not perform or request an investigation you cannot interpret.
▶ Similarly, always look at, interpret, and act on any investigations you have performed.

Temperature, pulse, blood pressure, and respiratory rate These are the nurses' stock in trade. You need to be able to interpret the results.

Temperature (35.5–37.5°C) ↑ physiologically post-operatively for 24 h, otherwise may indicate infection or a transfusion reaction. ↓ in hypothermia or shock.

Pulse Adult (60–80 beats/min; child is higher (up to 140 beats/min in infants). Should be regular.

Blood pressure (120–140/60–90 mmHg) ↑ with age. Falling BP may indicate a faint, hypovolaemia, or other form of shock. High BP may place the patient at risk from a GA. An ↑ BP + ↓ pulse suggests ↑ intracranial pressure (p. 490).

Respiratory rate (12–18 breaths/min) ↑ in chest infections, pulmonary oedema, and shock.

Urinalysis is routinely performed on all patients admitted to hospital. A positive result for:

Glucose or ketones may indicate diabetes.

Protein suggests renal disease especially infection.

Blood suggests infection or tumour.

Bilirubin indicates hepatocellular &/or obstructive jaundice.

Urobilinogen indicates jaundice of any type.

Blood tests (sampling techniques, p. 590) Reference ranges vary.

Full blood count (EDTA, pink tube) measures:

Haemoglobin (M 13–18 g/dl, F 11.5–16.5 g/dl) ↓ in anaemia, ↑ in polycythaemia and myeloproliferative disorders.

Haematocrit (packed cell volume) (M 40–54%, F 37–47%). ↓ in anaemia, ↑ in polycythaemia and dehydration.

Mean cell volume (76–96 fl) ↑ in size (macrocytosis) in vitamin B12 and folate deficiency, ↓ (microcytosis) iron deficiency.

White cell count ($4–11 \times 10^9/1$) ↑ in infection, leukaemia, and trauma, ↓ in certain infections, early leukaemia and after cytotoxics.

Platelets ($150–400 \times 10^9/1$) See also p. 528.

Biochemistry Urea and electrolytes are the most important:

Sodium (135–145 mmol/l) Large fall causes fits.

Potassium (3.5–5 mmol/l) Must be kept within this narrow range to avoid serious cardiac disturbance. Watch carefully in diabetics, those in IV therapy, and the shocked or dehydrated patient. Suxamethonium (muscle relaxant) ↑ potassium.

Urea (2.5–7 mmol/l)   Rising urea suggests dehydration, renal failure, or blood in the gut.

Creatinine (70–150 micromol/l)   Rises in renal failure. Various other biochemical tests are available to aid specific diagnoses, e.g. bone, liver function, thyroid function, cardiac enzymes, folic acid, vitamin B_{12}, etc.

Glucose (fasting 4–6 mmol/l)   ↑ suspect diabetes, ↓ hypoglycaemic drugs, exercise. Competently interpreted proprietary tests, e.g. 'BMs' = well to blood glucose (p. 576).

Virology   Viral serology is costly and rarely necessary. If you must, use 10 ml clotted blood in a plain tube.

Immunology   Similar to above but more frequently indicated in complex oral medicine patients; 10 ml in a plain tube.

Bacteriology

Sputum and pus swabs   are often helpful in dealing with hospital infections. Ensure they are taken with sterile swabs and transported immediately or put in an incubator.

Blood cultures   are also useful if the patient has septicaemia. Taken when there is a sudden pyrexia and incubated with results available 24–48 h later. Take two samples from separate sites and put in paired bottles for aerobic and anaerobic culture (i.e. four bottles, unless your lab indicates otherwise).

Biopsy   See p. 410.

Cytology   With the exception of smears for candida and fine-needle aspiration, cytology is little used and not widely applicable in the dental specialties.

Investigations—specific

Sensibility testing It must be borne in mind when vitality testing that it is the integrity of the nerve supply that is being investigated. However, it is the blood supply which is of more relevance to the continued vitality of a pulp. Test the suspect tooth and its neighbours.

Application of cold This is most practically carried out using ethyl chloride on a pledget of cotton wool.

Application of heat Vaseline should be applied first to the tooth under test to prevent the heated GP sticking. No response suggests that the tooth is non-vital, but an ↑ response indicates that the pulp is hyperaemic.

Electric pulp tester The tooth to be tested should be dry, and prophy paste or a proprietary lubricant used as a conductive medium. Most machines ascribe numbers to the patient's reaction, but these should be interpreted with caution as the response can also vary with battery strength or the position of the electrode on the tooth. For the above methods misleading results may occur:

False-positive	*False-negative*
Multi-rooted tooth with vital + non-vital pulp	Nerve supply damaged, blood supply intact
Canal full of pus	Secondary dentine
Apprehensive patient	Large insulating restoration

Test cavity Drilling into dentine without LA is an accurate diagnostic test, but as tooth tissue is destroyed it should only be used as a last resort. Can be helpful for crowned teeth.

Percussion is carried out by gently tapping adjacent and suspect teeth with the end of a mirror handle. A positive response indicates that a tooth is extruded due to exudate in apical or lateral periodontal tissues.

Mobility of teeth is ↑ by ↓ in the bony support (e.g. due to peridontal disease or an apical abscess) and also by # of root or supporting bone.

Palpation of the buccal sulcus next to a painful tooth can help to determine if there is an associated apical abscess.

Biting on to gauze or rubber can be used to try and elicit pain due to a cracked tooth.

Radiographs (pp. 20, 752)

Area under investigation	**Radiographic view**
General scan of teeth and jaws (retained roots, unerupted teeth)	DPT
Localization of unerupted teeth	Parallax periapicals
Crown of tooth and interdental bone (caries, restorations)	Bitewing

Root and periapical area	Periapical
Submandibular gland	Lower occlusal view
Sinuses	Occipito-mental, DPT
TMJ	DPT, trans-pharyngeal
Skull and facial bones	Occipito-mental
	PA and lateral skull
	Submento-vertex

Local anaesthesia can help localize organic pain.

Radiology and radiography

Radiography is the taking of radiographs, **radiology** is their interpretation. Referring to a radiologist as a radiographer ensures upset.

Radiographic images are produced by the differential attenuation of X-rays by tissues. Radiographic quality depends on the density of the tissues, the intensity of the beam, sensitivity of the emulsion, processing techniques, and viewing conditions.

Intra-oral views

Uses a stationary anode (tungsten), direct current ↓ dose of self-rectifying machines. Direct action film (↑ detail) using D or E speed. E speed is double the speed of D hence ↓ dose to patient. Rectangular collimation ↓ unnecessary irradiation of tissues.

Periapical shows all of tooth, root, and surrounding periapical tissues. Performed by:

1 Paralleling technique Film is held in a film holder parallel to the tooth and the beam is directed (using a beam-aligning device) at right angles to the tooth and film. Focus-to-film distance is increased to minimize magnification; the optimium distance is 30 cm. Most accurate and reproducible technique.

2 Bisecting angle technique Older technique which can be carried out without film holders. Film placed close to the tooth and the beam is directed at right angles to the plane bisecting the angle between the tooth and film. Normally held in place by patient's finger. Not as geometrically accurate a technique as more coning off occurs and needlessly irradiates the patient's finger.

Bitewings shows crowns and crestal bone levels, used to diagnose caries, overhangs, calculus, and bone loss < 4 mm. Patient bites on wing holding film against the upper and lower teeth and beam is directed between contact points perpendicular to the film in the horizontal plane. A 5° tilt to vertical accommodates the curve of Monson.

Occlusals demonstrate larger areas. May be oblique, true, or special. Used for localization of impacted teeth, salivary calculi. Film is held parallel to the occlusal plane. Oblique occlusal is similar to a large bisecting angle periapical. True occlusal of the mandible gives a good cross-sectional view.

Key points
- Use paralleling technique.
- Use film holders.
- Rectangular collimation.
- E speed film.

Extra-oral views

Skull and general facial views use a rotating anode and grid which ↓ scattered radiation reaching the film but ↑ dose to patient. Screen film is used for all extra-orals (intensifying screens are now rare earth, e.g. gadolinium and lanthanum). X-rays act on screen which fluoresces and the light interacts with emulsion. There is loss of detail but ↓ the dose to patient. Dark-room techniques and film storage are affected due to the properties of the film.

Lateral oblique   Largely superseded by panoramic but can use dental X-ray set.

PA mandible   Patient has nose to forehead touching film. Beam perpendicular to film. Used for diagnosing/assessing # mandible.

Reverse Townes   position, as above, but beam 30° up to horizontal. Used for condyles.

Occipitomental   Nose/chin touching the film beam parallel to horizontal unless OM prefixed by, e.g., 10°, 30°, which indicates angle of beam to horizontal.

Submentovertex   Patient flexes neck vertex touching film, beam projected menton to vertex. ↓ use due to ↑ radiation and risk to cervical spine.

Cephalometry   (pp. 142, 144) uses cephalostat for reproducible position. Use Frankfort plane or natural head position. Wedge (aluminium or copper and rare earth) to show soft tissues. Lead collimation to reduce unnecessary dose to patient and scatter leading to ↓ contrast. Barium paste can be used to outline soft tissues.

Panoramic   Generically referred to as DPT (dental panoramic tomograph), sometimes by make, e.g. OPT/OPG. The technique is based on tomography (i.e. objects in focal trough are in focus, the rest is blurred). The state of the art machine is a moving centre of rotation (previously two or three centres) which accommodates the horseshoe shape of the jaws. Correct patient positioning is vital. Blurring and ghost shadows can be a problem (ghost shadows appear opposite to and above the real image due to 5–8° tilt of beam). Relatively low-dose technique and sectional images can be obtained.

Lead aprons   (0.25 mm lead equivalent)
The 10-day rule is now defunct for dental radiology. In well-maintained, well-collimated equipment where the beam does not point to the gonads the risk of damage is minimal. Apply all normal principles to pregnant women (use lead apron if primary beam is directed at fetus), but otherwise do not treat any differently.

There is no risk in dentistry of deterministic/certainty effects (e.g. radiation burns). Stochastic/change effects are more important (e.g. tumour induction). The thyroid is the principal organ at risk. Follow principles of ALARP, p. 751.

Parralax technique   involves 2 radiographs with a change in position of X-ray tube between them (eg DPT and periapical). The object furthest from the X-ray beam will appear to move in the same direction as the tube shift.

Advanced imaging techniques

Computed tomography (CT)

Images are formed by scanning a thin cross-section of the body with a narrow X-ray beam (120 kV), measuring the transmitted radiation with detectors and obtaining multiple projections, which a computer then processes to reconstruct a cross-sectional image ('slice'). Three-dimensional reconstruction is also possible on some machines. Modern scanners consist of either a fan beam with multiple detectors aligned in a circle, both rotating around the patient, or a stationary ring of detectors with the X-ray beam rotating within it. The image is divided into pixels which represent the average attenuation of blocks of tissue (voxels). The CT number (measured in Hounsfield units) compares the attenuation of the tissue with that of water. Typical values range from air at −1000 to bone at +400 to +1000 units. As the eye can only perceive a limited gray scale the settings can be adjusted depending on the main tissue of interest (i.e. bone or soft tissues). These 'window levels' are set at the average CT number of the tissue being imaged and the 'window width' is the range selected. The images obtained are very useful for assessing extensive trauma or pathology and planning surgery. The dose is, however, higher compared with conventional films and the NRPB recommends that all radiologists be made aware of the high-dose implications.

Magnetic resonance imaging (MRI)

The patient is placed in a machine which is basically a large magnet. Protons then act like small bar magnets and point 'up' or 'down', with a slightly greater number pointing 'up'. When a radio-frequency pulse is directed across the main magnetic field the protons 'flip' and align themselves along it. When the pulse ceases the protons 'relax' and as they re-align with the main field they emit a signal. The hydrogen atom is used because of its high natural abundance in the body. The time taken for the protons to 'relax' is measured by values known as T1 and T2. A variety of pulse sequences can be used to give different information. T1 is longer than T2 and times may vary depending on the fluidity of the tissues (e.g. if inflamed). MRI is not good for imaging cortical bone as the protons are held firmly within the bony structure and give a 'signal void', i.e. black, although bone margins are visible. It is useful, however, for the TMJ and facial soft tissues.

Problems are: patient movement, expense, the claustrophobic nature of the machine, noise, magnetizing, and movement of instruments or metal implants and foreign bodies. Cards with magnetic strips (e.g. credit cards) near the machine may also be affected.

Digital imaging

This technique has been used extensively in general radiology, where it has great advantages over conventional methods in that there is a marked dose reduction and less concentrated contrast media may be used. The normal X-ray source is used but the receptor is a charged coupled device linked to a computer or a photo-stimulable phosphor plate which is scanned by a laser. The image is practically instantaneous and eliminates the problems of processing. However, the sensor is difficult to position and smaller than normal film, which means the dose reduction is not always obtained. Gives ↓ resolution. Popular in some European countries and gaining popularity in the UK.

Ultrasound (US)

Ultra-high frequency sound waves (1–20 MHz) are transmitted through the body using a piezoelectric material (i.e. the material distorts if an electric field is placed across it and vice versa). Good probe/skin contact is required (gel) as waves can be absorbed, reflected, or refracted. High-frequency (short wavelength) waves are absorbed more quickly whereas low-frequency waves penetrate further. US has been used to image the major salivary glands and the soft tissues.

Doppler US is used to assess blood flow as the difference between the transmitted and returning frequency reflects the speed of travel of red cells. Doppler US has also been used to assess the vascularity of lesions and the patency of vessels prior to reconstruction.

Sialography

This is the imaging of the major salivary glands after infusion of contrast media under controlled rate and pressure using either conventional radiographic films, or CT scanning. The use of contrast media will reveal the internal architecture of the salivary glands and show up radiolucent obstructions, e.g. calculi within the ducts of the imaged glands. Particularly useful for inflammatory or obstructive conditions of the salivary glands. Patients allergic to iodine are at risk of anaphylactic reaction if an iodine-based contrast medium is used. Interventional sialography is now possible, e.g. for stone retrieval.

Arthrography

Just as the spaces within salivary glands can be outlined using contrast media, so can the upper and lower joint spaces of the TMJ. Although technically difficult, both joint compartments (usually the lower) can be injected with contrast media under fluoroscopic control and the movement of the meniscus can be visualized on video. Stills of the real-time images can be made although interpretation is often unsatisfactory.

Differential diagnosis and treatment plan

Arriving at this stage is the whole point of taking a history and performing an examination, because by narrowing down your patient's symptoms into possible diagnoses you can, in most instances, formulate a series of investigations &/or treatment that will benefit them.

Suggested approach

1 History and examination (as above).
2 Preliminary investigations.
3 Differential diagnosis.
4 Specific investigations which will confirm or refute the differential diagnoses.
5 Ideally, arrive at the definitive diagnosis(es).
6 List in a logical progression the steps which can be undertaken to take the patient to oral health.
7 Then carry them out.

Simple really!

This is the ideal, but life, as you are no doubt well aware, is far from ideal, and it is not always possible to follow this approach from beginning to end. The principles, however, remain valid and this general approach, even if much abbreviated, will help you deal with every new patient safely and sensibly.

An example

Mr Ivor Pain, 25, an otherwise healthy young man has 'toothache'.

C/O Pain, left side of mouth.

HPC Lost large amalgam $\overline{5}$ 3 weeks ago. Had twinges since then which seemed to go away, then 2 days ago tooth began to throb. Now whole jaw aches and can't eat on that side. The pain radiates to his ear and is worse if he drinks tea. He has a foul taste in his mouth. Little relief from analgesics.

PMH Well. Medical history NAD, i.e. no 'alarm bells' on questionnaire.

PDH Means well, but is an irregular attender, 'had some bad experiences', 'don't like needles'.

O/E

EO Medical examination inappropriate in view of PMH. Some swelling left side of face due to left submandibular lymphadenopathy. Looks distressed and anxious.

IO Moderate OH, generalized chronic gingivitis, no mucosal lesions, caries

$$\frac{7\,6\quad|\quad4\,6}{7\,6\,5\quad|\quad5\,7},$$

partially erupted $\overline{8}$ with pus exuding, $\overline{5}$ large cavity, but seems periodontally sound, no fluctuant soft tissue swelling. Otherwise complete dentition with Class I occlusion.

General investigations Temperature 38°C.

Differential diagnoses
1 Acute apical abscess 5˥ .
2 Acute pericoronitis 8˥ .
3 Chronic gingivitis? Periodontitis.
4 Caries as charted.

Specific investigations
1 Vitality test ˥5 (non-vital).
2 Periapical X-ray ˥5 (patent canal, apical area).

Rx plan
1 Drain ˥5 via root canal (does not require LA as pulp is necrotic, hence won't unduly distress anxious patient, but will relieve pain and infection).
2 Irrigate operculum of 8˥ .
3 Antibiotics (as patient is pyrexic with two sources of infection: usually due to mixed anaerobic/aerobic organisms ∴ use amoxycillin and metronidazole) and analgesics (NSAID for 24–48 h).
4 Explain the problems and arrange a review appointment for OHI, periodontal charting, and a DPT.

Future plan
5 OHI, scaling.
6 RCT ˥5 .
7 Plastic restorations as indicated.
8 Post/core crown ˥5 .
9 Remove third molars as indicated (clinically and from DPT).

Treatment at the first visit is kept at a minimum to relieve patient's pain and thereby gain his trust and future attendance.

Preventive and community dentistry

Relevent pages in other chapters   Plaque control, p. 226; prevention of secondary caries, p. 266; prevention of trauma to anterior teeth, p. 105.

Principal sources: J. J. Murray 1996 *Prevention of Dental Disease*, OUP. E. A. M. Kidd 1987 *Essentials of Dental Caries: The Disease and Its Management*, Wright R. J. Elderton 1987 *Positive Dental Prevention*, Heinemann. R. J. Elderton 1990 *Clinical Dentistry in Health and Disease*, Vol. 3, *The Dentition and Dental Care*, Heinemann. A. Rugg-Gunn 1993 *Nutrition and Dental Health*, OUP.

Dental caries

Dental caries is a sugar-dependent infectious disease.[1] Acid is produced as a by-product of the metabolism of dietary carbohydrate by plaque bacteria, which results in a drop in pH at the tooth surface. In response, calcium and phosphate ions diffuse out of enamel, resulting in demineralization. This process is reversed when the pH rises again. Caries is ∴ a dynamic process characterized by episodic demineralization and remineralization occurring over time. If destruction predominates, disintegration of the mineral component will occur, leading to cavitation.

Enamel caries The initial lesion is visible as a white spot. This appearance is due to demineralization of the prisms in a sub-surface layer, with the surface enamel remaining more mineralized. With continued acid attack the surface changes from being smooth to rough, and may become stained. As the lesion progresses, pitting and eventually cavitation occur. The carious process favours repair, as remineralized enamel concentrates fluoride and has larger crystals, with a ↓ surface area. Fissure caries often starts as two white spot lesions on opposing walls, which coalesce.

Dentine caries comprises demineralization followed by bacterial invasion, but differs from enamel caries in the production of secondary dentine and the proximity of the pulp. Once bacteria reach the ADJ, lateral spread occurs, undermining the overlying enamel.

Rate of progression of caries Although it has been suggested that the mean time that lesions remain confined radiographically to the enamel is 3–4 years,[2] there is great individual variation and lesions may even regress.[3] The rate of progression through dentine is unknown; however, it is likely to be faster than through enamel. Progression of fissure caries is usually rapid due to the morphology of the area.

Arrested caries Under favourable conditions a lesion may become inactive and even regress. Clinically, arrested dentine caries has a hard or leathery consistency and is darker in colour than soft, yellow active decay. Arrested enamel caries can be stained dark-brown.

Susceptible sites The sites on a tooth which are particularly prone to decay are those where plaque accumulation can occur unhindered, e.g. approximal enamel surfaces, cervical margins, and pits and fissures. Host factors, e.g. the volume and composition of the saliva, can also affect susceptibility.

Saliva and caries Saliva acts as an intra-oral antacid, due to its alkali pH at high flow-rates and buffering capacity. In addition saliva:
- ↓ plaque accumulation and aids clearance of foodstuffs.
- Acts as a reservoir of calcium, phosphate, and fluoride ions, thereby favouring remineralization.
- Has an antibacterial action because of its IgA, lysozyme, lactoferritin, and lactoperoxidase content.

1 E. A. M. Kidd 1987 *Essentials of Dental Caries: The Disease and its Management*, Wright.
2 N. B. Pitts 1983 *Comm Dent Oral Epidemiol* **11** 228.
3 N. B. Pitts 1991 *BDJ* **171** 313.

An appreciation of the importance of saliva can be gained by examining a patient with a dry mouth.

Some manufacturers are now promoting the remineralizing potential of chewing gum, effected by an increase in salivary production. Chewing sugar-free gum regularly after meals does appear to ↓ caries, but the reduction is small.[1]

Root caries With gingival recession root dentine is exposed to carious attack. Rx requires, first, control of the aetiological factors and for most patients this involves dietary advice and OHI. Topical fluoride may aid remineralization and prevent new lesions developing. However, active lesions will require restoration with GI cement (p. 274).

Caries prevention

Classically three main approaches are possible:
1 Tooth strengthening or protection.
2 Reduction in the availability of microbial substrate.
3 Removal of plaque by physical or chemical means.

In practice this means dietary advice, fluoride, fissure sealing, and regular toothbrushing (which is also important in the prevention of periodontal disease). The relative value of these varies with the age of the individual.

Of equal importance with the prevention of new lesions is a preventive philosophy on the part of the dentist, so that early carious lesions are given the chance to arrest and a minimalistic approach is taken to the excision of caries where primary prevention has failed.

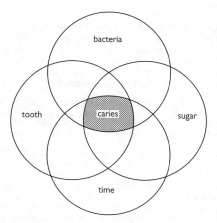

Diagram to show the factors involved in the development of caries.

1 *Drug and Therapeutics Bulletin* 1992 **30** 23.

Caries diagnosis

As caries can be arrested or even reversed, early diagnosis is important.

Aids to diagnosis

- Good eyesight (and a clean, dry, well-illuminated tooth). Magnification between ×2 and ×6 (leaning forward with the naked eye magnifies the image but you can only get so close to your patient); loupes are better!
- A blunt probe should only be used to horizontally dredge plaque away form the fissures (as a sharp probe may actually damage an incipient lesion).
- Bitewing radiographs are useful in the detection of occlusal and approximal caries. They are best approached systematically viewing 'approximal–occlusal–approximal' surface for each tooth, first in enamel then dentine, first with the naked eye and then with a viewing box (magnification and external light blackened out). The clinical situation is more advanced than the radiographic appearance. However, it is thought that the probability of cavitation is low when a lesion is confined to enamel on X-ray.
- Fibreoptic transillumination (FOTI) probes with a 0.5 mm tip are useful for detecting dentinal lesions at approximal sites. FOTI is considered to be an adjunct to bitewing radiographs.[1]
- Diagnodent is a laser-based instrument which uses fluorescent properties of the carious lesion to produce a quantitative reading of infected carious tissue, particularly dentine caries. Diagnodent should be used with care—it can produce false positives due to stain or dental materials.

Diagnosis and its relevance to management

▶ Remember: precavitated lesion—prevention
                cavitated lesion—prevention and restoration
▶ Counsel the patient that if the lesion is not cavitated it has the potential to arrest. This makes the preventive advice very relevant to the patient, increasing the chance of that patient acting on the advice.

Smooth surface caries is relatively straightforward to diagnose. The chances of remineralization are ↑ as it is obvious, and accessible for cleaning. Restoration is indicated if prevention has failed and the lesion is cavitated, or if the tooth is sensitive or aesthetics poor.

Pit and fissure caries is difficult to diagnose reliably, especially in the early stages. A sharp probe is of limited value as stickiness could be due to the morphology of the fissure. The anatomy of the area also tends to favour spread of the lesion, which often occurs rapidly. As fissure caries is less amenable to fluoride and OH, fissure sealing is preferable to watching and waiting. Occlusal caries evident on b/w radiographs should not always be excised. If the tooth is fissure-sealed or restored, check the margins very carefully, and if intact monitor the lesion radiographically. If marginal

---

1 *Selection Criteria for Dental Radiography.* Faculty of General Dental Practitioners RCS (Eng) 1998.

integrity not intact, investigate the area with a small round bur. The 'cavity' can be aborted if no caries found and the surface sealed.

Approximal caries   Currently accepted practice:
- If lesion confined to enamel on b/w, institute preventive measures and keep under review.
- If lesion has penetrated dentine radiographically, a restoration is indicated unless serial radiographs show that it is static.

If in doubt whether an approximal lesion has cavitated or not, fit an elastic orthodontic separator for 3–7 days so the surfaces can be visualized.

Recall intervals[1]

This subject has evoked considerable controversy, some arguing that regular attendance puts a patient more at risk of receiving replacement fillings, while others contend that regular and frequent check-ups are necessary to monitor prevention. In fact, it would appear that only a minority of the British public attend for 6-monthly check-ups. The available evidence suggests that there is no clear benefit for recall intervals of less than 1 yr for *healthy* patients, although the at-risk patient often needs to be seen more frequently.[2] In addition, as changing dentist ↑ the likelihood of replacement restorations the profession has to re-examine its criteria for replacement.

In the UK, guidance from the National Institute of Clinical Excellence (NICE) recommends that dental recall intervals ("oral health review" intervals) should be determined by the needs of the individual patient. For adult patients this interval can be between 3 and 24 months and for children 3 and 12 months.[3]

1 BASCD 1988 *The desirable frequency of attendance for dental clinical examination—a policy statement.*
2 N.B. Pitts 1992 *BDJ* **172** 225.
3 NICE 2004 Clinical guideline on dental recall.

Fluoride

The history of fluoride is covered well in other texts.[1]

Mechanisms of the action of fluoride in reducing dental decay

Enamel deposition and calcification	→	Enamel maturation	→	Eruption into oral environment
↑		↑		↑
Fluoride in blood		Fluoride in tissue fluid		Fluoride in saliva and cervicular fluid

The concentration of fluoride in enamel ↑ with ↑ fluoride content of water supply and ↑ towards the surface of enamel.

Pre-eruptive effects Enamel formed in the presence of fluoride has:
• Improved crystallinity and ↑ crystal size, and ∴ ↓ acid solubility.
• More rounded cusps and fissure pattern, but the effect is small.

Discontinuation of systemic fluoride results in an ↑ in caries, ∴ pre-eruptive effects must be limited.

Post-eruptive effects **NB** Newly erupted teeth derive the most benefit.
• Inhibits demineralization and promotes remineralization of early caries. Fluoride enhances the degree and speed of remineralization and renders the remineralized enamel more resistant to subsequent attack.
• Decreases acid production in plaque by inhibiting glycolysis in cariogenic bacteria.
• An ↑ concentration of fluoride in plaque inhibits the synthesis of extra-cellular polysaccharide.
• It has been suggested that fluoride affects pellicle and plaque formation, but this is unsubstantiated.

At higher pH fluoride is bound to protein in plaque. A drop in pH results in release of free ionic fluoride, which augments these action.

NB Fluoride is more effective in ↓ smooth surface than pit and fissure caries.

Safety and toxicity of fluoride

Fluoride is present in all natural waters to some extent. Many simple chemicals are toxic when consumed in excess, and the same is true of fluoride.

Fluoride is absorbed rapidly mainly from the stomach. Peak blood levels occur 1 h later. It is excreted via the kidneys, but traces are found breast in milk and saliva. The placenta only allows a small amount of fluoride to cross, ∴ pre-natal fluoride is relatively ineffective.

Fluorosis (or mottling) occurs due to a long-term excess of fluoride. It is endemic in areas with a high level of fluoride occurring naturally in the water. Clinically, it can vary from faint white opacities to severe pitting and discoloration. Histologically, it is caused by ↑ porosity in the outer third of the enamel.

1 J. J. Murray 1996. *Prevention of Oral Disease* 3rd edn, OUP.

Concentration of fluoride (ppm) in water supply	Degree of mottling
<0.9	+
0.9	+
2	++
>2	++++

Toxicity

Safely tolerated dose (STD)   Dose below which symptoms of toxicity are unlikely = 1 mg/kg body weight

Potentially lethal dose (PLD)   Lowest dose associated with a fatality. Patient should be hospitalized = 5 mg/kg body weight

Certainly lethal dose (CLD)   Survival unlikely = 32–64 mg/kg body weight

Fluoride concentration in various products
Standard adult fluoride toothpaste 1000 ppm F (parts per million fluoride) = 1 mg F/ml
Daily fluoride mouthrinse 0.05% NaF = 0.023% F=0.23mg F/ml
APF gel 1.23% F = 12.3 mg/ml
Fluoride varnish 5% NaF = 2.26% F = 22.6 mg/ml

To reach the 5 mg F/kg threshold (requiring hospitalization) a 5 yr-old (about 19 kg) would have to ingest 95 (1 mg F) tablets, 95 ml of toothpaste, or 7.6 ml of 1.23% of APF gel.

Antidotes: <5 mg F/kg body weight—large volume of milk. >5 mg F/kg body weight—refer to hospital quickly for gastric lavage. If any delay give IV calcium gluconate and an emetic.

Cancer   There is no evidence to support the contention that fluoridated communities experience a higher incidence of cancer.

▶ Advice about managing fluoride overdose can be sought from the National Poisons Information Service (0870 6006266)

Planning fluoride therapy

Many consider that the most important action of fluoride is to favour remineralization of the early carious lesion. Although fluoride incorporated within developing enamel results in a high local concentration following acid attack, the maximum benefit appears to be derived from frequent low-concentration topical administration.[1] Fluoridated water is the most effective method, as it provides both a systemic and topical effect.

Systemic fluoride

▶ To minimize the risk of mottling only one systemic measure should be used at a time.

Water fluoridation in a concentration of 1 ppm (1 mg F per litre) gives a caries reduction of 50%. The two main advantages of this measure are that no effort is required on the part of the individual, and the low cost. Yet despite the proven benefits only 10% of the UK population receive fluoridated water. In some countries school water has been fluoridated, but a concentration of 5 ppm is required to offset the less frequent intake.

Fluoride drops and tablets Regimen (mg F per day) depends upon drinking water content (see table opposite). This approach can be almost as effective as fluoridated water if the supplement is given regularly, but this requires a high level of parental motivation. Unfortunately, continued compliance has been shown to be generally poor, so the overall value of this approach on a population basis is questionable.

Milk with 2.5–7 ppm F has been tried successfully.

Salt is cheap and effective for rural communities in developing countries where water fluoridation is not feasible.

Topical fluoride

Professionally applied fluorides A wide variety of solutions, gels, and application protocols are available. Overall, caries reductions of 20–40% are reported. If these are applied in trays without adequate suction the systemic dosage can be high ∴ it is better to apply to a few, well-isolated teeth at a time. Fluoride varnish (e.g. Duraphat) is useful for applying directly to individual lesions to aid arrest, and regular site-specific application has been shown to be effective at reducing caries incidence. However, care is required and it should be applied sparingly, especially in young children as it contains 23 000 ppm fluoride.

Rinsing solutions Mouthrinses are C/I in children <7 yrs. The concentration prescribed depends upon the frequency of use: 0.2% fortnightly/weekly or 0.05% daily. Daily use is the most beneficial. Caries reductions of the order of 16–50% have been reported with rinsing alone. The most widely used solution is sodium fluoride.

Toothpastes aid tooth cleaning and polishing, but, most importantly, act as a vehicle for fluoride delivery. In the UK they contain abrasives (to

---

1 E. A. M. Kidd 1987 *Essentials of Dental Caries: The Disease and Its Management*, Wright.

a specified abrasivity standard), detergents, humectants, flavouring, binding agents, preservatives, and active agents, including:

1 Fluoride. Most toothpastes contain sodium monofluoro-phosphate &/or sodium fluoride, in concentrations of 1000–1450 ppm (i.e. 1–1.45 mg per 1 cm of paste). Caries reductions of 15% (in fluoridated areas) to 30% (in non-fluoridated areas) are reported. Low-dose formulations for children <7 yrs containing <500 ppm are available, to ↓ risk of mottling.

2 Anticalculus agents, e.g. sodium pyrophosphate, can ↓ calculus formation by 50%.

3 De-sensitizing agents, e.g. 10% strontium or potassium chloride, or 1.4% formaldehyde.

4 Antibacterial agents, e.g. triclosan.

Recommended daily fluoride supplementation (mg F)[1,2]

For children considered to be at high risk of caries and who live in areas with water supplies containing less than 0.3 ppm:

Age	mg F per day
6 months to 3 yrs	0.25
3 yrs to 6 yrs	0.5
>6 yrs	1.0

Suggested guidelines for children
Toothpaste

- Children should brush twice daily using a fluoride toothpaste.
- The most appropriate concentration is determined by the child's age and perceived risk of caries development (see table).
- Children under 6yrs of age should use a "smear", or no more than a small pea-size blob (<0.3 ml) of toothpaste.
- Children should spit out well, but not rinse, after brushing.
- Brushing using a fluoride toothpaste should start as soon as the first teeth erupt (about 6 months of age). Parents should supervise brushing up to at least 7 yrs of age to avoid over-ingestion of toothpaste and ensure adequate plaque removal.

Fluoride supplement (drops and tablets)

- May be prescribed for children deemed to be at risk of developing caries living in areas with less than optimal fluoride in the water supply.

Fluoridation of water still remains the most cost-effective method.

Table: Recommended fluoride concentration of toothpaste for children

Age (yrs)	Concentration of fluoride (ppm)	
	Low caries risk	High caries risk
0.5–5	<600	1000
6 +	1000	1500

1 BDA/BSPD/BASCD 1997 BDJ **182** 6.
2 R. Holt et al. Int J Paed Dent 1996 **6** 139.

Bacterial plaque and dental decay

Evidence for role of bacteria in dental caries

1 *In vitro*. Incubating teeth with plaque and sugar in saliva results in caries.
2 Animal experiments; e.g. germ-free rodents fed a cariogenic diet do not develop caries, but following the introduction of *Streptococcus mutans* caries occurs.
3 Epidemiological evidence showing that a supply of bacterial substrate results in caries.
4 Clinical experiments; e.g. stringent removal of plaque ↓ decay.

A correlation has been found between the presence of *Strep. mutans* and caries. This is not surprising, because this organism is acidophilic, can synthesize acid rapidly from sugar, and produces a sticky extracellular poly-saccharide which helps bind it to the tooth. However, caries can develop in the absence of *Strep. mutans*, and its presence does not inevitably lead to decay; e.g. root caries has been associated with *Strep. salivarius* and *Actinomyces* species. *Lactobacilli* are also acidophilic and have been implicated in fissure caries. In addition, plaque prevents acid diffusing away from the enamel and hinders the neutralizing effect of salivary buffers.

Methods of preventing caries by bacterial control

Physical removal of plaque

1 By a professional. If sufficiently frequent it can ↓ caries,[1] but rarely practical.
2 By the individual. Unfortunately, at the standard employed by the majority of the general public, toothbrushing per se is not an effective method of caries control. However, brushing with a fluoridated toothpaste provides regular topical fluoride. Also ↓ gingivitis.

Chemical removal of plaque   To achieve more than a transitory effect, an antiseptic needs to be retained in the mouth. The only chemical capable of this at present is chlorhexidine, a positively charged bactericidal and fungicidal antiseptic, which is attracted to the negatively charged proteins on the surface of teeth and oral mucosa, and in saliva from where it gradually leaches out. It is available as a 0.2% mouthwash and a 1% gel (Corsodyl) which are cheaper over the counter than by prescription. Although the main application of chlorhexidine is in the management of gingivitis, it has been shown to be effective at ↓ caries when used regularly.[2] While its widespread use for this purpose is not practical, it can be helpful in the management of handicapped patients or those with ↓ salivary flow. Unwanted effects include staining, disturbance of taste, and parotid swelling (which is reversible). It is less effective in the presence of a large build-up of plaque and is inactivated by commercial toothpastes.

1 J. Lindhe 1975 *Comm Dent Oral Epidemiol* **3** 150.
2 H. Loe 1972 *Scand J Dent Res* **80** 1.

A variety of pre-brushing rinses are now available. Research suggests that these do have a small beneficial effect if used in conjunction with toothbrushing.[1]

Immunization against caries   As no vaccine is completely safe, the ethics of vaccinating against caries, an avoidable non-lethal disease, have been hotly debated.[2] Yet despite considerable research, efforts to produce a viable vaccine have been unsuccessful due to a number of problems:

- Which species of *Strep. mutans* to target, and whether pathogenicity would then shift to another species.
- Differing modes of action in monkeys and rodents, ∴ ? relevance of experiments to humans.
- Cross-reactivity with heart muscle in animal experiments.
- Duration of effect and acceptance by public. Some patients may prefer caries to repeated injections of a vaccine.

1 H. V. Worthington 1993 *BDJ* **175** 322.
2 W. Sims 1985 *Comm Dent Health* **2** 129.

Fissure sealants

Pits and fissures in teeth provide a sheltered niche for bacterial proliferation. Toothbrush bristles are too wide to fit into these areas, making complete plaque removal impossible. A fissure sealant is a material that provides an impervious barrier to the fissure system to prevent the development of caries.

Historical   Several approaches to ↓ fissure caries have been tried:
- Chemical Rx of the enamel, e.g. with silver nitrate.
- Prophylactic odontotomy. This involved restoring the fissure with amalgam (hardly a preventive approach!).
- Sealing of the fissures. Several materials have been tried, including black copper cement (not retained), cyanoacrylate (toxic), polyurethane, and GI cement. The most common type of fissure sealant (f/s) is a composite resin used with an acid-etch technique.

Is there a need for sealants?   Although developed countries have enjoyed a reduction in dental decay in recent years this has not been uniform for all tooth surfaces. Given that part of this reduction is thought to be due to an increased availability of fluoride, it is not surprising that there has been a greater reduction in approximal, rather than in pit and fissure caries. If decay is to be eliminated, then the need for a method of ¬ occlusal caries is even more pressing.

Are sealants effective?   To be effective, sealants need to be carefully applied to susceptible teeth. Unfortunately, those situations where they are most valuable (recently erupted first molars) are often where moisture control is the most difficult; ∴ sealants should be monitored, and replaced if lost. For maximum benefit, teeth should be sealed as soon as practicable after eruption and certainly within 2 yrs. Guidelines for placement of f/s have been described.[1]

Patient selection   f/s should be provided for 6s in:
- children with impairments;
- those with extensive caries in the primary dentition (dmfs is 2 or more).

Children with caries-free primary dentitions do not need routine f/s of 6s but should be monitored regularly.

Tooth selection

For children who fulfil the criteria above:
- All susceptible fissures of permanent teeth should be sealed—occlusal, fissures and cingulum, buccal, and palatal pits. Teeth should be sealed as soon as sufficiently erupted for adequate moisture control.
- Where occlusal caries affects one 6 the remaining caries-free permanent molars (6s and 7s) should be f/s.
- f/s of primary molars is not normally recommended.

If there is doubt about a stained fissure, a bitewing radiograph should be taken. If the lesion is in enamel f/s and monitor clinically and radiographically. If in doubt carry out an enamel biopsy. If the lesion extends to dentine place a PRR, providing the cavity does not extend to more than one-third of the occlusal surface, in which case a conventional restoration is required.

The accepted figures for composite resin-based sealant retention are > 85% after 1 yr and > 50% after 5 yrs.[2]

Discussion of the cost-effectiveness of sealants compared to restoration has been well aired over the years, which is surprising given that the end results are not comparable. However, recent studies which have indicated that amalgam restorations have a rather more finite life than was once assumed (p. 278), has deflated this debate.

Types of fissure sealant Sealants can be classified by polymerization method (light- or self-cure), resin system (Bis-GMA or urethane diacrylate), colour (clear or tinted), and whether they are filled or unfilled. The choice is one of personal preference; however, it has been pointed out that coloured-/opaque sealants are more readily obvious to the patient (and the Dental Practice Board!). The retention rates of the different types are similar: success depends upon maintaining an absolutely dry field during application.

Glass ionomer sealants do release fluoride but have poorer retention than resin sealants. They are useful for high caries-risk children as a temporary sealant where adequate isolation for successful placement of resin-based sealants is not possible; e.g. partially erupted teeth/poor cooperation.

Fissure sealant technique
1 Prophylaxis (this may be omitted, if the tooth is already relatively free from plaque).
2 Isolate and dry the tooth.
3 Etch for the time recommended by the manufacturer (usually 20–40 sec) with 30–50% phosphoric acid.
4 Wash thoroughly, re-isolate, and dry very, very well. If salivary contamination occurs, re-etch.
5 Apply f/s (method depends upon delivery system).
6 After polymerization try to remove the sealant. If satisfactory, occlusal adjustment is usually not required unless a large volume has inadvertently been applied or a filled resin is used.

Follow up. f/s should be monitored clinically, and where appropriate, radiographically (bitewings). Defective sealants should be replenished in orders to maintain their marginal integrity.

2 National Institutes of Health 1984 *J Am Dent Assoc* **108** 233.

Sugar

The term, sugar, is commonly used to refer to the mono- and disaccharide members of the carbohydrate family. Monosaccharides include glucose (dextrose or corn sugar), fructose (fruit sugar), galactose, and mannose. Disaccharides include lactose (in milk), maltose, and sucrose (cane or beet sugar). Polysaccharides (starch) are composed of chains of glucose molecules and are not readily broken down by the oral flora. Dietary sugars have been classified as intrinsic when they are part of the cells in a food (vegetables and fruit) or extrinsic (milk sugar or, the real baddy, non-milk extrinsic sugar, e.g. table sugar). Both intrinsic and extrinsic sugars may cause decay, although non-milk extrinsic sugars are generally considered to be the most cariogenic.

Evidence for the role of sugar in dental caries[1]
1 Epidemiological evidence:
  - World-wide comparison of sugar consumption and caries levels.
  - Low caries experience of people on low-sugar diet, e.g. wartime diet; patients with hereditary fructose intolerance.
  - ↑ caries experience following ↑ availability of sugar, e.g. Eskimos.
  - Cross-sectional studies relating caries experience to sugar intake.
2 Clinical studies, e.g. Vipeholm study, Turku sugar study (Xylitol)
3 Plaque pH studies, *in vivo* and *in vitro*. See Stephan curve opposite.
4 Animal experiments e.g. rats fed by stomach tube do not develop caries.

Sucrose is considered a major culprit, due in part to being the most commonly available sugar, but also because of its ability to facilitate production of extracellular polysaccharide in plaque. However, other sugars can also cause caries. For example, frequent consumption of fruit-based drinks is known to be a key factor in the development of early childhood caries (ECC). In ↓ cariogenicity:
1 Sucrose, glucose, fructose, maltose (honey).
2 Galactose, lactose.
3 Complex carbohydrate (e.g. starch in rice, bread, potatoes).

The frequency of sugary intakes and the interval between them, the total amount of sugar eaten in the diet, and the concentration of sugar and stickiness of a food have been shown to be important. The acidogenicity of a sugar-containing food can be modified by other items in the food or meal. Foods that stimulate salivary flow can speed the return of plaque pH to normal, e.g. cheese, sugar-free gum, salted peanuts.

Sugar and health   In 1989 the COMA panel on Dietary Sugars and Human Disease reported that dental decay is positively associated with the frequency and amount of non-milk extrinsic sugar consumption. However, while sugar may contribute to the excess calorific intake which causes obesity and predisposes towards diabetes or coronary heart disease, there is no direct evidence linking sugar intake and these medical conditions.[2]

---

1 A. Rugg-Gunn 1993 In *Nutrition and Dental Health*, OUP.
2 COMA 1989 *Dietary Sugars and Human Disease*, HMSO.

Prevention of caries by ↓ the availability of microbial substrate
The following aims take into account the modern habit of 'snacking'
(also known as 'grazing'):
- Remove sugar from selected foods.
- Substitute non-cariogenic sweeteners.
- Modify sugar-containing foods so that they are less cariogenic.

Modification of only a restricted number of snack foods would probably
be to have a significant effect.

Diagram of a Stephan curve showing the pH drop that occurs after
a sugary drink is consumed (shown by arrow). The dashed line indicates
the critical pH; below this pH demineralization will occur. The shape of
the curve is affected by a number of factors, including the type of sugary
food, buffering potential of the saliva, and foods or drinks ingested after
the sugary challenge.

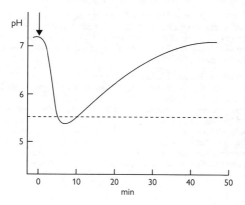

Alternative sweeteners
(In this table sweetness of sucrose = 1)

Sweetener	Type	Sweetness	Cariogenicity	Comments
Sorbitol	Bulk sweetener	0.5	Low	Isocalorific to sugar
Mannitol	Bulk sweetener	0.7	Low	
Xylitol	Bulk sweetener	1	None	Diarrhoea
Isomalt	Bulk sweetener	0.5	Low	
Lycasin*	Bulk sweetener	0.75	Low	
Acesulfame	Intense	130	None	
Aspartame	Intense	200	None	C/I in phenylketonuria
Saccharin	Intense	500	None	Bitter aftertaste
Thaumatin	Intense	4000	None	

* Lycasin is the trade name for hydrogenated glucose syrup (which didn't fit in the table!).

The bulk sweeteners (largely polyols) can cause osmotic diarrhoea if consumed in large amounts and are ∴ C/I in small children. However, it is probably wise to avoid all artificial sweeteners in pre-school children. The bulk sweeteners are isocalorific with sucrose, whereas the intense sweeteners are low calorie.

Recommendations for ↓ the risk of caries
- Reduce frequency of consumption of sugar-containing foods and drinks, especially between meals.
- Reduce frequency of consumption of fruit-based drinks, even those labeled "no added sugar".
- A few snack foods are "safe" (e.g. nuts and cheese), but foods containing artificial sweeteners may be less decay-producing.
- Foods containing starch and sugar in combination (e.g. cakes, biscuits) and carbonated sugary drinks are especially decay-producing.

Dietary analysis and advice

Diet can affect teeth:

Pre-eruptively   Fluoride is the most important. The effect of calcium, phosphate, vitamins, and sugar is unclear, but is unlikely to be great.

Post-eruptively   Again, fluoride is important, as is sugar. Acidic foods or drinks can cause erosion (p. 310).

Dietary analysis

Aim   To ↓ the time for which the teeth are at risk of demineralization and increase the potential remineralization period.

Indications   **1** high caries activity **2** unusual caries pattern **3** suspected dietary erosion.
Dietary advice should be tailored to the individual. This is most easily done after analysing the patient's present eating pattern.

Method   A consecutive 3- or 4- day analysis (including at least one weekend day) is the most widely used, with the patient recording the time, content, and quantity of food/drink consumed. In addition, tooth-brushing and bedtime should be indicated. When the form is returned the entries should be checked with the patient.

Analysis

1 Ring the main meals. If in any doubt, identify those snacks that contain complex carbohydrate. Assess nutritional value of meals.
2 Underline all sugar intakes in red.
3 Identify between-meal snacks and note any associations, e.g. following insubstantial meals or at school.
4 Decide on a maximum of three recommendations.

Dietary advice   should include an explanation of the effect of between-meals eating and sugary drinks. It must also be personal, practical, and positive! The suggestion that a child should select crisps when friends are buying sweets is more likely to be followed than total abstinence. Some helpful hints:

• Suggest saving sweets to be eaten on 1 day, e.g. Saturday dinnertime, or to be eaten at the end of a meal.
• All-in-one chocolate bars are preferable to packets of individual sweets.
• Foods which stimulate salivary flow (e.g. cheese, sugar-free chewing gum) can help to reverse the pH drop due to sugar, if eaten afterwards.
• Treacle, honey, and fruit (especially fruit juice) are cariogenic.
• Artificial sweeteners should be avoided in pre-school children.
• Fibrous foods, e.g. apples, are preferable to a sucrose snack, but they can still cause decay and there is no evidence that they can clean teeth.

Where the nutritional content of meals is inadequate considerable tact is necessary. It may be possible to suggest that larger meals would reduce the temptation to eat snacks. For children who are "picky" eaters snacks and sweets saved until the end of a meal can act as an encouragement to consume more food at mealtimes.

BUT Remember that while cheese, peanuts, and crisps may constitute a safe snack in dental terms, they are all high in fat, and peanuts can be inhaled by small children. Also,'diet' cola is sugar-free, but can still cause erosion if large quantities are drunk.

Therefore, dental dietary advice should be given in the wider context of the general health of the individual, i.e. ↓ consumption of sugars and fats, and ↑ consumption of fibre-rich starchy foods, fresh fruit, and vegetables. Meals provide a better nutritional balance than snacks. Hence good eating/drinking at mealtimes and ↓ avoiding in-between meals-snacking is healthy.

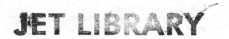

Dental health education

What is it? The objective of dental health education is to influence the attitude and behaviour of the individual to maintain oral health for life and prevent oral disease.

Primary prevention: seeks to prevent the initial occurrence of a disease or disorder and is aimed at healthy individuals.

Secondary prevention: aims to arrest disease through early detection and Rx.

Tertiary prevention: helps individuals to deal with the effects of the disease and to prevent further recurrence.

Who should give it? All health professionals. In practice, many patients relate better to advice from a hygienist or nurse.

What information should be given? It is important that the information given is factual and that different sources do not give conflicting advice. In order to unify the profession's approach, the Health Education Authority has published a policy document[1] laying out four simple messages:
- Restrict sugar-containing foods to mealtimes.
- Clean teeth and gums thoroughly twice daily with a fluoride toothpaste.
- Attend the dentist regularly.
- Water fluoridation is beneficial.

How? The way in which the advice is imparted is as important as its content. There are three main routes for dental health education:
1 The mass media. This is an expensive alternative and, whilst commercial advertisers tempt the consumer, the success of a dental health education which is exhorting the public to stop doing something they find pleasurable is not guaranteed.
2 Community programmes. These need to be carefully planned, targeted, and monitored.[2]
3 One-to-one in the clinical environment. This is usually the most successful approach, because the message can be tailored to the individual and reinforcement is facilitated. However, it is expensive in terms of manpower.

Individual dental health education Because many patients find the dental surgery threatening, it may be better to choose a more neutral environment, e.g. a dental health or preventive unit. It is important that the information is given by someone the patient trusts and can relate to—this is not always the dentist! It is important also to have adequate time, as a hurried approach is of dubious value, and to choose words that the patient will understand.

The following approach has been used successfully:
1 Define the problem and its aetiology. For example, poor OH which has resulted in periodontal disease—is it because the patient lacks

1 *The Scientific Basis of Dental Health Education* 3rd edn 1989 Health Education Authority, Hamilton House, Marbledon Place, London WC1H 9TX.
2 *Notes on Dental Health Education*, Scottish Health Education Group, Woodburn House, Canaan Lane, Edinburgh.

motivation or the appropriate skills? This stage includes questioning the patient to discover how often and for how long he brushes.

2 Set realistic objectives. It is better to start with trying to motivate the patient to brush well once a day rather than teaching them how to floss.

3 Demonstrate on the patient, as this makes the advice more relevant, and more likely to be remembered.

4 Monitor by comparing plaque scores before and after. This not only enables you to monitor improvement but also allows improvements in the patient's oral hygiene behaviour to be reinforced.

5 Remember that everyone responds well to praise, so if a patient is doing well, tell him.

Keys to successful dental health education
• Relevant to the individual, their life-style and problems.[1]
• Keep the message simple. Too much information may be counter-productive.
• Repetition of message.
• Positive reinforcement.

Where to go for help or information   Advice on preparing a talk on dental health education, setting up a preventive unit, or even a health programme can be obtained from:

1 Local Health Education (or Promotion) Unit. These centres will be happy to provide leaflets, educational packs, slides, videos, or just advice.

2 Consultant in Dental Public Health, or nearest Department of Postgraduate Dental Education.

1 A. S. Blinkhorn *BDJ* 1998 **184** 58.

Provision of dental care

Delivery of care

General Dental Service This is the main source of dental care for the majority of the population (whether NHS or private).

Community Service The Community Dental Service (CDS) was formed from the School Dental Service in 1974.

In 1989[1] the remit of the CDS was expanded (the guidance being updated in 1997)[2] to cover the following:
- Provision of oral health promotion.
- Rx for patients for whom there is evidence they would not otherwise seek Rx from the GDS, e.g. patients with special needs.
- Rx of patients who have experienced difficulty obtaining Rx from the GDS (normally termed the "safety net" function).
- Provision of Rx which may not be generally available in the GDS.
- Dental health screening of children in state schools and other vulnenerable groups with particular special needs.
- Epidemiology to assist the planning of local health services and as part of coordinated national surveys.

Hospital Service The role of the consultant service is to provide specialist advice and Rx, in addition to postgraduate training.

1 National Health Service 1989 *General Dental Services—The Future Development of the Community Dental Services*, FPN 468.
2 Department of Health HSC(97)4.

Receipt of care

Two factors are important:
1 Availability and accessibility of dental services. Research shows that a greater proportion of the public visit the dentist regularly where the dentist to population ratio is high. This ratio tends to follow a geographical pattern, with the greatest number of dentists in the south-east.
2 Social class affects both the incidence of dental disease and the uptake of dental care. Interestingly, the differences in caries experience between the social classes are much lower in fluoridated regions.

Because dentists have traditionally preferred to practise in leafy suburbs rather than poor inner city areas, these effects are often compounded.

As part of a government initiative in 1999, Dental Acess Centres were established in some areas with the aim of ensuring patients can access NHS dental care. Such development was reinforced in "Modernizing Dentistry—Implementing the NHS Plan".[1] Further changes outlined in the recent document "Options for Change"[2] may also help to address patient access issues.

Barriers to the uptake of dental care[3]

A survey found that the two main barriers to regular uptake of dental care by the general public were anxiety and cost.

Anxiety   This was manifest as fear of pain or a particular procedure, or a feeling of vulnerability brought about by relinquishing control to the dentist in the sensitive area of the mouth. The importance of first impressions was highlighted, because the reception received from staff and the environment in which the patient had to wait to be seen could either allay or reinforce their anxieties. The attitude of the dentist was also a significant factor: a 'good' dentist had a friendly, personal touch and explained what he was doing.

Cost   Respondents to the survey reported that they thought dental Rx was expensive, and the way in which the charges are calculated confusing, but welcomed an estimate of the costs prior to Rx.

The results suggested that the pattern of attendance varies throughout life, with children now enjoying a visit to the dentist, but adolescents breaking the habit of regular attendance due to apathy &/or other pressures on their time. A return to the dentist may be triggered by pregnancy and desire to provide a good example to the children, or a need for urgent Rx and a fear of becoming edentulous.

---

1 Department of Health 1999 "Modernizing Dentistry—Implementing the NHS Plan".
2 Department of Health 2002 "NHS Dentistry—options for Change".
3 Barriers to the receipt of dental care *BDJ* 1988 **164** 195.

Dentistry for the disabled

A disabled person is someone with a physical or mental impairment which has a substantial and long-term adverse effect on his ability to carry out normal day-to-day activities.

Intellectual impairment (mental handicap/learning difficulty) Prevalence 3%. Classified into mild (IQ 50–70) and severe (IQ <50).

Many cases lack well-defined aetiology but there are some subgroups where cause/Δ is known

- Down syndrome; Fragile–X syndrome.
- Cerebral palsy, birth anoxia.
- Meningitis, rubella.
- Autism, microcephaly.

Physical impairment Most common is cerebral palsy, which is the motor manifestation of cerebral damage. Many patients with cerebral palsy have normal IQs, but ↑ muscle tone and hyperactive reflexes can make Rx difficult. Many can be treated by GDS provided there is wheelchair access.

Medical impairment 1% of children have either heart disease, bleeding disorders, diabetes, or kidney disease.

Sensory impairment i.e. blindness, deafness.

Many have more than one type of impairment.

The above groups are general disabilities. We also need to consider those that are orally disabled, i.e. have gross oral problem or deficit which necessitates special dental Rx (e.g. cleft lip &/or palate).

Disability Discrimination Act 1995
This requires that:
- Employers must not discriminate against disabled employees.
- Service providers (including dentists) have to consider making reasonable adjustments to the way they deliver services so that disabled people can access them. Such adjustments need to be permanently in place by 2004.

Problems

It is difficult to generalize, but usually mental disability provides the biggest challenge. Difficulties ↑ in patients with > 1 impairment.
- Delivery of care. This has three aspects: **1** ¬ demand, due to low priority placed on dental health; **2** lack of provision made to provide the necessary care; **3** practical difficulties in carrying out dental work.
- In general, disabled patients have ¬ plaque control and ∴↑ periodontal problems.
- Although caries incidence is not significantly ↑ compared to the normal population, the amount of untreated caries is.
- Long-term sugared medications.
- Prevalence of hepatitis in institutionalized patients.
- Dentures may be impractical ∴ extractions not a realistic solution to the problems of providing dental Rx.
- Consent (see p. 708)

Management

Again, it is difficult to generalize. Patients with less severe disabilities can be treated in GDS along with other members of the family. Those with severe medical &/or mental impairments are probably best managed by a specialist who will have greater access to facilities. However, with the changing emphasis in the CDS, better care should become available to institutionalized patients and those living in the community.

Rx planning An initial plan should be formulated ignoring the disability. This can then be discussed with the patient, parent, or carer and modified for the individual. It is advisable to start with OHI and prevention, then re-assess Rx requirements in the light of the response. For those patients for whom a satisfactory standard of OH is not possible, restorative Rx should aim to ↓ plaque accumulation. Guidelines for the dental care of disabled patients have been produced by the British Society for Disability and Oral Health.[1]

OHI Those patients who can brush their own teeth should be encouraged to do so. Modification of toothbrush handles (p. 376) or purchase of an electric one may be helpful. Where patients are unable to brush their teeth, instruction should be given to their carer. The best method is to stand behind the patient and cradle the head with one arm, leaving the other free to brush. However, if possible this should be supplemented with regular professional cleaning. Chemical control of plaque with chlorhexidine may be helpful.

Restorative care Greatest problems are posed by mentally impaired. Kind but firm restraint may be necessary—ideally, get the patient's carer to help. A prop (e.g. McKesson rubber) may be needed. It is often easier to use intraligamentary LA technique. Sedation may help reduce the spontaneous movements of cerebral palsy. In some cases there is no alternative but to carry out examination and Rx under GA. In addition, for those patients who can tolerate out-patient Rx, but only a little at a time, it may be kinder to clear a backlog under GA, thus allowing concentration on prevention subsequently. However, this approach requires special facilities and no medical C/I.

Down syndrome, p. 757.

The Royal National Institute for the Deaf

STANDARD MANUAL ALPHABET

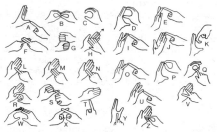

Reprinted by kind permission of the RNID (19–23 Featherstone Road, London EC1Y 8SL).

1 British Society for Disability and Oral Health. www.bsdh.org.uk

Professions Complementary to Dentistry

Dental auxiliary personnel (or Professions Complementary to Dentistry (PCD)) are becoming increasingly important as the skill mix of the dental team changes. Delegation of repetitive duties to trained PCDs allows the dentist to concentrate on Rx planning and management.

The WHO classify dental auxiliary personnel as follows:

1 Non-operating auxiliaries: Type I, dental technician; Type II, dental nurse; Type III, dental preventive worker.

2 Operating auxiliaries: Type IV, hygienist; Type V, dental therapist.

Hygienists in UK can carry out the following unsupervised procedures under the written direction of a dentist:

• Administering infiltration LA.
• Scaling and polishing.
• Application of topical fluoride and sealants.
• OHI and preventive advice, e.g. diet.
• Remove excess cement with instruments (including rotary instruments).
• Take impressions.
• Replace crowns with a temporary cement in an emergency.

Hygienists are also allowed to do the following under the direct supervision of a dentist:

• Inferior dental block.
• Treat patients under conscious sedation, provided a dentist remains in the room throughout Rx.

Therapists In addition to the duties of a hygienist, therapists in the UK are permitted to carry out primary tooth extraction, simple restorations, pulp Rx of primary teeth, and place preformed crowns on primary teeth.

Orthodontic auxiliaries This grade of auxiliary is widely employed in many countries, including the USA and Scandinavia. Their work includes placement of fixed appliances, changing archwires, and taking impressions.

The future—a dental team

With increasing demand for dental (and orthodontic) Rx and restraints on health care costs, the advantages of delegating more routine tasks to dental auxiliaries is obvious. There is also improved job satisfaction for all members of the dental team. In 1998 the GDC[1] advocated the introduction of expanded roles for nurses, hygienists, therapists, and technicians, and also the introduction of two new grades of clinical auxiliary, the orthodontic auxiliary and the clinical dental technician. Subsequently, the

1 GDC 1998 Professions Complementary to Dentistry—a consultation paper.

GDC established a register for PCDs in the UK. Eventually it is intended that all classes of PCD will be registered with the GDC.

With the introduction of more auxiliaries the role of the dentist will inevitably change, to become more centred on Δ and Rx planning, and more complex Rx, with team leadership skills becoming increasingly important.

Lies, damn lies, and statistics

Sugar

- The UK per capita consumption of sugar is 1 kg/week.
- UK children receive about 1/5 to 1/4 of their energy intake from sugars. Of these 2/3 are added sugars, > 2/3 of which come from sweets, table sugar, and soft drinks.[1]
- 65% of all soft drink sales are to < 15-yr-olds.
- Low-income families consume more sugar/person/day than higher-income families.

Fluoride

- Water fluoridation ↓ caries experience by about 50%.
- A cup of tea contains about 1 ppm. (1 in 3 people in UK take teabags abroad with them on holiday!)
- At equivalent concentrations there is no difference in the efficacy of sodium fluoride or sodium monofluorophosphate-containing toothpastes.[2]

Caries

- A reduction of 10–60% in the caries experience of developed countries has been widely reported. This is thought to be due to a variety of factors, including: fluoride toothpaste, increased public awareness, changes in infant feeding practices, ↓ sugar consumption, and antibiotics in the food chain.
- In addition, there has been a change in the pattern of carious attack, with a greater ↓ in smooth surface than fissure caries (perhaps reflecting the influence of fluoride).
- Small occlusal lesions appear to be becoming the predominant type of lesion.[3]
- **BUT**: there is some evidence to suggest that the ↓ in caries may have halted in Britain.[4]

Adult dental health 1988[5]

	1978	*1988*
Proportion of adults edentulous	30%	21%
Average condition of teeth:		
• Missing	9 teeth	7.8 teeth
• Decayed	1.9 teeth	1 tooth
• Filled	8.1 teeth	8.4 teeth
• Sound	13 teeth	14.8 teeth

A marked regional variation was noted, with Scotland and N. Ireland having the smallest number of sound untreated teeth (13 and 12.6, respectively). The average number of filled teeth was highest in southern England (9.1).

1 A. J. Rugg-Gunn et al.1986 *Human Nutrition: Applied Nutrition* **40A** 115.
2 *American Journal of Dentistry*, Special Issue, 1993.
3 A. Sheiham 1989 *BDJ* **165** 240.
4 R. Welbury (ed.) *Paediatric Dentistry*, OUP.
5 OPCS Monitor 1990 *Adult Dental Health United Kingdom*, HMSO.

Periodontal disease
- Prevalence in UK:

	17–24 yrs	25+ yrs
Gingivitis	77%	87%
Periodontitis	3%	64%

- Recent estimates indicate that approximately 10–15% of adults may be at high risk of developing progressive periodontal disease.

Child dental health

- The proportion of caries-free 5-yr-olds in England and Wales rose from 29% in 1973 to 55% in 1993, thus achieving one of the goals set by the WHO for the year 2000.[1] By 2001/02 60% of 5-yr-olds were caries free,[2] although the distribution of caries was highly skewed, with about 80% of caries occurring in 20% of the population.
- Reductions in levels of dental caries among children in the UK since 1983 were substantially greater in the permanent dentition than those found in primary dentition. However, levels of caries are still substantial. In 2000/01 38% of 12-yr-olds in England and Wales had caries experience in the permanent dentition[3].
- Overall, 54% of 9-yr-old children are in need of orthodontic Rx.

Indices

DMFT	decayed, missing, and filled permanent teeth.
dmft	decayed, missing, and filled deciduous teeth.
deft	decayed, exfoliated, and filled deciduous teeth.
dft	decayed and filled deciduous teeth.
DMFS	decayed, missing, and filled surfaces in permanent teeth.

1 M. O'Brien 1994 *Childrens' Dental Health in the UK*, 1993, HMSO.
2 N. B. Pitts *et al.* 2003. *Comm Dent Health* **20.** 45.
3 N. B. Pitts *et al.* 2002. *Comm Dent Health* **19.** 46.

Paediatric dentistry

Principal sources: R. Andlaw 1996 *A Manual of Paedodontics*, Churchill Livingstone. J. O. Andreasen 1981 *Traumatic Injuries of the Teeth*, Munksgaard. J. O. Andreasen 1992 *Atlas of Replantation and Transplantation of Teeth*, Mediglobe. G. J. Roberts and P. Longhurst 1996 *Oral and Dental Trauma in Children and Adolescents*, OUP. R. R. Welbury 2001 *Paediatric Dentistry*, 2nd edn., OUP. M. E. J. Curzon 1999 *Handbook of Dental Trauma*, Wright. M. S. Duggal *et al.* 2002 *Restorative Techniques in Paediatric Dentistry*, Dunitz. BSPD policy documents and clinical guidelines are available on the BSPD website: www.bda.org/bspd.

The child patient

! Treat the patient not the tooth.

Principal aims of Rx

Freedom from pain and infection.

- A happy and cooperative patient.
- Prevention.
- Development and maintenance of healthy and attractive primary and permanent dentitions.

Points to remember

- Praise good behaviour (reinforcement, p. 62), ignore bad.
- Involve parents (they determine whether child will return).
- Do not offer choice where there is none. Avoid rhetorical questions (Would you like to get into my chair?).
- Children have short attention spans (with age).
- Children have ↓ sensory acuity (may confuse pressure with pain, sensibility tests less reliable).
- Children have ↓ manual dexterity, ∴ need help with toothbrushing <7 yrs.
- Formulate a comprehensive Rx plan, which should address both operative and preventive care, at an early stage.
- Start with easy procedures (e.g. OHI) and progress, at child's pace, to more complicated Rx.
- Set attainable targets for each visit and attain them.

The first visit

- Children should first visit a dentist as soon as they have teeth (i.e. about 6 months of age). For young children, watching other members of the family receive Rx prior to their turn may be preferable.
- Let parent accompany child: check medical history and reason for attendance.
- Talk to child: communication is the key to success!
- Show patient chair, mirror, light, and explain purpose. (tell, show, do, p. 64).
- Count the patient's teeth.
- If good progress, polish a few teeth, but don't tire child by attempting too much.
- Show parent child's teeth and what has been done that visit.
- If child in pain, the source of this needs to be determined and dealt with as quickly as possible.
- Younger children can be more successfully examined if a parent sits with child facing and then lowers child back on to his/her arm or the dentist's lap.

Treatment planning for children

Diagnosis Dental caries is often a rapidly progressing condition in children. It is essential to secure an accurate Δ before making a Rx plan. This is achieved by taking a history, doing an examination, and, where possible, taking bitewing radiographs.

▶ Bitewings are essential for an accurate Δ unless all surfaces of the primary molars can be visualized (i.e. the dentition is spaced).

Rx plan The ultimate aim in dentistry for children is for the child to reach adulthood with good dental status and a positive attitude towards dental health and dental Rx. The final Rx plan will take into account the following considerations:

- Behaviour management (p. 64).
- Prevention (Chapter 2).
- Restorative Rx (p. 84).
- Developing occlusion.

▶ Remember to consider the developing occlusion:

- Long-term prognosis for first permanent molars (p. 154).
- Palpate for 3⊥3 at age 9–10 yrs (p. 162).
- Beware disturbances in eruption sequence (p. 66) and asymmetry.
- Early referral to specialist for skeletal discrepancies, and for any abnormal findings.

The Rx plan is drawn up visit by visit. Each visit has both a preventive and operative component (delivering one preventive message per visit).

As it is considered to be easier to administer LA for maxillary teeth, these teeth are usually treated before mandibular teeth.

Restorative care (i.e. repair) without prevention is of limited value.

Dental caries is treated by "preventive" measures; restoration purely repairs the damage caused by the carious process.

Children with caries in primary molars treated by prevention alone are likely to experience toothache/infection, especially if the child is young when the caries is first diagnosed. ∴ a combination of prevention and restoration/extraction is indicated for most children with caries in the primary dentition.

Other considerations

Pain or evidence of infection may influence the order of the Rx plan.

Temporization of open cavities at the start of Rx:

- gives a good introduction to dentistry;
- helps to minimize the risk of pain before Rx is completed;
- improves comfort (e.g. during brushing and eating);
- reduces salivary *Streptococcus mutans* count;
- produces a preliminary coronal seal, enhancing the chances of pulpal recovery and survival;
- may provide slow release of fluoride in the short term if a GI cement is used.

Delivery of care

Once the Rx plan has been decided upon, discuss appropriate delivery of care with the parent and child:

- Council parent and patient about the Rx options.
- LA/sedation/GA—consider and discuss risks vs. benefits of each (p. 63).
- Plan operative care at a pace appropriate to the child's ability to cope.
- Be prepared to reconsider method of delivery of care (e.g. sedation/GA) if patient proves unable to accept Rx using original delivery strategy.

Look out for any signs of underlying medical or social problems which may modify the Rx plan:

- small stature;
- failure to thrive;
- systemic disease;
- NAI (p. 106).

The anxious child

Techniques for behaviour management

Most of these are fancy terms to describe techniques that come with experience of treating children over a period of time. However, for the student they may prove useful for answering essay questions as well as for handling their first few child patients.

General principles
- Show interest in child as a person.
- Touch > facial expression > tone of the voice > what is said.
- Don't deny patient's fear.
- Explain—why, how, when.
- Reward good behaviour, ignore bad.
- Get child involved in Rx, e.g. holding saliva ejector.
- Giving the child some control over the situation will also help them to relax, e.g. raising their hand if they want you to stop for any reason.

Tell, show, do Self-explanatory, but use language the child will understand.

Desensitization Used for child with pre-existing fears or phobias. Involves helping patient to relax in dental environment, then constructing a hierarchy of fearful stimuli for that patient. These are introduced to the child gradually, with progression on to the next stimulus only when the child is able to cope with previous situation.

Modelling Useful for children with little previous dental experience who are apprehensive. Encourage child to watch other children of similar age or siblings receiving dental Rx happily.

Behaviour shaping The aim of this is to guide and modify the child's responses, selectively re-inforcing appropriate behaviour, whilst discouraging/ignoring inappropriate behaviour.

Reinforcement This is the strengthening of patterns of behaviour, usually by rewarding good behaviour with approval and praise. If a child protests and is uncooperative during Rx, do not immediately abandon session and return them to the consolation of their parent, as this could inadvertently reinforce the undesirable behaviour. It is better to try and ensure that some phase of the Rx is completed, e.g. placing a dressing.

Should parent accompany child into surgery? Essential on first visit, thereafter depends upon childs's age. If in doubt ask child's preference. However, if parent is dental phobic, their anxiety in the dental environment may adversely affect child, so in these cases it is probably wiser to leave mum or dad in the waiting room. Some children will play up to an over-protective parent in order to gain sympathy or rewards, and may prove more cooperative by themselves. However, many parents wish to be involved in, and informed about their child's Rx. Ideally parents should be motivated positively and instructed implicitly to act in the role of the 'silent helper'.

Sedation

Indicated for the genuinely anxious child who wishes to cooperate with Rx.

Oral: Drugs such as midazolam and chloral hydrate can be used, although specialized knowledge and skills are required.

Intramuscular: rarely used in children.

Intravenous: rarely used in children.

Per rectum: popular in some Scandinavian countries.

Inhalation: uses nitrous oxide/oxygen mixture to produce relative analgesia (RA) and is most popular technique for use with children. Effective for reducing anxiety and increasing tolerance of invasive procedures in children who wish to cooperate but are too anxious to do so without help. Technique, see p. 648. It is a good idea not to carry out any Rx during the visit when the child is introduced to 'happy air'. Let child position nose-piece themselves.

Hypnosis

Hypnosis produces a state of altered consciousness and relaxation, though it cannot be used to make subjects do anything that they do not wish. Although many good books[1] and articles are available, attendance at a course is necessary to gain experience with susceptible subjects, so the operator has confidence in his abilities. It can be described as either a way of helping the child to relax, or as a special kind of sleep.

General anaesthesia

Allows dental rehabilitation &/or dental extractions to be achieved at one visit. General anaesthesia should only be used for dental Rx when absolutely necessary (i.e. when other methods of management, e.g. local analgesia or sedation, are deemed unsuitable). Alternative strategies and the risks of general anaesthesia must be discussed to enable parents to make an informed decision. From December 2001 dental general anaesthesia in the UK can only be provided in a hospital setting.[2]

Risks

The risk of unexpected death of a healthy person:
- under general anaesthesia has been estimated to be about 3 in 1 million;
- under sedation has been estimated to be about 1 in 2 million.

Other behaviour problems and their management

- The questioner attempts to delay Rx by a barrage of questions. Firm but gentle handling is needed. Tell the patient that you understand their anxieties and that you will explain as you go along.
- The temper tantrum: Try to establish communication. Praise good and ignore bad behaviour. Set an easily achievable goal e.g. brushing teeth and make sure it is achieved—comment on the positive outcome, not what was not achieved.

1 J. Hartland 1982 *Medical and Dental Hypnosis*, Baillière Tindall.
2 'A Conscious Decision'—A Review of the Use of Dental General Anaesthetic and Sedation Services in Primary Dental Care. 2000, HMSO.

The child with toothache

When faced with a child with toothache the dentist has to use his clinical acumen to try and determine the pulpal state of the affected tooth/teeth, as this will decide the Rx required. To that end the following investigations may be employed:

History Take a pain history (see p. 260) from the child and parent. Beware of variations in accuracy; anxious children may deny being in pain when faced with an eager dentist, whereas parents who feel guilty for delaying seeking dental Rx may exaggerate pain. Remember some pathology is painless, e.g. chronic periradicular periodontitis.

Examination Swelling, temperature, lymphadenopathy. Intraorally look for caries, abscesses, chronic buccal sinuses, mobile teeth (? due to exfoliation or apical infection) and erupting teeth.

Percussion Can be unreliable in children. Care needed to establish a consistent response.

Sensibility testing Again, this is unreliable in primary teeth, but for permanent teeth a cotton-wool roll, ethyl chloride, and considerable ingenuity may provide some useful information. In older children electric pulp testing may be helpful.

Radiographs Bitewing radiographs are most useful, because not only are they less uncomfortable for small mouths than periapicals, but they also show up the bifurcation area where most primary molar abscesses start.

Remember, the only 100% accurate method is histological!

Diagnosis
Fleeting pain on hot/cold/sweet stimuli = Reversible pulpitis.
Longer-lasting pain on hot/cold/sweet stimuli = irreversible pulpitis.
Spontaneous pain with no initiating factor (no mobility, not TTP) = irreversible pulpitis.
Pain on biting and pressure &/or swelling and tenderness of adjacent tissues, mobility = acute periradicular periodontitis.
With a fractious child keep examination and operative intervention to a minimum, doing only what is necessary to alleviate pain and win child's trust.
If extractions under a GA are required consider carefully the long-term prognosis of remaining teeth to try and avoid a repeat of the anaesthetic in the near future.
Other common potential causes of toothache:
• Dentoalveolar trauma (p. 104).
• Mucosal ulceration (p. 440).
• Teething (p. 68).

Diagnosis	Emergency management	Definitive management
Reversible pulpitis	LA Excavate soft caries: If exposed and vital—dress ledermix/formocresol. Restore temporarily with a zinc oxide/eugenol cement	Pulpotomy or extraction
Irreversible pulpitis	LA Excavate soft caries: If exposed and vital—dress ledermix/formocresol. Restore temporarily with a zinc oxide/eugenol cement	Pulpotomy/pulpectomy or extraction
Acute periodontitis	LA (may not be necessary if loss of vitality is certain) Excavate soft caries until pulp chamber accessed—dress pulp chamber with formocresol or ledermix on cotton wool. Seal with temporary dressing	
Acute periodontitis with facial swelling If • No or mild pyrexia (<38 °C) • Localized acute erythematous tender soft tissue swelling • No significant involvement of 'danger areas' (see below) • Not otherwise systemically unwell	Antibiotics and analgesics Ensure adequate fluid intake Establish drainage via tooth (and dress) if possible Review every 24 h to ensure resolution	Extraction of tooth (or pulpectomy in selected cases) once acute phase has resolved
If: • Signifcant pyrexia >38 °C • Poorly localized, spreading infection • Systemically unwell: dehydration, lethargy, nausea, and vomiting • Swelling involving a 'danger area', i.e. floor of mouth, submandibular/neck, infraorbital region	Aggressive antibiotic Rx (e.g. amoxicillin and metronidazole) Immediate referral to specialist centre	Extraction of tooth &/or intra-/extra-oral drainage

Abnormalities of tooth eruption and exfoliation

Natal teeth are usually members of the primary dentition, not supernumerary teeth, and so should be retained if possible. Most frequently affect mandibular incisor region and, because of limited root development at that age, are mobile. If in danger of being inhaled or causing problems with breast-feeding, they can be removed under local analgesia.

Teething As eruption of the 1° dentition coincides with a diminution in circulating maternal antibodies, teething is often blamed for systemic symptoms. However, local discomfort, and so disturbed sleep, may accompany the actual process of eruption. A number of proprietary 'teething' preparations are available, which usually contain a combination of an analgesic, an antiseptic, and anti-inflammatory agents for topical use. Having something hard to chew may help, e.g. teething ring.

Eruption cyst is caused by an accumulation of fluid or blood in the follicular space overlying an erupting tooth. The presence of blood gives a bluish hue. Most rupture spontaneously, allowing eruption to proceed. Rarely, it may be necessary to marsupialize the cyst.

Failure of/delayed eruption It must be remembered that there is a wide range of individual variation in eruption times. Developmental age is of more importance in assessing delayed eruption than chronological age.

▶ Disruption of normal eruption sequence and asymmetry in eruption times of contralateral teeth >6 months warrants further investigation.

General causes Hereditary gingival fibromatosis, Down syndrome, Gardner syndrome, hypothyroidism, cleido-cranial dysostosis, rickets.

Local causes
- Congenital absence. Is the most likely cause for failure to appearance of 2 (p. 70).
- Crowding. Rx: extractions.
- Retention of primary tooth. Rx: extraction of 1° tooth.
- Supernumerary tooth. Is the most likely reason for failure of eruption of 1 (p. 70).
- Dilaceration (p. 74).
- Dentigerous cyst.
- Trauma to primary tooth leading to apical displacement of permanent incisor.
- Abnormal position of crypt. Rx: extraction or orthodontic alignment. See options for palatally displaced 3 (p. 162).
- Primary failure of eruption usually affects molar teeth. The aetiology is not understood. Although bone resorption proceeds above the unerupted tooth, they appear to lack any eruptive potential. Rx: keep under observation, but ultimately extraction may be necessary.

Infraoccluded (ankylosed) primary molars Occur where the primary molar has failed to maintain its position relevant to the adjacent teeth in the developing dentition and is ∴ below the occlusal level of adjacent teeth.

Caused by preponderance of repair in normal resorptive/repair cycle of exfoliation. This is usually self-correcting (if the permanent successor is present and not ectopic) and the affected tooth is exfoliated at the normal time.[1] However, where the premolar is missing or where the infraoccluded-molar appears in danger of disappearing below the gingival level, extraction may be indicated.

Ectopic eruption of the upper first permanent molars resulting in an impaction of the tooth against the E occurs in 2–5% of children. It is an indication of crowding. In younger patients (<8 yrs) it may prove self-correcting ('jump'). If still present after 4–6 months ('hold') or in older children, insertion of an orthodontic separating spring (or a piece of brass wire tightened around the contact point) may allow the 6 to jump free. More severe impactions should be kept under observation. If the E becomes abcessed or the 6 is in danger of becoming carious then the primary tooth should be extracted. The resulting space loss can be dealt with as part of the overall orthodontic Rx plan later.

Premature exfoliation Most common reason for early tooth loss is extraction for caries. Traumatic avulsion is less common. More rarely, systemic disease such as leukaemia, congenital or cyclic neutropenia, diabetes, hypophosphatasia, Langerhans cell hystiocytosis, Papillon–Lefevre syndrome, Chediak–Higashi syndrome, or Down syndrome may result in an abnormal periodontal attachment and thus premature tooth loss (p. 224). Alveolar bone loss in a young child is a serious finding and warrants referral.

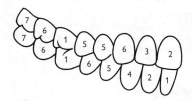

Normal sequence of eruption (permanent dentition)

1 J. Kurol 1985 *Am J Orthod* **87** 46.

Abnormalities of tooth number

Anodontia
Means complete absence of all teeth. Rare. Partial anodontia is a misnomer.

Oligodontia
American term indicating absence of one or more teeth.

Hypodontia
British equivalent of oligodontia.

Prevalence 1° dentition 0.1–0.9%, 2° dentition 3.5–6.5%.[1] In Caucasians most commonly affected teeth are 8 (25–35%), 2 (2%), +5 (3%). Affects F > M and is often associated with smaller than average tooth size in remainder of dentition. Peg-shaped 2 often occurs in conjunction with absence of contralateral 2 **NB** 3 migrates down guided by the distal aspect of 2. When 2 is absent, peg-shaped, or small-rooted, it is important to monitor the upper 3 for signs of ectopic eruption.

Aetiology *Often* familial—polygenic inheritance. Also associated with ectodermal dysplasia and Down syndrome.

Rx: 1° dentition—none. 2° dentition—depends on crowding and maloccusion.
8—none.
2—see p. 122.
5—(**NB** late development of 5̄ not unknown). If patient crowded, extraction of Ē, either at around 8 yrs for spontaneous space closure or later if space is to be closed as a part of orthodontic Rx. If lower arch well-aligned or spaced, consider preservation of E, and bridgework later.

Hyperdontia
Better known as supernumerary teeth.

Prevalence 1° dentition 0.8%, 2° dentition 2%.[1] Occurs most frequently in premaxillary region. Affects M > F. Associated with cleido-cranial dysostosis and CLP. In about 50% cases $ in 1° dentition followed by $ in 2° dentition, so warn mum!

Aetiology Theories include: offshoot of dental lamina, third dentition.

Classification either by

Shape	or	Position
Conical (peg-shaped)		Mesiodens
Tuberculate (barrel-shaped)		Distomolar
Supplemental		Paramolar
Odontome		

Effects on dentition and Rx
- No effect. If unerupted keep watch if erupts—extract.
- Crowding. Rx: extract; if supplemental, extract tooth with most displaced apex.

1 A. H. Brooks 1974 *J Int Assoc Dent Child* **5** 32.

- Displacement. Can cause rotation &/or displacement. Rx: extraction of $ and fixed appliance, but tendency to relapse.
- Failure of eruption. Most likely cause of 1 to fail to erupt. Rx: extract $ and ensure sufficient space for unerupted tooth to erupt. May require extraction of primary teeth &/or permanent teeth and appliances. Then *wait*. Average time to eruption in these cases is 18 months.[1] If after 2 yrs unerupted tooth fails to erupt despite sufficient space may require conservative exposure and orthodontic traction.

1 D. DiBiase 1971 *Dental Practitioner* **22** 95.

Abnormalities of tooth structure

Disturbances in structure of enamel

Enamel usually develops in two phases, first an organic matrix and second mineralization. Disruption of enamel formation can ∴ manifest as:

Hypoplasia

Caused by disturbance in matrix formation and is characterized by pitted grooved, or thinned enamel.

Hypomineralization

hypocalcification is a disturbance of calcification. Affected enamel appears white and opaque, but post-eruptively may become discoloured. Affected enamel may be weak and prone to breakdown. Most disturbances of enamel formation will produce both hypoplasia and hypomineralization, but clinically one type usually predominates.

Aetiological factors   (not an exhaustive list)

Localized causes: Infection, trauma, irradiation, idiopathic (see enamel opacities, p. 74).

Generalized causes:
1 Environmental (chronological hypoplasia).
    (a) Pre-natal, e.g. rubella, syphilis.
    (b) Neo-natal, e.g. prolonged labour, premature birth.
    (c) Post-natal, e.g. measles, congenital heart disease, fluoride, nutritional.
2 Hereditary
    (a) Affecting teeth only—amelogenesis imperfecta.
    (b) Accompanied by systemic disorder, e.g. Down syndrome.

Chronological hypoplasia

So called because the hypoplastic enamel occurs in a distribution related to the extent of tooth formation at the time of the insult. Characteristically, due to its later formation, 2̲ is affected nearer to its their incisal edge than 1̲ or 3̲.

Fluorosis, p. 32.

Rx of hypomineralization/hypoplasia depends on extent and severity:

Posterior teeth   Small areas of hypoplasia can be sure-sealed or restored conventionally, but more severely affected teeth will require crowning. SS crowns (p. 90) can be used in children as a semi-permanent measure.

Anterior teeth   Small areas of hypoplasia can be restored using composites, but larger areas may require veneers (p. 288) or crowns. For Rx of fluorosis, see p. 74.

Molar incisor hypomineralization (MIH)

- Aetiology unknown, but prevalence appears to have ↑ over the past two decades in developed countries.
- Primarily affected 1st permanent molars but significant proportion of affected individuals have defects on permanent incisors.
- Affected 6 have hypomineralized defects of enamel, which vary from discoloration to severe enamel dysplasia exhibiting post-eruptive breakdown. Sensitivity↑, secondary caries↑. Defects may affect anything from one to all 6s.

- Yellow/white opacities on buccal surface of affected incisors.
  Distribution often asymmetrical. No clear chronological pattern.
  Incisors less prone to enamel breakdown than 6.

Rx options include intracoronal restoration, stainless steel crowns, or extraction (p. 154). Opacities in anterior teeth can be improved by partial composite veneering.

Amelogenesis imperfecta

Many classifications exist, but generally these are classified by the type of enamel defect &/or the mode of mode of inheritance.

Main types

Hypoplastic—The enamel may be thin (smooth or rough) or pitted. Most commonly autosomal dominant inheritance.

Hypocalcified—Enamel is dull lustreless, opaque white, honey, or brown coloured. Enamel may breakdown rapidly in severe case. Sensitivity↑, calculus↑ common. May be autosomol dominant or recessive.

Hypomaturation— mottled or frosty looking white, opacities, sometimes confined to incisal third of crown ("snow-capped teeth").

Usually both 1° and 2° dentitions and all the teeth are affected. The different subgroups give rise to a wide variation in clinical presentation, ranging from discoloration to soft &/or deficient enamel. It is ∴ difficult to make general recommendations, but it is wise to seek specialist advice for all but the mildest forms. Rx: in more severe cases, SS crowns and composite resin can be used to maintain molars and 2° incisors, prior to more permanent restorations when child is older.

Disturbances in the structure of dentine

Disturbances in dentinogenesis include dentinal dysplasias (types I and II), regional odontodysplasia, vitamin D-resistant rickets, and Ehlers–Danlos syndrome—all of which are rare. A commoner defect is hereditary opalescent dentine, referred to as dentinogenesis imperfecta (II). Main types of dentinogensis imperfecta:
I—associated with osteogenesis imperfecta.
II—teeth only.

Dentinogenesis imperfecta affects 1 in 8000 people. Both 1° and 2° dentitions are involved, although later-formed teeth less so. Affected teeth have an opalescent brown or blue hue, bulbous crowns, short roots, and narrow flame-shaped pulps. The ADJ is abnormal, which results in the enamel flaking off, leading to rapid wear of the soft dentine. Rx: along similar lines as for severe amelogenesis.

▶ Early recognition and Rx of amelogenesis and dentinogenesis imperfecta important to prevent rapid tooth wear.

Disturbances in the structure of cementum

Hypoplasia and aplasia of cementum are uncommon. The latter occurs in hypophosphatasia and results in premature exfoliation. Hypercementosis is relatively common and may occur in response to inflammation, mechanical stimulation, or Paget's disease, or be idiopathic. Concrescence is the uniting of the roots of two teeth by cementum.

Abnormalities of tooth form[1]

Normal width $\underline{1}$ = 8.5 mm, $\underline{2}$ = 6.5 mm.

Double teeth

Gemination

Occurs by partial splitting of a tooth germ. *Fusion* occurs as a result of the fusion of two tooth germs. As fusion can take place between either two teeth of the normal series or, less commonly, with a $ tooth, then counting the number of teeth will not always give the correct aetiology.

As the distinction is really only of academic interest, the term 'double teeth' is to be preferred. Both 1° and 2° teeth may be affected and a wide variation in presentation is seen. The prevalence in the 2° dentition is 0.1–0.2%.

Rx for aesthetics should be delayed to allow pulpal recession. If the tooth has separate pulp chambers and root canals, separation can be considered. If due to fusion with a $ tooth, the $ portion can be extracted. Where a single pulp chamber exists either the tooth can be contoured to resemble two separate teeth or the bulk of the crown reduced.

Macrodontia/megadontia

Generalized macrodontia rare, but is unilaterally associated with hemifacial hypertrophy. Isolated megadont teeth are seen in 1% of 2 dentitions.

Microdontia

Prevalence   1° dentition < 0.5%. In 2° dentition overall prevalence is 2.5%. Of this figure 1–2% is accounted for by diminutive $\underline{2S}$ Peg- shaped $\underline{2S}$ often have short roots and are thought to be a possible factor in the palatal displacement of $\underline{3S}$ (p. 156). $\underline{8}$ also commonly affected.

Dens in dente

This is really a marked palatal invagination, which gives the appearance of a tooth within a tooth. Usually affects $\underline{2}$, but can also affect premolars. Where the invagination is in close proximity to the pulp, early pulp death may ensue. Fissure sealing of the invagination as soon as possible after eruption may prevent this, but is often too late. Conventional RCT is difficult and extraction is usually required.

Dilaceration

Describes a tooth with a distorted crown or root. Usually affects $\underline{1}$. Two types seen, dependent upon aetiology.

Developmental[2]	*Traumatic*
Crown turned upward and labially	Crown turned palatally
Regular enamel and dentine	Disturbed enamel and dentine
Usually no other affected teeth	formation seen
Affects F > M	No sex predilection

1 A. H. Brooks 1974 *J Int Assoc Dent Child* **5** 32.
2 D. J. Stewart 1978 *BDJ* **145** 229.

The traumatically induced type is caused by intrusion of the 1° incisor, resulting in displacement of the developing 2° incisor tooth germ. The effects depend upon the developmental stage at the time of injury.

Rx: depends upon severity and patient cooperation. If mild it may be possible to expose crown and align orthodontically provided the apex will not be positioned against the labial plate of bone at the end of the Rx, otherwise extraction indicated.

Turner tooth

Term used to describe the effect of a disturbance of enamel and dentine formation by infection from an overlying 1° tooth ∴ usually affects premolar teeth. Rx: as for hypoplasia, p. 70.

Taurodontism

Of academic interest only, but seems to crop up on X-rays in exams much more frequently than in clinical practice. Means bull-like, and radiographically an elongation of the pulp chamber is seen. Rx: none required.

Abnormalities of tooth colour

Extrinsic staining By definition this is caused by extrinsic agents and can be removed by prophylaxis. Green, black, orange, or brown stains are seen, and may be formed by chromogenic bacteria or be dietary in origin. Chlorhexidine mouthwash causes a brown stain by combining with dietary tannin. Where the staining is associated with poor oral hygiene, demineralization and roughening of the underlying enamel may make removal difficult. Rx: a mixture of pumice powder and toothpaste or an abrasive prophylaxis paste together with a bristle brush should remove the stain. Give OHI to prevent recurrence.

Intrinsic staining This can be caused by:
- Changes in the structure or thickness of the dental hard tissues, e.g. enamel opacities.
- Incorporation of pigments during tooth formation, e.g. tetracycline staining (blue/brown), porphyria (red).
- Diffusion of pigment into hard tissues after formation, e.g. pulp necrosis products (grey), root canal medicaments (grey).

Enamel opacities are localized areas of hypomineralized (or hypoplastic) enamel. Fluoride (p. 32) is only one of a considerable number of possible aetiological agents.

Rx: four possible approaches:

1 Acid pumice abrasion technique is used only for surface enamel defects. Hydrochloric acid technique (quicker), or phosphoric acid technique (slower but potentially safer). Pre-up photos are helpful to assess improvement

▶ Rubber dam, protective eyewear, bicarbonate of soda placed around teeth to be treated, and care, essential.

Hydrochloric acid technique
A mixture of 18% hydrochloric acid and pumice is applied to the affected area using a wooden stick. The mixture is rubbed into the surface for 5 sec and then rinsed away. These two steps are repeated (max. 10 times—removing <0.1 mm enamel) until the desired colour change is achieved. The enamel is then polished and a fluoride solution applied.[1]

Phosphoric acid technique
Etch with 30–50% orthophosphoric acid for 1 min, wash, then pumice slurry (pumice and water) on rubber prophy cup for 1 min (take care not to overheat the tooth). Wash. Repeat etch and pumice stage twice more, washing between. Dry tooth and apply topical fluoride solution (avoid pigmented varnishes). May be repeated up twice more, but leave at least 6 weeks before each repeat to check for improvement.
2 Bleaching, p. 316.
3 Veneers, p. 292.
4 Crowns, p. 284.

1 T. P. Croll 1986 *Quintessence Int* **17** 81.

Anatomy of primary teeth (and relevance to cavity design)

Primary teeth differ in several respects from permanent teeth, affecting both the sequelae of dental disease and its management.

Thinner enamel (1) Enamel in 1° teeth is approximately 1mm thick, which is 1/2 that of 2° teeth.

Larger pulp horns (2) The pulp chamber in 1° teeth is proportionately larger, with more accentuated pulp horns. D̲E̲—three pulp horns MB, DB, and palatal. D̅E̅—four pulp horns MB, ML, DB, and DL. These features mean that caries will affect the pulp sooner and there is a greater likelihood of pulp exposure during cavity preparation. Aim for 0.5–1.0mm penetration of dentine only.

Pulpal outline (3) follows the amelo-dentinal junction more closely in 1° teeth, ∴ cavity floor should follow external contour of tooth sinuously to avoid exposure.

Narrower occlusal table Greater convergence of the buccal and lingual walls results in a proportionately narrower occlusal table. This is more pronounced in D than E. ∴, over-extension of an occlusal cavity or lock can lead to weakening of the cusps.

Broad contact points (4) This makes detection of interproximal caries more difficult, and means that in 1° molars divergence of the buccal and lingual walls towards the approximal surface is necessary to ensure cavity margins are self-cleansing. Isthmus should not extend >1/2 intercuspal distance.

Bulbous crown (5) 1° molars have a more bulbous crown form than 2°, molars, making matrix placement more difficult.

Inclination of the enamel prisms (6) In the cervical 1/3 of 1° molars the enamel prisms are inclined in an occlusal direction so there is no need to bevel the gingival floor of a proximal box.

Cervical constriction (7) is more marked in 1° molars, ∴ if the base of the proximal box is extended too far gingivally it will be difficult to cut an adequate floor without encroaching on the pulp.

Alveolar bone permeability This is increased in younger children, thus it is usually possible to achieve local anaesthesia of 1° mandibular molars by infiltration alone, up to 6 yrs of age.

Thin pulpal floor and accessory canals (8) may explain the greater incidence of inter-radicular involvement following pulp death.

Root form (9) 1° molars have proportionately longer roots than their permanent counterparts. They are also more flared to straddle the developing premolar tooth. The roots are flattened MD, as are canals within.

Radicular pulp (10) follows a tortuous and branching path, making complete cleansing and preparation of the root canal system almost

impossible, although instrumenting canals is often easier than suggested in some texts. In addition, as the roots resorb, a different approach to RCT is needed for the 1° dentition, pure zinc oxide and eugenol being the obturation material of choice.

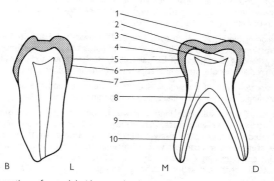

Cross-sections of second deciduous molar showing features of anatomy of primary molars.

Extraction versus restoration of primary teeth

Despite a welcome reduction in the prevalence of dental decay, the dilemma of whether to restore or extract a primary tooth is still all too familiar. In making a decision a number of factors should be considered:

Age   This will influence the likely cooperation for restorative procedures, the expected remaining length of service of the affected tooth, and the severity of sequelae following early tooth loss (as the earlier the tooth is lost the greater the potential for space loss).

Medical history   Possible sources of recurrent bacteraemia should be avoided in patients with a history of cardiac disease and in the immuno-compromised. (Hence pulp therapy is inappropriate and extractions should be carried out under antibiotic cover). In haemophiliacs, extractions should be avoided and 1° teeth preserved, if possible, until their exfoliation. Prevention is particularly important in these patients.

Motivation and cooperation of parents   As it is the parents that bring the child to the surgery, we must explain to them the benefits of maintaining the primary dentition. Unfortunately, a small proportion of the population still regard a dentist that fills primary teeth with suspicion—after all, everyone knows that baby teeth fall out!

Caries rate   In a child with an otherwise caries-free mouth every attempt should be made to preserve an intact dentition. Where there is extensive caries, restoration of 2nd primary molars and loss of first Primary molars can be an acceptable compromise.

Pain   If a child is suffering pain from one or more teeth, this needs to be alleviated as soon as possible. If symptom-free, then the dentist will have more time to explore the extent of the lesion(s) and the child's cooperation.

Extent of lesion(s)   In 1° molars destruction of the marginal ridge indicates a high probability of pulpal involvement.[1] If several 1° molars require pulp therapy, and cooperation/motivation is poor, serious thought should be given to extraction rather than restoration.

Position of tooth   Although early loss of 1° incisors will have little effect, extraction of C, D, or E will, in a crowded patient, lead to localization of the crowding. Extraction of Es, particularly in the upper arch, should be deferred, if possible, until the first permanent molar has erupted.

Presence/absence of permanent successor   Bear in mind the amount of crowding present and the likelihood of spontaneous space closure.

Malocclusion   If still undecided, it is worth considering the occlusion. In a particularly crowded case, restoration of a decayed tooth may be indicated if further space loss would mean that extraction of more than one premolar per quadrant would be required. Much has been written about compensating (same tooth in opposing arch) and balancing (contralateral tooth) extractions, although this is still an area of an area of

1 M. S. Duggal 2002 *Eur J Paed Dent* **3** 112.

some controversy.[1] The rationale is that a symmetrical problem is easier to deal with later, but if taken to its logical conclusion, gross caries of D̲ and E̲ will result in a clearance!, In general, loss of C̲, C̅, or D̅ in a crowded patient should be balanced to prevent a centre-line shift.

So much for the theory; in practice, it should be remembered that a happy and cooperative patient is more important long term. For some children this may mean that the extraction of several carious teeth at the one visit is preferable to prolonged open combat in the dental chair. For most, restoration is better than running the risk of a GA, which in itself may be a distressing experience. Inevitably, the wrong decision will sometimes be made, but we are all human.

1 W. P. Rock 2002 *Int J Paed Dent* **12** 151.

Local analgesia for children

Although there is no scientific evidence to suggest that 1° teeth are less sensitive than 2° teeth, clinically it is often possible to complete cavity preparation without LA, provided extensive dentine removal is not required. However, Walls et al. found that restorations placed without LA did not survive as long as those where LA was used.[1]

General principles
- Explain to patient in terms they will understand what you are trying to do and why.
- Use flavoured topical anaesthesia (20% benzocaine).
- Warm anaesthetic solution to room temperature only.
- Use fine-gauge disposable needle.
- Always have DN to assist.
- Hold mucosa taut.
- Use slow rate of injection.
- Warn about post-op numbness and avoidance of self-infected trauma (e.g. lip chewing).

Choice of anaesthetic agent
First choice: lignocaine 2% with 1:80 000 adrenaline.
Second choice: prilocaine 3% with felypressin (0.31 IU/ml)—gives less profound anaesthesia.
Dosage
Lignocaine maximum dose = 4.4 mg/kg. Prilocaine maximum dose = 6.6 mg/kg
In both cases this equates to a maximum of 2.2 ml for a 10 kg, 1.5-yr-old child and 4.4 ml for a 20 kg, 5-yr-old.

Infiltration injection
Used for maxillary teeth, mandibular incisors, and lower primary molars before 6 has erupted. After 6 yrs of age bone permeability is reduced and an IDB is required. Technique as for adults (p. 644). In children, the malar buttress overlies 6, so it is often advisable to deposit some solution over the more permeable bone mesial and distal to this tooth.

Block injection
Inferior dental block   Using thumb and forefinger, find the shortest width of ramus. Penetrate about 1 cm into lingual tissues from internal oblique ridge, on a line between thumb and finger. An aspirating syringe is essential.

Posterior superior alveolar block   is rarely required in children. If necessary due to failure of infiltration for 6, the technique should be modified by depositing solution distal to the zygomatic buttress and massaging it backwards towards the posterior superior alveolar foramen (maxillary molor block).[2]

Alternative techniques
Intraligamentary injection   These purpose-designed syringes have an ultra-short needle and a 'gun' or 'pen' appearance. This makes it helpful for children with a needle phobia, or as a more acceptable alternative or

1 A. W. G. Walls 1985 *BDJ* **158** 133.
2 A. K. Adatia 1976 *BDJ* **140** 87–92

adjunct to an IDB. In addition, as the lips and tongue are not anaesthetized it is useful for young or disabled children, in whom there is a greater risk of post-operative soft-tissue trauma.

Jet injection   In this technique a jet syringe (e.g. Syrijet or Injex) is used to inject LA solution under pressure through mucosa and bone to a depth of about 1 cm. Useful for producing soft-tissue analgesia prior to conventional LA injection or for infiltration analgesia, and for patients who will not contemplate LA using a needle.

Computer-controlled delivery (e.g. The Wand)   Allows carefully controlled slow delivery via a line and needle resembling an IV giving set. Especially useful for direct palatal analgesia.

Restoration of carious primary teeth

Making an accurate pre-operative Δ (including appropriate radiographs) and Rx plan is essential. This will enable Rx to be provided as efficiently as possible (p. 62)

Local anaesthesia, p. 82.

Isolation   Ideally, rubber dam should be used routinely for all restorative procedures. It not only protects the airway, but also improves moisture control and visibility, and aids in patient management. It is essential for all root canal and pulp therapy for permanent teeth, and advisable for restoration of primary teeth. If placement of rubber dam is not possible, plastic disposable salivary ejectors are better tolerated than the metal flange type.

Instruments

Burs   High-speed; pear-shaped bur numbers 330 and 525, and short fissure bur number 541. Slow-speed: a selection of pear-shaped and round burs are most useful. For access use a small bur, and for caries removal use the largest round bur which fits into the cavity.

Handpiece   A miniature-head handpiece is invaluable. Some children are apprehensive of the aspirator tip, making use of a high-speed, water-cooled handpiece difficult; others find the vibration of the slow-speed handpiece distressing, and may confuse it with pain. In these cases a vivid imagination and considerable ingenuity help. It is possible, but time-consuming, to complete cavity preparation with hand instruments.

Material selection for intracoronal restorations

Amalgam   In spite of concerns about toxicity and environmental pollution, this still remains an acceptable and durable material for class I and II restorations in primary molars.

GI cement   Has advantages of adhesion and fluoride release, but more technique sensitive that amalgam and less wear resistant. Most useful in non-load bearing class III and V catives, temporization of primary teeth in young, pre-cooperative children, or teeth within a year or so of exfoliation.

Compomer   A modified composite-type material with some of the properties of GI cement. More technique and moisture sensitive than amalgam, but studies suggest similar longevity.

Composite resin   Early studies suggested poor performance in primary teeth, but modern materials placed with good isolation (i.e. rubber dam) should perform similarly to compomers, although little recent data on performance in primary molars exists.

▶ Plastic, intracoronal restorations perform best in primary molars with small class I and II cavities. Stainless steel crowns (p. 90) give superior longevity where lesions are more extensive.

Principles of cavity design

Outline form   should include any undermined enamel. Extension for prevention is now outmoded, but any suspect adjacentfissures should be included. Do not cross transverse marginal ridges unless they are undermined.

Caries removal   Caries should be excavated from the ADJ first. If necessary, you may need to re-establish outline form to improve access to ensure ADJ is caries free. Then progress to carefully removing caries from floor.

Resistance form/retention form The completed restoration must be able to adequately resist dislodgement. Usually a 90° cavosurface angle and caries removal suffice.

Reasons for failure of restorations in primary teeth

- Recurrent caries, often due to failure to adequately complete caries removal because of flagging patient cooperation or failure to use adequate local analgesia. If unable to finish cavity it is better to place a temporary dressing and try again at another visit.
- Cavity preparation does not satisfy the mechanical requirements of the filling material.
- Inadequate moisture control, especially true of GI cements, compomers, and composites.
- Presence of occlusal high spot.

Many others, but these are the most common.

Useful tips

- Let the child participate by 'looking after' the saliva ejector or cotton wool.
- If the child is nervous give them some control by asking them to signal, e.g. by raising their hand, if they want you to stop.
- If the child's cooperation runs out before the cavity is completed, try and ensure all caries is removed from the amelo-dentinal junction and place a dressing of either ZnO or GI cement. This can then be left for several visits, until you are ready to try again.
- Vibration is less of a problem with lower teeth, ∴ if possible start with a lower tooth.
- However, giving LA is easier in the maxilla.
- Don't try to do too much at one visit; quadrant conservation is not really feasible in an 8-yr-old!

Communication

▶ It is important to explain to the child what you are trying to do, and why, in terms they can understand.

It may be helpful to describe some of the instruments we use in ways that can make them seem less threatening to a child, e.g.

slow-speed handpiece	Mr Buzz/buzzy bee/bumble bee
high-speed handpice	Mr Spray/wizzy brush/tooth tickler
handpiece and prophylaxis cup	electric toothbrush/tooth polisher
aspirator tip	vacuum cleaner/hoover
rubber dam	tooth raincoat
saliva ejector	straw
	curly-wurly (coiled type only)
air from 3-in-1	wind
fissure sealan	plastic coating
etchant solution	tooth shampoo/cleaner
	lemon juice
cotton wool roll	snowman
dental light	the sun/car light

Class I in primary molars

See p. 78 for anatomy of 1° molars and effect upon cavity design. Have all necessary instruments and filling materials ready so that appointment is kept as short as possible.

- Explain and show child (and parent) what you are trying to do.
- LA if required (p. 82).
- In small cavity will need to gain access and this is most easily done with a high-speed handpiece and pear-shaped bur. The outline can then be established and caries removed.
- In larger cavities an excavator or large round bur can be used to start caries removal from the walls. Any undermined enamel should be cut back.
- If caries deep, stop and re-assess whether pulpotomy (p. 96) required.
- Check retention and walls are caries free.
- Wash and dry cavity.
- Line with hard-setting calcium hydroxide if using amalgam.
- Place amalgam incrementally. GI or composite are also acceptable.
- Check occlusion
- This is usually a good opportunity to reinforce any preventive advice, but keep it brief.

▶ Praise child, and if bribery has not been used don't forget the sticker/ badge/toothbrush.

Polishing of amalgam restorations in 1° molars is unnecessary.

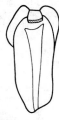

Cross-sectional view of class I restoration (bucco-lingually).

Class II in primary molar—amalgam

See p. 78 for anatomy of 1° molars and effect upon cavity preparation. Class II cavities are designed for the Rx of inter proximal caries and consist of three parts.

Occlusal key is designed to retain the restoration and eliminate any occlusal caries. Should be prepared first and is identical to class I cavity preparation, p. 84. This component is essential for class II amalgam restorations, but can be omitted for minimal cavities restored with adhesive materials.

Isthmus joins the occlusal key with the interproximal box. It is the part of the filling most prone to fracture. Dimensions of the isthmus are a balance between:

adequate depth without risking pulpal exposure (1.5–2 mm)	adequate width without weakening cusps (1/3 – 1/2 distance between cusps)

▲

Approximal box To allow access for caries removal. Ideally should just extend into embrasures and walls should converge occlusally.

Minimal caries with marginal ridge intact (usually diagnosed on pre-operative b/w radiographs).
- Follow steps for small occlusal cavity.
- When occlusal cavity (key) complete, extend it towards approximal surface. Most texts advise retaining some enamel inter-proximally to protect adjacent tooth, but this is often easier said than done.
- Establish floor of box, taking care not to extend beyond maximum bulbosity of tooth.
- Fracture away remaining approximal enamel with hand instruments.
- Complete preparation of box following external contours of tooth and 90° cavosurface angle.
- Remove all caries. If exposure, then pulp Rx.
- Check retention.
- If amalgam, place hard-setting lining; if adhesive material, no lining needed.
- Position narrow matrix band and wedge.
- Place material and shape/carve with matrix in place. Light cure if necessary.
- Check occlusion.

More advanced approximal caries (marginal ridge broken down—likelihood of pulpal involvement).
Plastic restorations perform best in class I and small class II cavities. In extensive cavities &/or where pulp Rx is necessary, stainless steel crowns provide a more durable restoration.

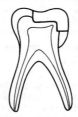

Cross-section of $\overline{D}$|mo restoration (mesio-distally).

Stainless steel crowns

▶ SS crowns are the most durable restoration for primary molars with extensive caries, caries on three or more surface, and those where pulp Rx has been performed.

▶ Although made of stainless steel, SS crowns do contain small traces of nickel and are therfore not suitable for patients with a known nickel allergy.

Indications

- Badly broken down 1° molar.
- After pulp therapy in 1° molars.
- As interim measure for 2° molars, where crowns are required but the patient is too young.
- Temporary coverage during preparation of cast crown for pre molar or 2° molar.
- Developmental anomalies.
- Severe tooth loss due to bruxism/erosion.

Instruments High-speed tapered diamond bur (e.g. 582) and diamond occlusal wheel. Straight handpiece and a stone. Slow-speed handpiece and burs as required. Crown scissors, dividers, selection of suitable crowns, and Adam's pliers. Johnstone contouring pliers (number 114) and Abel pliers (number 112) are also useful for making accurate adjustments.

Technique

SS crowns rely for retention only on a tight adaptation at the gingival margin of the preparation, ∴ taper of preparation walls is not critical.

- LA, and if possible rubber dam.
- Measure M–D length with dividers to aid crown selection.
- Remove caries.
- Occlusal reduction (approx 1 mm) with occlusal wheel, roughly following cuspal planes.
- Approximal reduction (approx 20° from vertical) using tapered diamond, without producing a ledge at gingival margin.
- Remove buccal and lingual bulbosities only sufficient to set crown (often little/no reduction required).
- Select crown. Correct size will be a 'click' fit (like a press-stud).
- Check height and occlusion. Minor prematurity is not a problem. If extensive blanching of surrounding tissues or over-extended, trim crown. With modern crowns this step will usually not be necessary.
- Use Adams or 112/114 pliers to adapt contact points to crimp margins, and smooth trimmed margins with stone.
- Cement with zinc polycarboxylate or glass ionomer cement.

Technique for 2° molars is similar but more careful adjustment is necessary.

Success rates

A number of studies have demonstrated that SS crowns have a far superior longevity to other types of restoration in primary molars.

Further reading Stainless steel crowns. RCS clinical guideline. *Int J Paed Dent* 1999 **9** 311. M. S. Duggal *et al.* 2002 *Restorative Techniques in Paediatric Dentistry*, Dunnitz.

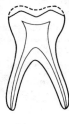

Occlusal reduction

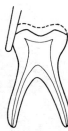

Mesial (and distal) reduction

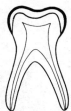

Completed crown

Preparation for stainless steel crown.

Classes III, IV, and V in primary teeth

Carious 1° incisors and canines are seen less frequently than molars and are ∴ indicative of a high caries rate (see Severe Early Childhood Caries p. 94).

Management   Objectives are relief of pain and prevention. Aesthetics are less important.

Rx options include
- Extraction.
- Topical fluoride (2% sodium fluoride) and observation. Intervene if caries progresses.
- Discing (safer to use flat fissure No. 1 bur, than disc) plus topical fluoride.
- Restoration; usually there is insufficient hard tissue for adequate retention, ∴ adhesive materials are preferable.

Class III restoration   Similar technique to that used for permanent incisors, but omit incisal retention groove.

Class IV restoration   If restoration is essential the greater strength of composite is required. Polycarboxylate (strip) crowns are advocated by some paedodontists, for the well-motivated child.

Class V restoration   Remove caries with inverted cone and restore with GI.

Composite strip crowns   Cellulose acetate crown forms for primary incisors. Enable restoration of primary incisors using composite resin.

Severe early childhood caries

Aetiology   Frequent ingestion of sugar &/or reduced salivary flow.

Nursing bottle or bottle mouth caries   Associated with frequent consumption of a sugar-containing drink, especially from a feeding-bottle. Also attributed to prolonged on-demand breast-feeding, especially at night, due to the lactose in breast milk.[1] Characteristically, starts with the maxillary 1° incisors, but in more severe cases the first primary molars are also involved. The mandibular incisors are relatively protected by the tongue and saliva.

Rampant caries   A term often used to describe extensive, rapidly progressing caries affecting many teeth in the primary &/or permanent dentition.

Severe early childhood caries may also be caused by the prolonged and frequent intake of sugar-based medications; however, both pharmaceutical companies and doctors are more aware of the problem and the number of alternative sugar-free preparations is increasing. See p. 126 for list.

Management
- Removal of aetiological factors (education, artificial saliva).
- Fluoride rinses for older age groups (daily 0.05%).
- 1°dentition—may need to extract teeth of poor prognosis and concentrate on prevention for permanent dentition.
- 2°dentition—need assessment of long-term prognosis for teeth. Final Rx plan should be drawn up in consultation with orthodontist.

Radiation caries   Radiation for head and neck cancer may result in fibrosis of salivary glands and salivary flow. Patients often resort to sucking sweets to alleviate their dry mouth, which exacerbates the problem.

1 G. J. Roberts 1982 *Journals of Dentistry* **10** 346.

Primary molar pulp therapy

NB Primary molar roots resorb
Where the carious process has jeopardized pulpal sensibility there are two alternatives: (1) extraction; (2) pulp therapy.

Indication and contraindications See Extraction versus restoration, p. 78.

▶ Any medical condition where a focus of infection is potentially dangerous (e.g. congenital heart disease, rheumatic fever) is an absolute contraindication to pulp therapy. Extraction under antibiotic cover as advised by the child's physician is necessary.

Pulp therapy is preferable to extraction in children with bleeding disorders. Tooth must be restorable following pulp therapy.

Diagnosis of pulpal state can be difficult, as not only is a child's perception of pain less precise than an adult's, but the clinical picture may also be complicated by death of one root canal whilst the other(s) remain vital.

Indicators of possible pulp involvement
- Breakdown of marginal ridge.
- Symptoms.
- Tenderness to percussion, ↑mobility, buccal swelling/sinus.
- Inter-radicular radiolucency seen radiographically.

Definitions
Pulpotomy: removal of coronal pulp and Rx of radicular pulp.
Pulpectomy: removal of entire coronal and radicular pulp.

Principles of Rx Attempting to retain the sensibility of the pulp in 1° molars is not recommended because (1) pulpal involvement is more likely, (2) it is difficult to accurately determine the likely condition of the pulp, and (3) calcium hydroxide frequently leads to internal resorption. ∴, direct pulp capping is only advisable for small traumatic exposures. Pulpotomy remains the Rx of choice for 1° molars:

VITAL PULP ⟨ one-visit pulpotomy (procedure of choice)

two-visit pulpotomy or (only used when one visit not possible)

NON-VITAL PULP ⟨ non-vital pulpotomy

pulpectomy

Materials The most commonly used medicaments are
Formocresol (for one-visit pulpotomy), which can be mixed by a pharmacist (a 1 to 5 dilution is almost universally used) formalin 19 ml, creosol 35 ml, glycerin 25 ml, water 21 ml.
Devitalizing paste
paraformaldehyde 1 g, lignocaine 0.06 g, carmine (colour) 0.01 g, carbowax 1500 1.3 g, propylene glycol 0.5 ml.
Beechwood creosote (for non-vital pulpotomy), standard British Pharmacopeia preperation.

▶ These materials are caustic, ∴ take care.

Success rates vary from 50% for non-vital teeth to over 90% for vital pulps.[1]

Because of concerns about potential toxicity of formocreosol, numerous other medicaments have been tried. The most promising is 15.5% ferric sulfate (Astringident–Optident) which appears to have a similar success rate to formocreosol. Other potentially viable alternatives include calcium hydroxide (difficult to use successfully) and MTA (very expensive).

1 M. E. J. Curzon 1986 *Dental Advertiser* **51** 14.

Pulpotomy techniques for vital pulps

In 1° molars the relatively larger pulps result in earlier pulpal involvement; ∴ devitalization and fixation of the pulpal tissues gives more consistent results than techniques that attempt to retain vitality, e.g. indirect pulp capping. There are two alternative approaches:

- one-visit formocreosol pulpotomy;
- two-visit devitalization pulpotomy.

The choice of technique depends upon the status of the pulp, and the cooperation of the child. The generally accepted pulpotomy Rx for 1° molars is the one-visit formocreosol pulpotomy.

One-visit formocreosol pulpotomy

This method fixes most of the radicular pulp, but the apical part may be unaffected by the medicament.

- Give LA and place rubber dam.
- Complete cavity preparation and excavate caries.
- Remove roof of pulp chamber.
- Amputate coronal pulp with a large excavator or sterile round bur.
- Wash chamber and arrest bleeding with damp cotton wool.
- Place cotton wool pledget dampened with formocreosol on exposed pulp stumps for 5 min, then remove.
- Apply dressing of reinforced ZOE cement.
- Restore tooth, usually with a stainless steel crown.

Problems

Inadequate LA: repeat LA or use a two-visit technique.

Necrotic pulp: proceed with non-vital technique.

Profuse haemorrhage: indicates more serious inflammation of the radicular pulp. Formocreosol can be sealed in the canal for 1 week, then continue the procedure as above.

Alternative medicaments Ferric sulphate.

Two-visit devitalization pulpotomy

Sometimes there are occasions where it is not possible to obtain anaesthesia of a vital pulp, or cooperation is difficult and a two-visit devitalization technique may be justified. Devitalizing paste is applied to the exposure on cotton wool and sealed tightly in place for 2 weeks. On re-opening the pulp should be non-vital and Rx can proceed as for a non-vital tooth.

Non-vital pulp techniques

There are two methods used for Rx of the non-vital pulp:

Pulpotomy

This method removes infected coronal pulp and disinfects radicular pulp, so allowing normal root resorption to proceed. It is still practised in some centres, but carries a relatively low success rate (50%).

First visit

- LA will be required as part of pulp could still be vital.
- Complete cavity preparation and removal of caries.
- Remove roof of pulp chamber and excavate pulpal debris.
- Place pledget of cotton wool moistened with beechwood creosote or formocreosol in pulp chamber.
- Seal with temporary dressing (GI or ZOE).
- Arrange next appointment for 1–2 weeks later.

Second visit

- Enquire re symptoms; if none, proceed.
- Remove temporary dressing and cotton wool.
- Place antiseptic dressing (50:50 formocreosol and eugenol mixed with zinc oxide powder) and press down into root canals.
- Restore tooth.

Problems   Vital &/or sensitive tissue encountered: place devitalizing paste and seal for 1–2 weeks, before proceeding with non-vital pulpotomy.
Abscess formation during Rx: either repeat (consider whether need to incise abscess), carry out pulpectomy, or extract tooth.

Alternative medicaments   Formocreosol, and 'Kri' liquid have been suggestsed.

Technique for abscessed teeth   Acute abscesses require drainage to relieve symptoms. This can be achieved either by leaving tooth on open drainage for 1 week before proceeding as above (this is more applicable to upper teeth), or by incising abscess under topical LA. Chronic abscess drainage may be occurring through a sinus; if so, proceed straight to first-visit technique. If drainage occurring through occlusal cavity, placement of a seal may lead to an exacerbation in symptoms; ∴ always warn parents to return if any problems.

Pulpectomy

A pulpectomy is often considered difficult in primary molars because of the complexity of ribbon-shaped canals (although instrumentation is often easier than some texts might suggest). The risk of damage to the permanent successor also needs to be considered, but if conditions are favourable it is the Rx of choice for non-vital pulps.[1] The technique can be carried out in one or two visits.

- LA and rubber dam.
- Remove the necrotic pulp, locate and file canals.
- Radiograph to show position of files is desirable but not essential.

1 M. D. Duggal 1989 *Dental Update* **16** 26.

- Fill canal with plain ZOE paste with a spiral filler.
- Restore with SS crown.

If there is evidence of any infection or there is bleeding from the radicular pulp, a two-stage Rx is recommended, leaving formocreosol on a pledget of cotton wool in the canal for 1–2 weeks prior to filling.

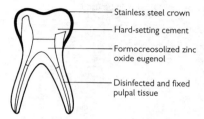

Stainless steel crown

Hard-setting cement

Formocreosolized zinc oxide eugenol

Disinfected and fixed pulpal tissue

Non-vital pulpotomy.

Pulp therapy for primary anterior teeth

Usual Rx is extraction, as $\underline{A}$ and $\underline{B}$ are exfoliated before patient is able to cooperate satisfactorily with more complicated Rx. However, $\underline{C}$ is exfoliated later and unilateral loss may result in centre-line shift, ∴ pulp Rx is indicated for some patients. The root canal morphology is amenable to pulpectomy and the canal should be cleaned using files, with care (remember underlying successor). A resorbable filling material, e.g. calcium hydroxide or ZOE, should be used.

Dental trauma

▶ If evidence of head injury, transfer patient to hospital immediately.

Note
- By 15 yrs of age 33% of children have experienced at least one episode of dental trauma.[1]
- Prognosis ↑ with good immediate Rx, ∴ see patient as soon as possible.
- Avulsed permanent teeth should be re-planted immediately.
- Child and parent may be upset, ∴ handle accordingly and defer any non-urgent Rx.
- Take good notes for future reference and medico-legal purposes.
- If crown # this will have dissipated most of the energy of impact, ∴ root # less likely.

History
Take a structured history as an aide memoire and for medico-legal purposes.

▶ Loss of consciousness? Concussion/headache (p. 490)? Refer immediately to hospital.

Accompanied by? Parent/teacher? Consider consent issues.
When? Time interval between injury and Rx affects prognosis.
Where? Does patient need a tetanus booster? If so, refer to GMP or Hospital.
How? Be alert to the possibilities of other injuries and NAI.
Tooth fragments? These may have been inhaled or embedded in soft tissues (e.g. lip). If fragment/tooth not accounted for &/or loss of consciousness, a CXR is mandatory.
PDH? Previous trauma may affect prognosis, cooperation in the dental setting.
PMH? Risk of infective endocarditis/bleeding disorder/allergy to penicillin.

Aims of Rx
1° dentition: (1) preserve integrity of permanent successor; (2) preserve primary tooth if cooperation good and compatible with first aim.
2° dentition: (1) preserve vitality of the tooth to allow maturation of the root; (2) restore the crown to prevent drifting, tilting, and overeruption.

Principles of Rx
Emergency Rx
- Elimination of pain.
- Protection of pulp.
- Reduction and immobilization of mobile teeth.
- Suturing of soft tissue lacerations (IO—3/0 resorbable suture (Dexon, Vicryl); EO—refer to hospital).
- ? antibiotics, ? tetanus, ? analgesics, ? chlorhexidine mouthwash.

1 J. E. Todd 1985 *Children's Dental Health in the UK*, HMSO.

Intermediate Rx

- Pulp therapy.
- Consider orthodontic requirements and long-term prognosis of damaged teeth.
- Semi-permanent restorations.
- Keep under review, usually 1 month, 3 months, and then 6-monthly for 2 yrs.

Permanent Rx

- Usually deferred until > 16 yrs (to allow pulpal and gingival recession and ↓ likelihood of further trauma); e.g. PJC, post and core crown.

Classification of tooth injuries

Several exist; some use roman numerals, others describe the injuries sustained (WHO system):

Complicated #—pulp exposed.

Uncomplicated #—pulp intact.

Prevention

- Prevalence ↑ as the o/j ↑ (> 9 mm prevalence doubles), ∴ ? early orthodontics.
- Mouthguard for sports (vacuum-formed thermoplastic vinyl best, triple thickness).
- ▶ Be alert for evidence of non-accidental injury (p. 106).

Non-accidental injury (NAI)

All professionals involved with children need to be alert to the possibility of NAI (a term which is now favoured over 'child abuse').

The following signs are associated with NAI:

- Usually younger children are involved.
- The presenting injuries may not match the parent's account of how they were sustained.
- Attendance at a surgery or clinic for Rx of the injury is often delayed.
- Bruises of different vintages are found on examination.
- Ear pinches, and frenal tears in children < 1 yr old are highly suspicious.
- 50% of abused children will have signs on the head &/or neck.

Management

In most areas local guidelines will have been drawn up. These can usually be obtained from Social Services or the Paediatric Department at the local hospital. A copy of these should be kept in every practice. The BDA has also included advice about handling NAI in its advice sheet *Ethical and Legal Obligations of Dental Practitioners*.[1]

If an NAI is suspected, the practitioner should refer to the local protocol, or contact either a local Paediatrician or the duty social worker at the local services department for advice. If the referral is made to the Social Services Department this will need to be confirmed in writing. The child's medical practitioner should also be informed. If a child presents with serious injuries which are suspicious, they should be referred to the nearest accident and emergency department, with the department informed of the situation before the child's arrival.

Tact is required in dealing with the patient's family. It is better to concentrate on treating the patient's injuries, referring them on to the experts who will fully evaluate the case before making a Δ of NAI.

---

1 BDA advice sheet *Ethical and Legal Obligations of Dental Practitioners*.

Injuries to primary teeth

Eight per cent of 5-yr-olds have experienced dental trauma,[1] mainly at toddler stage. As alveolar bone is more elastic the younger the child, the most common injuries are loosening &/or displacement. Crown and root # are rare.

Management

If radiographs are required, you may have to get mother to hold child and film. Alternatively, try placing a periapical film between the teeth (like an occlusal view) and angle the beam at 45°.

Need to consider the effect of any proposed Rx upon permanent successor. Splinting of 1° incisors is exceedingly difficult and not indicated. When in doubt, extract 1° tooth! (For definitions, see p. 114.)

Concussion of tooth   Rx: reassurance and soft diet.

Subluxation   If tooth near to exfoliation, extract. Otherwise, soft diet (for about 1 week). May become non-vital, ∴ keep under observation.

Luxation   Extraction indicated unless crown is displaced palatally (away from permanent tooth), tooth is not in danger of being inhaled, and tooth does not interfere with occlusion. If crown displaced labially, risk of damage to underlying 2° incisor.

Intrusion   Most common injury (> 60%).[2] If X-ray confirms that tooth has been forced into follicle of 2° tooth, extract 1° incisor. Otherwise leave tooth and wait to see if spontaneous eruption will occur (between 1 and 6 months). Unfortunately, pulpal necrosis often follows, necessitating either pulp Rx (p. 96) or extraction. Should the tooth fail to erupt, then extraction is indicated. It is prudent to warn parents about possible damage to underlying permanent tooth.

Extrusion   If > 1–2 mm, extract, as difficult to splint and will probably become non-vital.

Avulsion Do not replant.

Crown #   Rare. Minimal # can be smoothed and left under observation. Larger #:   either restore with composite &/or RCT if pulp involved, or extract.

Root #   Provided not displaced and little mobility, advise soft diet and keep under review. If coronal fragment displaced or mobile, extract, but leave apical portion as it will usually resorb.

Sequelae of trauma

Primary dentition

Discoloration   It becomes grey in early post-trauma period, pulp may be vital and discoloration reversible. Greying later indicates pulp necrosis. Yellowing of tooth is suggestive of calcification of pulp— no Rx required.

---

1 J. E. Todd 1985 *Children's Dental Health in the UK*, HMSO
2 J. O. Andreasen 1981 *Traumatic Injuries of the Teeth*, Munksgaard.

Ankylosis Rx: extraction to prevent displacement of 2° incisor.

Pulp death Rx: RCT or extraction.

Permanent dentition

In about 60% of children <4 yrs trauma to 1° tooth affects underlying developing successor.[1] Effect depends upon stage of development, type of injury and severity, Rx, and pulpal sequelae. Can cause hypomineralization, hypoplasia (likelihood <4 yrs and more severe injury), dilaceration, severe malformation, and arrest of development.

1 G. Roberts 1996 *Oral and Dental Trauma in Children and Adolescents*, OUP.

Injuries to permanent teeth—crown fractures

Prevalence: 26–76% of injuries.

Enamel only

For small enamel #, smooth with white stone.

Enamel and dentine

Need to protect exposed dentine, preferably with a hard-setting calcium hydroxide cement and an acid-etch retained composite. If time permits, this can be done with a crown former to restore tooth contour. Keep under review. Veneer or PJC can be considered later. If # near to pulp, treat as for pulp involvement.

Acid-etch composite tip technique

- Place rubber dam, if possible.
- Place hard-setting calcium hydroxide on exposed dentine. No need to bevel enamel.
- Using contralateral tooth as guide, select a cellulose acetate crown former.
- Trim crown former to within 1–2 mm of # line.
- Etch enamel for 20 sec, wash, and dry.
- Place bonding resin and cure.
- Put sufficient composite and a little extra into crown former and position.
- Allow to cure and remove crown former.
- Trim, using soflex discs. Shofu points are useful for palatal aspect.
- Check occlusion.

Enamel, dentine, and pulp

Rx depends upon size of exposure, state of root development (1 root radiographically complete 10–11 yrs, histologically 14–15 yrs), time since injury, and other injuries (e.g. root #). If apex open blood supply to pulp, ∴ likelihood of pulp death. This is advantageous as Rx should be directed towards retaining vitality of radicular pulp to allow root closure to continue. If pulp non-vital, see p. 120. Otherwise, Rx alternatives are:

Pulp cap with non-setting calcium hydroxide (mixed with water) followed by hard-setting calcium hydroxide (e.g. Dycal), and place composite tip. Review vitality.

Partial (Cvek) pulpotomy

Indications Exposure >1 mm; up to 4 days old; complete or incomplete root development.

- LA and rubber dam.
- Slightly enlarge access at site of exposure with high speed and amputate pulp to a depth of 2–4 mm into healthy pulp tissue.
- Arrest bleeding with sterile, moist cotton wool (usually takes several minutes).
- Cover amputation site with non-setting calcium hydroxide.

- Seal with GI cement.
- Restore crown.

Full coronal pulpotomy

Indications Large, contaminated exposures; long duration; incomplete root development.

- LA and rubber dam.
- Open up pulp chamber and amputate coronal pulp to cervical construction with sterile bur/sharp excavator.
- Wash with sterile water.
- Place non-setting calcium hydroxide and restore tooth with polycarboxylate or GI cement and composite.
- Leave 6–8 weeks, then review symptoms and vitality. Investigation of the presence or not of a calcific barrier is not necessary.
- If tooth becomes non-vital, see p. 120.

All pulpotomized teeth should be kept under long-term review as pulp necrosis and calcification are common sequelae. Success rates of 72% for cervical pulpotomies and 96% for minimal pulpotomies have been reported.[1]

1 M. E. J. Curzon 1999 *Handbook of Dental Trauma*, Wright.

Root fractures

Prevalence: <10% of injuries to permanent dentition.

NB Where root # is suspected, two radiographic views at different angulations in the vertical plane are advisable to improve chances of visualizing the # line.

The prognosis for this type of injury depends upon whether the # line communicates with the gingival crevice. Actual Rx depends on position of #.

Apical 1/3 Usually no Rx required unless mobility↑ significantly. However, tooth should be kept under observation as death of coronal 2/3 of pulp may occur. Only need to prepare canal to # line as apical 1/3 usually retains vitality. Prognosis good. If extraction required, apical 1/3 can be left *in situ* to preserve bone.

Middle 1/3 In majority of cases tooth is loosened, ∴ in order to achieve repair of # line with hard-tissue union, the tooth should be splinted rigidly for 8–12 weeks. If coronal part not displaced loss of vitality unlikely. Where coronal fragment displaced, re-position, splint, and if loss of vitality occurs, RCT to # line. Calcium hydroxide should be used as an interim dressing to limit inflammation and resorption. Delay in Rx ↓ prognosis. If extraction required, consider leaving apical portion *in situ*.

Coronal 1/3 By definition, # in this group communicate with the gingival crevice, allowing ingress of bacteria into pulp. Emergency Rx consists of a choice between either extraction of both parts of tooth or, preferably, removal of the coronal fragment, RCT of remainder, and then placement of a dressing which will prevent gingival tissues overgrowing root surface. This can be achieved by placing a temporary post-retained crown, but replacement of the coronal fragment using a dentine-bonding agent has been described. For permanent Rx, can place a post and core crown. However, if # extends below alveolar crest, need improved access for crown fabrication; there are two alternatives:

Ostectomy/gingivectomy	*Orthodontic extrusion*
Gives quicker result	Cervical circumference of
Needs post and diaphragm	crown ↓ compared to
Tend to get perio pocket	contralateral tooth
Leads to ↓ gingival width	Better crown : root ratio
	May attached gingiva

Orthodontic extrusion can be accomplished, using a URA with a buccal arm which engages either an attachment bonded on to labial surface of temporary post and core crown or any available enamel. Forces of 50–100 g should be used. When sufficient extrusion has been achieved, retain for at least 3–6 months before fabricating a permanent restoration.

If tooth extracted, a P/- will need to be fabricated (p. 336).

Oblique Provided # extends <4 mm below alveolar crest, can treat as coronal #. Otherwise, if possible, extract coronal portion only, leaving apical portion *in situ* to preserve bone.

Vertical Extract.

Luxation, subluxation, intrusion, and extrusion

Prevalence: 15–40% of injuries.

Definitions

Concussion Injury to supporting tissues of tooth, without displacement.

Luxation Displacement of tooth (laterally, labially, or palatally).

Subluxation Actually means partial displacement, but commonly used to describe loosening of a tooth without displacement.

Intrusion Displacement of tooth into its socket. Often accompanied by # of alveolar bone.

Extrusion Partial displacement of tooth from its socket.

Rx

Concussion Reassurance and soft diet.

Luxation Need to reposition tooth as soon as possible. Give LA and use fingers to push back into place. Then tooth should be splinted flexibly 2–3 weeks. If there has been a delay of more than 24 h since the injury, manual reduction is unlikely to be successful. In these cases the tooth can be repositioned orthodontically. If the displaced tooth is interfering with the occlusion an URA, with buccal capping, should be fitted as soon as possible. If root development is complete loss of vitality is a common sequelae following luxation, leading to inflammatory resorption (p. 120). Teeth with immature apices have a much better chance of pulp survival External or internal resorption and pulp canal obliteration may also occur, ∴ keep under review.

Subluxation If minor, no Rx other than advising a soft diet is necessary. If mobile, splint for 1–2 weeks and watch vitality.

Intrusion[1] Teeth with immature roots are likely to erupt and ∴ no immediate Rx is required although consideration should be given to surgical repositioning is displacement is severe (i.e. > 6 mm intrusion). However, teeth with closed apices have a limited potential for re-eruption and will need orthodontic extrusion. This should be started as soon as possible to facilitate access for RCT. Again, surgical repositioning may be indicated when instrusion is severe. Surgically repositioned teeth require flexible splinting for 1–2 weeks. Pulp death &/or root resorption can ensue rapidly after injury and early pulp extirpation, and placement of the calcium hydroxide dressing is advisable. In immature teeth the—blood supply means that loss of vitality is less likely, but not impossible.

Extrusion The affected tooth should be repositioned under LA with digital pressure and splinted for 1–2 weeks. Again, loss of vitality is a common sequela, so the tooth should be observed for any signs of resorption or pulp death.

If any of the above occur in conjunction with # of the alveolar bone, the splinting period should be ↑ to 3–4 weeks to aid bony healing. If, however, the socket is comminuted, splinting needs to be extended to 6–8 weeks.

1 M. J. Kinirons 1998 *Int J Paed Dent* **8** 165.

Splinting

Indications

- To stabilize a loosened tooth to promote periodontal healing and improve patient comfort. To encourage fibrous rather than bony healing (ankylosis), a short splinting time with a flexible is recommended (avulsion = 7–10days. luxation = <3 weeks).
- To stabilize a root # and encourage healing with calcified tissue. Rigid splinting for 12 weeks is generally indicated.

Methods

Direct Constructed on patient. An almost infinite variety have been described, but the following are the most popular:
- Acid-etch splint with composite/acrylic/epimine resin &/or wire/orthodontic attachments.
- Lone standing teeth can be supported by sling suture.
- Interdental wiring of historical interest.
- Lead foil &/or cement. Useful in Australian Outback, but better alternatives available in most dental surgeries!

Indirect This type of splint is removable, allowing an assessment of mobility or firmness, which is valuable in cases of reimplantation. The more common types are:
- URA with cribs 6|6 and occlusal coverage.
- Vacuum-formed thermoplastic polyvinylacetatepolyethylene (!) 'Drufomat' type.

However, this approach requires an impression of traumatized mouth and involves some delay (few h/days) before splint can be fitted, so in practice direct splinting is usually preferred.

Factors affecting choice of splint

- Type of injury and ∴ length of time splint required. For example, root # will need 8–12 weeks of splinting, ∴ composite and wire splint advisable. For re-planted tooth prolonged splinting should be avoided as may lead to ankylosis.
- Dental status of patient, e.g. if 6EDC|CDE6 present and both 1|1 traumatized need full coverage acrylic splint.
- Facilities and time available.
  Number of teeth injured and availability of uninjured adjacent teeth.
- Luxated or replanted teeth can be held in place with sling sutures if no adjacent teeth to splint to.

Management of the avulsed tooth

Exarticulation = avulsion. Prevalence: 0–16% of injuries.

Factors affecting prognosis Success depends upon re-establishment of a normal periodontium.

- *Time from loss to re-implantation.* As PDL cells rarely survive > 60 min extra-orally, immediate replacement (by whoever is available at the scene) is the Rx of choice.
- *Storage medium.* Prognosis saliva > milk >water > air. (Dry storage rapidly damages periodontal cells.)
- *Splinting time* 7–10 days flexible splinting. Prolonged splinting will promote ankylosis.
- *Viability of pulp.* Seepage of pulp breakdown products into PDL will contribute to the development of inflammatory resorption. Although re-vascularization is possible in a tooth with an open apex which is replaced within 30 min, those teeth with closed apices and longer extra-alveolar times should be considered non-vital.

Immediate Rx (if avulsed tooth not already replaced)
- Avoid handling root surface. If tooth contaminated, hold crown and agitate gently in saline.
- Place tooth in socket. If does not readily seat, get patient to bite on gauze for 15–20 min.
- Compress buccal and lingual alveolar plates.
- Splint a curved piece of light wire(a light twist-flex type wire is ideal) to acid-etched enamel of affected and adjacent teeth using temporary crown material as this is less traumatic to remove than composite.
- Prescribe antibiotics, chlorhexidine mouthwash, and arrange tetanus booster if necessary.

Intermediate Rx (7–10 days later)
- Review splinting. Stop if tooth appears firm, continue for further week if still mobile. (If still mobile after 2 weeks, check nothing has been overlooked, e.g. root # or loss of vitality—in these cases prognosis is poor).
- If apex closed (or tooth with open apex, but extra-alveolar period > 30 min) extirpate pulp, clean canal, and place an initial intra-canal dressing of calcium hydroxide. An intermediate dressing of polyantibotic/steroid paste may be placed for 1–2 weeks prior to placement of calcium hydroxide.
- Keep teeth with open apices under close observation, so that at the first sign of pulp death RCT can be instituted. Waiting for radiographic evidence of inflammatory resorption is too late.
- Keep tooth under review. If calcium hydroxide placed in canal, should be renewed every 3 months until apical barrier formed and then GP filling placed.

Prognosis If above procedure followed, medium-term survival is relatively good:[1]
- Incomplete root formation: 66% survive 5 yrs.
- Complete root formation: 90% survive 5 yrs.

---

1 J. O. Andreaen 1992 *Atlas of Replantation and Transplantation of Teeth*, Mediglobe.

Long-term survival is closely related to extra-alveolar dry-storage time. Teeth stored dry for > 30 min have a very poor long-term prognosis, but replantation may still be worthwhile, as failure is usually by replacement resorption which is slow (i.e. tooth may last several years) and maintains bulk of alveolus (facilitates future prosthetic replacement).

Where prognosis is deemed to be poor, premolar transplant can be considered at 10–12 yrs old.

Sequelae

Surface resorption occurs as a result of minor trauma to PDL cells. Usually is self-limiting and affected areas are repaired by cementum. No Rx.

Replacement resorption (ankylosis) caused by damage to PDL cells during extra-alveolar period and promoted by prolonged splinting. It appears that the absence of vital periodontal ligament allows resorption of the root and replacement by bone. In growing child results in infra-occlusion of affected tooth. Once started is usually progressive, resulting in the eventual loss of the tooth.

Inflammatory resorption Development of inflammatory resorption is dependent upon the presence of both damage to the periodontal ligament and breakdown products from pulp necrosis diffusing through the dentinal tubules to the PDL. Occurs rapidly, as soon as 1–2 weeks after injury. Once evident radiographically prognosis is poor, as it is progressive and Rx is not always successful. Inflammatory resorption can be prevented by extirpation of the pulp as soon as is practicable after injury and placement of non- setting calcium hydroxide. If resorption is halted a GP root filling can be placed.

Delayed presentation Where viability of PDL cells doubtful, Andreasen has suggested chemical Rx of the root surface with F to limit resorption.[1] Following RCT with GP, the tooth is immersed in 2.4% sodium fluoride solution for 20 min. Then tooth is replanted and splinted for 6 weeks. As some replacement resorption is inevitable, perhaps best limited to adults. If the extra- alveolar period is greater than 24 h, leave and consider instead whether the resulting space should be maintained with a P/- (p. 336).

Pulpal sequelae following trauma

Damage to the pulp can occur as a result of disruption of the apical vessels or exposure of the pulp by a crown or root #, or be caused by haemorrhage and inflammation of coronal pulp, resulting in strangulation.

Pulp death   Remember that no response to vitality testing indicates damage to the nerve supply of a tooth, but not necessarily to the blood supply. ∴ following trauma, you should assess vitality in the light of symptoms, tooth colour, mobility, presence of buccal swelling, and radiographic evidence. Except where a tooth has been re-planted, it is best to adopt a wait and see approach if in doubt about vitality. When pulp death has occurred, subsequent Rx depends upon whether the apex is closed (p. 110) or open.

RCT of teeth with immature apices   As achievement of an apical seal is difficult in a tooth with an open apex, Rx should aim to allow apexification to continue. Under rubber dam, the necrotic pulp should be extirpated. The working length is set 1–2 mm short of the radiographic apex (unless vital pulp tissue is encountered earlier) and narrow files are used in order to negotiate any undercuts. The canal should then be filled with a radiopaque non-setting calcium hydroxide, e.g. Reogan (alternatively, use the catalyst from Dycal), to the apex and sealed. The calcium hydroxide should be replaced every 3 months, until a calcific apical barrier is detectable by gentle probing with a paper point. Then the canal can be filled. Usually, because of the width of the canal, a large GP point a conventional point upside down) is required. This should be warmed in a flame before pressing into place and then lots of laterally condensed points used to obtain a good seal. The average time for a calcific barrier to be formed is 9 months.[1] A 5-yr survival rate of 86% has been reported.[2] Clinical experience would suggest that RCT of incisors in children is often complicated by intractable infection of the canal. This may be due to the patency of the dentinal tubules. Polyantibiotic pastes can be tried, but a cheaper alternative is to crush metronidazole tablets with saline and place in the canal for 1 week.

Resorption   (commonly seen after avulsion, luxation, intrusion, or extrusion)
Internal resorption   is associated with chronic pulpal inflammation, which results in resorption of dentine from the pulpal surface. Is progressive, ∴ the pulp needs to be carefully extirpated. Dressing the tooth with calcium hydroxide appears to help arrest the resorption and, once controlled, a GP filling may be placed. If perforation has occurred the prognosis is ↓ considerably. Raising a flap, removal of granulation tissue, and placement of an amalgam seal are indicated.
External resorption   Three types are seen: surface, replacement, and inflammatory (p. 119).

Calcification   occurs in 6–35% of luxation-type injuries. Prophylactic endodontic Rx is not necessary as pulp necrosis occurs in only 13–16% of cases. A high rate of success (80%) has been reported for subsequent RCT, despite a hairline or no root-canal detectable on X-ray.

1 I. C. Mackie 1988 *Dental Update* **15** 155.
2 I. C. Mackie 1993 *BDJ* **175** 99.

Management of missing incisors

1 Rarely congenitally absent; usually lost following trauma or because of dilaceration.

2 Congenitally absent in approx. 2% of population (with likelihood of displacement **3**), but may also be lost following trauma.

Both can occur unilaterally, bilaterally, or together.

Missing upper anterior teeth are noticed by the general public before other types of malocclusion, e.g. o/j. ∴ the aim of Rx is to provide $\underline{321|123}$ smile. Although Cary Grant did well enough with a missing upper central incisor, symmetry is usually preferable. The management of missing incisors involves either recovery or maintenance of space for a prosthetic replacement, or orthodontic space closure. Nordquist[1] found that space closure was better aesthetically and periodontally than prosthetic replacement; however, with the introduction of newer materials and techniques this finding may be outdated. For each patient a number of factors need to be considered:

Skeletal relationship   In a class III case, space closure in the upper arch could compromise the incisor relationship, whereas in a class II/1 it would facilitate o/j ↓. Consider also the vertical relationship, as space closure is easier in patients with ↑ LFH and vice versa in ↓ LFH.

Crowding/spacing   In a patient with no crowding, space closure is difficult and requires prolonged retention. Before opening space it is important to ensure that sufficient will be available at the end of Rx for an aesthetic replacement (minimum width for **2** is 5 mm), for which a Kesling set-up is useful.

Colour and form of adjacent teeth   Although much can be done with composite additions and grinding, if **3** is significantly darker &/or caniform in shape, it will be difficult to turn it into convincing **2** if space closure planned. **2** can only be used to mimic **1** if root length and circumference at gingival margin are not significantly shorter.

Inclination of adjacent teeth   This will influence the type of appliance required to open or close space. The final axial inclination of the teeth will determine the aesthetics of the finished result.

Buccal occlusion   If a good buccal interdigitation exists this may C/I bringing the posterior teeth forward to close space.

Unilateral loss   A symmetrical result is more pleasing, ∴ maintenance or opening of space is preferable. If a **2** is missing and the contralateral tooth is peg-shaped, thought should be given to extracting this tooth to achieve symmetry.

Gingival level   Can alter with periodontal surgery.

Patient's wishes and cooperation   Only after assessing the above factors can the patient be given an informed choice. If the patient refuses fixed appliances this may alter the Rx plan.

1 G. G. Nordquist 1975 *J. Periodont* **46** 139.

Kesling set-up   Requires duplicate models of both arches, including at least two of the upper arch. Using a small hacksaw, the teeth which will require orthodontic movement are removed from the model and repositioned using wax. As many alternatives as desired can be tried to find the best result.

Space closure   This can be facilitated by early extraction of the primary teeth on the affected side; ∴ the earlier the decision is made to close space, the better. Almost invariably involves the use of fixed appliances, as even though spontaneous space closure may occur in a crowded mouth, over-correction of the axial inclination is advisable. It is better to carry out any masking procedures before orthodontic Rx, e.g. contouring 3 to resemble 2 (by removal of enamel incisally, interproximally, and from the palatal aspect &/or composite addition) as this will facilitate final positioning and occlusion. Retain with a bonded retainer.

NB the average difference in width between 3 and 2 is 1.2 mm, which can easily be removed mesially and distally from 3. If the lower arch is crowded extraction of a lower premolar will allow a class I buccal segment relationship to be established.

Space-maintenance/opening   If an incisor is selectively extracted and space maintenance is desired, a P/- or acid-etch bridge should be fitted immediately. Where a 2 is congenitally missing, this will not be possible and space may need to be opened orthodontically. The inclination of the teeth to be moved will determine whether fixed or removable appliances will be required. Following tooth movement, retention with a P/- for 3–6 months is advisable to allow the teeth to settle. If an acid-etch retained prosthesis is planned, ensure that there is sufficient room occlusally for the wings.

Resin bonded bridge, p. 308

Transplantation   of a lower premolar into the socket of an extracted incisor can be considered if lower arch is crowded.

Implant   when growth complete becoming more widely available (p. 428).

Common childhood ailments affecting the mouth

▶ Refer any patient with an ulcer that doesn't heal within 3 weeks or with any soft-tissue lesion of unknown aetiology.

See chapter on oral medicine.
Most common disease is gingivitis (p. 212).

Viral

Primary herpetic gingivostomatitis Occurs >6 months of age. *Symptoms*: febrile, cervical lymphadenitis, vesicles → ulcers on gingiva and oral mucosa. Rx: soft diet with plenty of fluids. Self-limiting, lasts for approximately 10 days.

Secondary herpes labialis Vesicles form around the lips, and crust. Self-limiting, but 5% aciclovir cream will speed healing.

Hand, foot, and mouth disease Rash on hands and feet plus ulcers on oral mucosa and gingiva. Little systemic upset. Self-limiting.

Herpangina Febrile illness with sore throat due to ulcers on Soft palate and throat. Usually lasts about 3–5 days. Rx: soft diet.

Warts Check hands. Usually self-limiting.

Also chickenpox (vesicles → ulcers), mumps (inflamed parotid duct), glandular fever (ulcers), measles.

Bacterial

Impetigo Very infectious staphylococcal (&/or streptococci) rash. Starts around mouth and may be mistaken for 2° herpes.

Streptococcal sore throat Can contract associated streptococcal gingivitis.

Necrotising ulcerative gingivitis Rare <16 yrs (p. 222).

Fungal

Candida Commensal of the mouth, which may become pathogenic when oral environment favours its proliferation. Two types of manifestation are seen in children. **Acute pseudo-membraneous candidiasis** (thrush) Seen in newborn, under-nourished infants after prolonged use of antibiotics or steroids. Presents as white patches that rub off. Rx: miconazole (25 mg/ml) and correct underlying problem. **Chronic atrophic candidiasis** Most commonly URA and poor OH &/or high sugar intake. Rx: OHI for appliance and teeth. Chlorhexidine mouthwash or miconazole gel.

Miscellaneous

Aphthous ulceration,[1] p. 440.

Common causes of oral ulceration in children (in order of frequency) aphthous; trauma; acute herpetic gingivostomatitis; herpangina; hand, foot, and mouth disease; glandular fever. If in doubt refer.

Common causes of soft-tissue swellings in children Abscess; mucocele; eruption cyst; epulides; papilloma.

▶ Oral cancer does occur in children, ∴ if in doubt refer to biopsy.

1 E. A. Field 1992 *Int J Paed Dent* **2** 1.

Sugar-free medications

The cariogenic effect of long-term medication sweetened with sugar is now well-recognized. As the Medicines Commission has instructed that liquid formulations for use in chronic conditions in children should be free of cariogenic sugars, the future looks bright, particularly as progress has been made on the reformulation of commonly used drugs. Unfortunately, there is no evidence that rinsing out or brushing the teeth after use of a sugar-based medicine will significantly↓ the incidence of caries. Current medical advice is for liquid medicines to be given to children by disposable syringes. This approach has the advantage that an accurate dose can be directed at the back of the mouth.

Below is a list of some sugar-free medicines. It is not exhaustive and where required reference should be made to the *British National Formulary* or ISD Scotland website (www.isdscotland.org)

Analgesics

Aspirin (> 12 years)	Dispersible aspirin tablets
Paracetamol	Disprol paediatric
	Junior Disprol suspension/tablets
	Junior Q-Panol
	Panadol baby and infant elixir
	Panadol Junior sachets
	Panadol soluble
	Junior Panaleve/Panaleve elixir
Paracetamol and codeine	Panadeine soluble
	Paracodol dispersible tablets
	Solpadeine
Ibuprofen	Ibuprofen oral suspension SF

Antacids

Aluminium and magnesium	Mucogel
	Maalox suspension
Cimetidine	Dyspamet chewable tablets/suspension
Ranitidine	Zantac dispersible tablets
	Zantax suspension

Anticonvulsants

Carbamazepine	Tegretol liquid
Phenobarbitone	Phenobarbitone elixir 30 mg/10 ml
Sodium valproate	Epilim crushable tablets/elixir

Anti-infectives

Aciclovir	Zovirax suspension
Amoxyiillin	Amoxil dispersible tablets SF
	Amoxil sachets SF
Amphotericin	Fungilin oral suspension/lozenges
Ampicillin and cloxacillin	Ampiclox neonatal suspension

Co-trimoxazole	Bactrim dispersible tablets/SF syrup
	Dispersible co-trimoxazole tablets
	Septrin dispersible tablets/
	suspension
Erythromycin	Erythroped sachets
Miconazole	Daktarin oral gel

Respiratory agents

Salbutamol	Cobutolin syrup
	Salbutamol syrup (Evans)
	Ventolin syrup

Miscellaneous

Choline salicylate	Teejel
	Bonjela
Folic acid	Lexpec syrup
Iron edetate	Sytron
Vitamins A, B, C, D, and E	Boots' Plurivite syrup for children

Calculating drug dosages

Age (yrs)	Average weight (kg)	Percentage of adult dose
1	10	25
3	14	33
5	18	40
7	23	50
12	37	75

Orthodontics

Relevant pages in other chapters   Surgical management of CLP, p. 506; abnormalities of eruption, p. 68; supernumerary teeth, p. 70; orthognathic surgery, p. 508.

Further reading   British Orthodontic Society 1996 *Young Practitioners Guide to Orthodontics*. M. L. Jones and R. G. Oliver 1995 *Walther and Houston's Orthodontic Notes*, Wright. F. McDonald and A. J. Ireland *Diagnosis of the Orthodontic Patient*, OUP. W. R. Proffitt 2000 *Contemporary Orthodontics*, Mosby.

It has been said that orthodontists forget to ask the patient to open wide, thus missing any dental pathology, whilst generalists forget to ask the patient to close together, thus missing any malocclusion! The aim of this chapter is to help ensure that this is not true. A problem-orientated approach has been used (rather than by classification) for simplicity.

What is orthodontics?

Orthodontics has been defined as that branch of dentistry concerned with growth of the face, development of the dentition, and prevention and correction of occlusal anomalies.[1]

Prevalence of malocclusion Crowding approx. 60%; Class II/1 15–20%; Class II/2 approx. 10%; Class III approx. 3%.

Why do orthodontics? Research shows that individual motivation has more effect upon the presence of plaque than alignment of the teeth. ∴, the main indications for orthodontic Rx are aesthetics and function. Functional reasons for Rx include crossbites (as associated occlusal interferences may tend to pre-dispose towards TMPDS); deep traumatic overbite; increased overjet (↑ risk of trauma), and labial crowding of a lower incisor (as this reduces periodontal support labially). While it is accepted that severe malocclusion may have a psychologically debilitating effect, the impact of more minor anomalies and, indeed, perceived need, are influenced by social and cultural factors. The Index of Orthodontic Rx Need (IOTN) has been developed to try to standardize and quantify this difficult issue (p. 134).

It is important that patients realize that orthodontic Rx is not without its disadvantages. Even with good OH, a small loss of periodontal attachment and root resorption is common and in susceptible patients this may be significant. With poor OH, greater loss of periodontal support and decalcification may result. ∴, the potential benefit to the patient must be sufficient to counter-balance these drawbacks.

Who should do orthondontics? All dentists should be concerned with growth and development. Unless anomalies are detected early and any necessary steps taken at the appropriate time, then provision of the best possible outcome for that patient is less likely. Most orthodontic Rx in Europe is now carried out by trained specialist orthodontic practitioners. In the UK the hospital consultant service acts as a source of advice and a referral point for more complex and multidisciplinary problems.

When should we do orthodontics? This depends upon the particular anomaly. In the early mixed dentition, Rx is only indicated to correct incisor Xbites and posterior Xbites with displacement. Functional appliance Rx may be started in the mixed dentition to coincide with the pubertal growth spurt; however, the majority of orthodontic Rx is not started until the 2° dentition has erupted. Rx during the early teens is preferable because the response to orthodontic forces is more rapid, appliances are better tolerated, and, most importantly, growth can be utilized to help effect sagittal or vertical change. In adults, tooth movement is slower and lack of growth will limit the type of malocclusion that can be tackled by orthodontics alone. But because of the ↑ acceptability of appliances, more adults are seeking Rx.

▶ If in doubt, refer a patient earlier rather than later, especially in cases with marked skeletal discrepancies.

---

1 W. J. B. Houston 1986 *A Textbook of Orthodontics*, Wright.

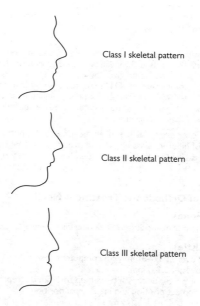

Class I skeletal pattern

Class II skeletal pattern

Class III skeletal pattern

The Index of Orthodontic Treatment Need

The IOTN was developed to quantify and standardize an individual patient's need for orthodontic Rx, so that the potential benefits can be weighed against the possible disadvantages.[1] The Index consists of two components:

The dental health component was developed from an index used by the Swedish Dental Health Board (which was used to determine the amount of financial help that would be given by the state towards Rx costs). The Dental Health Component of IOTN (reproduced by kind permission of VUMAN Ltd) has five categories of Rx need, ranging from little need to very great need. A patient's grade is determined by recording the single worst feature of their malocclusion.

The aesthetic component is based on a series of 10 photographs of the labial aspect of different class I or class II malocclusions, which are ranked according to their attractiveness. A patient's score is determined by the photograph, which is deemed to have an equivalent degree of aesthetic impairment.

The Index of Orthodontic Treatment Need

Grade 1 (None)

1 Extremely minor malocclusions including displacements less than 1 mm.

Grade 2 (Little)

2a Increased overjet 3.6–6 mm with competent lips.
2b Reverse overjet 0.1–1 mm.
2c Anterior or posterior crossbite with up to 1 mm discrepancy between retruded contact position and intercuspal position.
2d Displacement of teeth 1.1–2 mm.
2e Anterior or posterior openbite 1.1–2 mm.
2f Increased overbite 3.5 mm or more, without gingival contact.
2g Pre-normal or post-normal occlusions with no other anomalies. Includes up to half a unit discrepancy.

Grade 3 (Moderate)

3a Increased overjet 3.6–6 mm with incompetent lips.
3b Reverse overjet 1.1–3.5 mm.
3c Anterior or posterior crossbites with 1.1–2 mm discrepancy.
3d Displacement of teeth 2.1–4 mm.
3e Lateral or anterior openbite 2.1–4 mm.
3f Increased and complete overbite without gingival trauma.

Grade 4 (Great)

4a Increased overjet 6.1–9 mm.
4b Reversed overjet greater than 3.5 mm with no masticatory or speech difficulties.

1 W. C. Shaw 1991 *BDJ* **170** 107.

4c Anterior or posterior crossbites with greater than 2 mm discrepancy between retruded contact position and intercuspal position.
4d Severe displacement of teeth, greater than 4 mm.
4e Extreme lateral or anterior openbites, greater than 4 mm.
4f Increased and complete overbite with gingival or palatal trauma.
4h Less extensive hypodontia requiring pre-restorative orthodontic space closure to obviate the need for a prosthesis.
4l Posterior lingual crossbite with no functional occlusal contact in one or both buccal segments.
4m Reverse overjet 1.1–3.5 mm with recorded masticatory and speech difficulties.
4t Partially erupted teeth, tipped and impacted against adjacent teeth.
4x Supplemental teeth.

Grade 5 (Very great)

5a Increased overjet greater than 9 mm.
5h Extensive hypodontia with restorative implications (more than one tooth missing in any quadrant) requiring pre-restorative orthodontics.
5i Impeded eruption of teeth (with the exception of third molars) due to crowding, displacement, the presence of supernumerary teeth, retained deciduous teeth, and any pathological cause.
5m Reverse overjet greater than 3.5 mm with reported masticatory and speech difficulties.
5p Defects of cleft lip and palate.
5s Submerged deciduous teeth.

Definitions

Ideal occlusion   Anatomically perfect arrangement of the teeth. Rare.

Normal occlusion   Acceptable variation from ideal occlusion.

Competent lips   Lips meet together at rest.

Incompetent lips   Lips do not meet together at rest.

Frankfort plane   Line joining porion (superior aspect of external auditory meatus) with orbitale (lowermost point of bony orbit).

Lower facial height (LFH)   Clinically it is the distance from the base of the nose to the point of the chin, and in a normally proportioned face is equal to the middle facial third (eyebrow line to base of nose). Cephalometrically, it is the distance from anterior nasal spine to menton as a percentage of the total face height (from nasion to menton).

Class I   The lower incisor edges occlude with, or lie immediately below the cingulum of upper incisors.

Class II   The lower incisor edges lie posterior to the cingulum of the upper incisors. *Division I* the upper central incisors are upright or proclined and the overjet is ↑. *Division 2* the upper central incisors are retroclined and the overjet is usually ↓ but may be ↑.

Class III   The lower incisor edges lie anterior to the cingulum of the upper incisors and the overjet is ↓ or reversed.

Bimaxillary proclination   Both upper and lower incisors are proclined.

Overjet   Distance between the upper and lower incisors in the horizontal plane.

Overbite   Overlap of the incisors in the vertical plane.

Complete overbite   The lower incisors contact the upper incisors or the palatal mucosa.

Incomplete overbite   The lower incisors do not contact the upper incisors or the palatal mucosa.

Anterior open bite   When the patient is viewed from the front and the teeth are in occlusion, a space can be seen between the upper and lower incisor edges.

Crossbite   A deviation from the normal bucco-lingual relationship. May be anterior/posterior &/or unilateral/bilateral.

Buccal crossbite   Buccal cusps of lower premolars or molars occlude buccally to the buccal cusps of the upper premolars or molars.

Lingual crossbite   Buccal cusps of lower molars occlude lingually to the lingual cusps of the upper molars.

Dento-alveolar compensation   The position of the teeth has compensated for the underlying skeletal pattern, so that the occlusal relationship between the arches is less severe.

Leeway space   The difference in diameter between C, D, E, and 3, 4, 5. Greater in lower than upper arch.

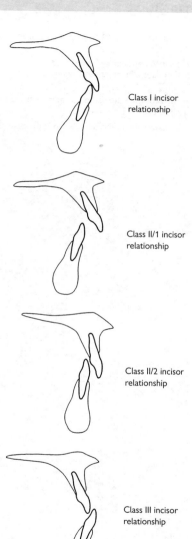

Class I incisor
relationship

Class II/1 incisor
relationship

Class II/2 incisor
relationship

Class III incisor
relationship

Mandibular deviation Path of closure starts from a postured position of the mandible.

Mandibular displacement When closing from the rest position, the mandible displaces (either laterally or anteriorly) to avoid a premature contact.

Balancing extraction Extraction of the same (or adjacent) tooth on the opposite side of the arch to preserve symmetry.

Compensating extraction Extraction of the same tooth in the opposing arch.

Orthodontic assessment

Equipment A mirror, probe, a small engineer's SS rule, and 'sharp' eyes.

Brief screening procedure

The purpose of this is to ensure early detection and Rx of any abnormality, prepare the patient for any later Rx and influence the management of any teeth of poor prognosis.

At every visit Once the 2° incisors have erupted and until 2°dentition is established (if in doubt refer).
1 Keep the eruption sequence in mind (p. 68). Any deviations from this should be observed for a few months only and then investigated.
2 Failure of a tooth to appear >6 months after the contralateral tooth has erupted should ring alarm bells.
3 Ask child to close together and look for Xbites, reverse or ↑ o/j.

Consider the long-term prognosis of the first permanent molars (p. 154).

From age 9 and until they erupt, palpate for 3 in the buccal sulcus. A definite hollow &/or asymmetry warrants further investigation.

Detailed orthodontic examination

Should be carried out in a logical sequence so that nothing is missed.
• Who wants Rx (patient or parent) and what for?
• What complexity of Rx is patient prepared to accept. Have the patient's peers worn braces and if not, will the child make a good pioneer?
• Enquire about any previous extractions and orthodontic Rx.

EO examination (with Frankfort plane horizontal)
• Assess skeletal pattern:
  1 antero-posteriorly (max = mand Class I, max>mand Class II, max<mand Class III);
  2 vertically (Frankfort–mandibular planes angle approx. 28°, lower 1/3 face usually 50% of total face height);
  3 transversely (? asymmetry).
• Soft tissues: Lips are only competent if they meet at rest. Check the position of the lower lip relative to the <u>inc</u> and how the patient achieves an oral seal (? lip to lip, lip to tongue, or by the lower lip being drawn up behind the incisors). Note also the length of the upper lip, the amount of <u>inc</u> seen, and lip tonicity.
• Check rest position of mandible and for any displacement on closure.
• Habits? Does patient suck a thumb/finger, bite fingernails or brux?

IO examination

• Record OH, gingival condition, and teeth present. Any of poor prognosis?
• LLS: Inclination to mandibular base, crowding/spacing, displaced teeth, angulation of 3|3.
• ULS: Inclination to maxillary base, crowding/spacing, rotations, displaced teeth, presence and angulation of 3|3.
• Measure o/j (mm), o/b (↑ or ↓, complete or incomplete). Check centre lines coincident and correct within face.

- Buccal segments: crowding/spacing, displaced teeth.
- Check molar and canine relationship. Any Xbites?

X-rays   Usually require a DPT and if not clearly visible on the DPT, an intraoral of the <u>inc.</u> A lateral skull view is indicated if the patient has a skeletal discrepancy or A–P movement of the incisors is anticipated).

- Look for unerupted, missing, or $ teeth, root resorption, or other pathology.
- Cephalometric analysis, p. 142.

Summary   should include a description of the patient's incisor relationship and skeletal pattern, and the main points of the malocclusion, e.g. crowding, Xbites. This gives a 'problem list' from which the aims of Rx can be derived (p. 146).

Study models   are not obligatory for orthodontic Δ, but they certainly help. Taking models allows you to mull over the possibilities at leisure and more accurately assess space requirements. If no Rx is planned unless the malocclusion deteriorates, give the models to the patient, who will usually guard them well.

▶ It is important to take models before and after orthodontic Rx so that progress can be monitored and for medico-legal purposes.

Overjet   Overbite

Cephalometrics

Cephalometric analysis is the interpretation of lateral skull radio- graphs. It is not obligatory for orthodontic Δ, and where no A–P change in incisor position is planned the X-ray exposure is not justified for the information gained. However, where A–P movement is required, a lateral skull radio- graph will back-up the clinical assessment of skeletal pattern, and help to determine the degree of difficulty and type of appliance indicated. Serial lateral skulls allow assessment of growth.

Tracing

Although this has been done using grease-proof paper and a TV as back- ground illumination (yes, really!), the quality of diagnostic information so obtained is limited. Tracing paper (secured to the film with masking tape), a sharp pencil (a 0.5 mm propelling-pencil is ideal), and good background illumination are essential. Spotting orthodontic landmarks is infinitely easier if carried out in a darkened room. If a point is hard to see, block off the rest of the film so that only that area is illuminated. If this fails, try holding up to a bright spotlight, but if still not clear, make a guesstimate! Due to the slight magnification (7–8%), two images of the mandibular border are usually seen. Both should be traced and an average taken for gonion. The most prominent image should be traced, i.e. the most ante- rior in the face so that the difficulty of Rx is not underestimated.

Pitfalls

- Consider the cephalometric values for a particular patient in conjunc- tion with the clinical assessment, as variation from the normal in a mea- surement may be compensated for elsewhere in the face or cranial base.
- Angle ANB varies with the relative prominence of nasion and the lower face. If SNA significantly ↑ or ↓ this could be due to the position of nasion, in which case an additional analysis should be used, e.g. Wits analysis.
- For landmarks which are bilateral (unless superimposed exactly) the midpoint between the two should be taken to correspond with those reference points which are in the midline.
- Tracing errors; with careful technique these should be of the order of ±0.5° and 0.5 mm. Errors are compounded when comparing tracings, ∴ changes of 1 or 2° should be interpreted with caution.

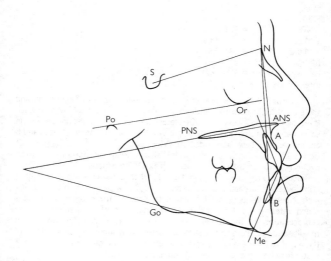

Most commonly used cephalometric points:
S   = Sella: mid-point of sella turcica.
N   = Nasion: most anterior point on fronto-nasal suture.
Or = Orbitale: most inferior anterior point on margin of orbit
      (take average of two images).
Po = Porion: uppermost outermost point on bony external
      auditory meatus.
ANS = Anterior nasal spine.
PNS = Posterior nasal spine.
Go = Gonion: most posterior inferior point on angle of mandible.
Me = Menton: lowermost point on the mandibular symphysis.
A   = A point: position of deepest concavity on anterior profile
      of maxilla.
B   = B point: position of deepest concavity on anterior profile of
      mandibular symphysis.
Frankfort plane = Po–Or.
Maxillary plane = PNS–ANS.
Mandibular plane = Go–Me.

More cephalometrics

Analysis and interpretation

The analysis of lateral skull tracings is carried out by comparing a number of angular measurements and proportions with average values for the population as a whole. Normal values for Caucasians (UK),[1] standard deviations in parentheses:

SNA	= 81° (±3)
SNB	= 79° (±3)
ANB	= 3° (±2)
<u>1</u>-Max	= 109° (±6)
1̄-Mand	= 93° (±6) or 120 minus MMPA
MMPA	= 27° (±4)
Facial proportion	= 55% (±2)
Inter-incisal angle	= 133° (±10)

If SNA or SNB are more than 3 standard deviations from the normal (and the patient looks human), check your tracing! However, the ANB difference is not an infallible assessment of skeletal pattern as it assumes (incorrectly in some cases) that there is no discrepancy in the cranial base and that A and B are indicative of basal bone position. When a cephalometric tracing seems at odds with your clinical impression it is worth doing another analysis which avoids reliance on the cranial base, such as a Wits analysis.

Before deciding on a Rx plan it is helpful to consider what factors have contributed to a particular malocclusion, e.g. in a patient with a Class II/1 incisor relationship on a Class I skeletal pattern, the prognosis for Rx is much better if the ↑ o/j is due to proclination of the upper rather than retroclination of the lower incisors. The relative contribution of the maxilla and mandible to the skeletal pattern may indicate possible lines of Rx; e.g. if an increased o/j is due to a retrusive mandible, a better aesthetic result may be achieved by use of a functional appliance.

As a rough guide can assume that there is 2.5° of angular movement for every millimetre of linear movement of the incisor edge.

1 J. R. E. Mills 1987 *Principles and Practice of Orthodontics*, Churchill Livingstone.

Wits analysis
Used to assess antero-posterior skeletal pattern

Method:
- Construct the functional occlusal plane (FOP) by drawing a line through the cusp tips of the molars and premolars or deciduous molars.
- Drop perpendiculars to the FOP from A point (to give AO) and B point (to give BO).
- Measure the distance from AO to BO.

In Class I AP relationship:
Males: BO is 1 mm ($\pm$1.9 mm) ahead of AO Females: BO=AO ($\pm$1.77 mm)

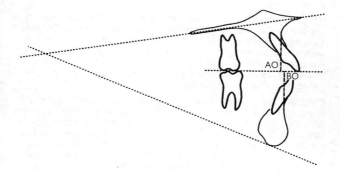

Treatment planning

Problem list Following the assessment of the patient a summary should be made of the main features of the malocclusion (p. 140). The problem list can then be drawn up; e.g.

- Crowding
- Posterior crossbite
- Increased overjet

Aims of Rx This is derived from the above problem list; e.g.

- Relieve crowding
- Correct crossbite
- Align arches
- Maintain overbite
- Reduce overjet

Plan lower arch The lower arch lies in a zone of stability between the lips, cheeks, and tongue; ∴ it is safer to consider it as immutable. This gives a starting point around which to plan Rx. The first step is to decide if the lower arch is sufficiently crowded to warrant extractions. If the crowding is likely to ↑ (patient in early teens, 8/8 present), then extractions may be indicated (p. 152). In Class 11/2 cases it may be advisable to accept a little crowding (p. 170). If in doubt refer for advice.

Plan upper arch In most cases planning will be to a Class I incisor and buccal segment relationship. ∴ it may be helpful, in the mind's eye, to correct the upper canine into a Class I relationship with $\overline{3}$ (in corrected position if LLS crowded). This will give an indication of the space required and the amount and type of movement necessary. In the upper arch space for retraction of $\underline{3}$ can be gained by (1) extractions, (2) expansion (only indicated if a Xbite exists), (3) distal movement of the upper buccal segments (p. 156). (4) a combination of these. Should extractions be indicated in both arches, mechanics are often easier if the same tooth is extracted in the upper as in the lower. However, in Class II cases it may be advantageous to extract further forward in the upper arch and vice versa in Class III.

Final Rx plan The next step is to plan what tooth movements need to be carried out, including which appliances are to be used and in what sequence. E.g. if distal movement is to be carried out it may be wise to fit the headgear first and review in the light of progress before embarking on extractions. Retention of the final result also needs to be included in the Rx plan, especially when the Rx is being explained to the patient and consent sought.

The practicalities of providing Rx also warrant consideration. In some cases more than one Rx plan can be offered to the patient, with a hierarchy of complexity and finished result. If a compromise plan is chosen by the patient this should be noted in their records.

The final plan for the example above may be:

- Quad helix appliance to expand upper arch.
- Extraction of all four first premolars.
- Lower fixed appliance.

- Upper fixed appliance once crossbite corrected.
- Reduce overjet.
- Retain corrected tooth movements.

Prognosis Will the proposed Rx be stable? Beware of o/j ↓ in a patient with grossly incompetent lips, or proclination of upper incisors in a Class III where there is no o/b to hold the corrected position.

Consent The risks and benefits of the proposed plan should be carefully explained to the patient/parent It is advisable to get written consent, including for specific details of the Rx.

▶ *Beware* If the malocclusion under consideration contains one of the following features:
- Marked skeletal discrepancy, anteroposteriorly (II or III), or vertically.
- If the o/j is increased and the upper incisors are upright.
- If the o/j is reversed and there is no o/b to retain correction of the incisor relationship.
- Severe Class II/2 malocclusions.
- Class II/l incisor relationship, with molars a full unit Class II and a crowded lower arch.

Rx planning is the most important, and most difficult, part of orthodontics. All but the trained orthodontist are advised to seek specialist advice.

Management of the developing dentition

See also delayed eruption, p. 68.

The way in which mixed dentition problems are approached will often affect the ease or difficulty of subsequent Rx.

Normal development of dentition The 1° incisors are usually upright and spaced. If there is no spacing warn the parents that the 2° incisors will probably be crowded. Overbite reduces throughout the 1° dentition until the incisors are edge to edge. All 2° incisors develop lingual to their predecessors, erupt into a wider arc, and are more proclined. It is normal for 1|1 to erupt with a median diastema which reduces as 2|2 erupt. Later, pressure from the developing canines on the roots of 2|2 results in their being tilted distally and spaced. This has been called the 'ugly duckling stage', but it is better to describe it as normal development to parents. As the 3 erupts the 2 upright and the spaces usually close.

The majority of Es erupt so that their distal edges are flush. The transition to the normal stepped (Class I) molar relationship usually occurs during the 1° dentition as a result of greater mandibular growth &/or the leeway space.

Development of dental arches In the average (!) child, the size of the dental arch is more or less established once the 1° dentition has erupted, except for an increase in inter-canine width (2–3 mm up to age 9) which results in a modification of arch shape.

Retained deciduous teeth—if deflecting eruption of 2° tooth, extract.

Submerging deciduous molars Prevalence 8–14%. Provided there is a successor, a submerged 1° molar will probably be exfoliated at the same time as the contralateral tooth.[1] Extraction is only indicated if there is no successor or the submerged tooth is likely to disappear below the gingival margin.

Impacted upper first permanent molars Prevalence 2–6%. Indicative of crowding. Spontaneous disimpaction rare after 8 yrs. Can try dislodging 6 by tightening a piece of brass wire round the contact point with E over several visits. Otherwise just observe, extracting E if unavoidable and dealing with resultant space loss in 2° dentition.

Habits Effects produced depend upon duration of habit and intensity. It is best not to make a great fuss of a finger-sucking habit. If parents concerned, reassure them (in presence of child) not to v orry, as only little girls/boys suck their fingers. Appliances to break the habit may help, but most children will stop when they are ready. However, this is no reason to delay the start of Rx for other aspects of the malocclusion.

1 J. Kurol 1985 Am *J Orthod* **87** 46.

Effects of premature loss of deciduous teeth

Unfortunately, when a child attends with toothache, in the rush to relieve pain it is all too easy to extract the offending tooth without consideration of the consequences. The major effect of early 1° tooth loss is localization of crowding, in crowded mouths. The extent to which this occurs depends upon the patient's age, degree of crowding, and the site. In a crowded mouth the adjacent teeth will move round into the extraction space, ∴ unilateral loss of a C (and to a lesser degree a D) will result in a centre-line shift. This is also seen when a C is prematurely exfoliated by an erupting 2. As correction of a centre-line discrepancy often involves fixed appliances, prevention is better than cure, so loss of Cs should always be balanced. If Es are lost the 6 will migrate forward. This is particularly marked if it occurs before eruption of the permanent tooth, so if extraction of an E is unavoidable try to defer until after the 6s are in occlusion and do not balance or compensate. The effect of early loss of 1° teeth on the eruption of the permanent successor is variable.

Timely loss of Cs is indicated for

- $\underline{2}$ erupting palatally due to crowding. Extraction of $\underline{C|C}$ as the $\underline{2}$ erupting may <u>allow</u> the tooth to escape labially and prevent a Xbite.
- Extraction of $\overline{C|C}$ when a lower incisor is being crowded labially will help to ↓ loss of periodontal support.

Extractions

In orthodontics, teeth are extracted either to relieve crowding or to provide space to compensate for a skeletal discrepancy.

▶ Before planning the extraction of any permanent teeth a thorough orthodontic and radiographic examination should be carried out.
▶ In a Class I or II, should extract at least as far forward in the upper arch as the lower; vice versa in a Class III.

Lower incisors Following the extraction of a $\overline{\text{inc}}$, the LLS tends to tilt lingually followed by the ULS. In addition, it is difficult to arrange 6 ULS teeth around 5 LLS teeth, ∴ try to avoid. However, if indicated, will need -/FA.

Upper incisors are never the teeth of choice for extraction, but if traumatized or dilacerated, there may be no alternative (p. 122).

Lower canines should only be extracted if severely displaced, as the resulting contact between $\overline{2}\ \overline{4}$ is unsatisfactory.

Upper canines, p. 160

First premolars are the most popular choice, due to their position in the arch and because a good contact point between the canine and second premolar is more likely. For maximum spontaneous improvement 4s should be extracted just as the 3s are appearing, but if appliance therapy is planned, defer until the canines have erupted.

Second premolars Preferred in cases with mild crowding, as their extraction alters the anchorage balance, favouring space closure by forward movement of the molars. FAs are required, especially in the lower arch. If 5s hypoplastic or missing there may be no choice. Early loss of an E will often lead to forward movement of the 6 and lack of space for 5s. In the upper arch this results in $\underline{5}$ being displaced palatally, and provided $\underline{4}$ is in a satisfactory position, extraction of $\underline{5}$ on eruption may ↓ the need for appliance therapy. In the lower arch $\overline{5}$s are usually crowded lingually. Extraction of $\overline{4}$ is easier and will give $\overline{5}$ space to upright spontaneously.

First permanent molars, p. 154

Second permanent molars Extraction of $\overline{7}$ will not alleviate incisor crowding but may relieve mild lower premolar crowding and avoid difficult extraction of impacted $\overline{8}$.
   To increase likelihood of $\overline{8}$ erupting successfully to replace $\overline{7}$, need: posterior crowding and $\overline{8}$ formed to bifurcation and at an angle of between 15° and 30° to long axis $\overline{6}$. Even so, may still require appliance therapy to align $\overline{8}$ on eruption.
   In the upper arch extraction of $\underline{7}$ often limited to facilitating distal movement of the upper buccal segments.

Third permanent molars Early extraction of these teeth used to be advocated to prevent LLS crowding, but as this can occur even in their absence, wisdom teeth are only a part of the aetiology. In addition, extraction of symptomless $\overline{8}$ is not advisable.

Space can also be provided in selected cases by:
1 expansion (only in upper arch with a Xbite, otherwise not stable);
2 distal movement of the upper buccal segments (p. 156);
3 reducing the width of the teeth approximally (usually limited to LLS in selected cases).

Extraction of the first permanent molars

First permanent molars are never the first choice for extraction, as even if removed at the optimal time a good spontaneous alignment of the remaining teeth is unlikely. However, when a two-surface (or more) restoration is required in a molar tooth for a child, the long-term prognosis should be considered. A well-timed extraction may be better for the child (and your BP) than heroic attempts to restore hopeless molars. Equally well, placing a dressing and maintaining a poor-quality 6 until the 7 has erupted and the extraction can be incorporated into an orthodontic plan, may keep you on the specialist orthodontists' christmas card list. Points to note:

- Check the remaining teeth are present and in a good position. If not, avoid extraction of 6 in affected quadrant.
- In the lower arch good spontaneous alignment is more likely following extraction 6 if: **1** 7|7 development has reached bifurcation; **2** angulation between crypt 7 and 6 is < 30°; **3** 7|7 crypts overlap 6|6 roots.
- There is a greater tendency for mesial drift in the maxilla, ∴ the timing of loss of 6 is less critical.
- Assess the prognosis for remaining 6s. If they are all restored then extraction of all four is probably indicated. If only one poor 6, do not extract corresponding lower tooth. If 6 of poor prognosis it is advisable to extract opposing 6 as otherwise this tooth will overerupt and prevent 7 moving forward. Balancing with extraction of a corresponding sound 6 is inadvisable; better to deal with other side of arch on its merit.
- In Class I with anterior crowding and Class II, 6|6 should, if possible, be preserved until 7|7 have erupted, and can be held back by an appliance and the extraction space utilized.
- In Class III, if 6|6 of poor prognosis try to preserve until incisor relationship corrected (to provide retention for appliance). In cases with poor quality 6|6, extract at optimal time to aid space closure.
- If the dentition is uncrowded, avoid extraction of 6s as space closure will be difficult.
- Extraction of 6s will relieve buccal segment crowding, but will have little effect on labial segment crowding. Impaction of 8s less likely but not impossible.

▶ In a child with poor quality 6s, remember that the premolars may well be in a similar condition 6 yrs on unless the caries rate is stabilized.

Distal movement of the upper buccal segments

This is usually thought of as an alternative to extraction, but in practice often results in the crowding being shifted distally, requiring the loss of 7 or 8. It is only applicable to the upper arch, in the following situations:

- Either Class I with mild upper-arch crowding, or Class II/1 with well-aligned lower arch and molars <1 unit Class II.
- Where extraction of 4|4 do not provide sufficient space to align upper arch.

Can be achieved either by a screw appliance, or more usually by EOT directly to molar bands on 6|6. As 6|6 move distally, will need some expansion. Greater chance of success with growing child. Can expect 1/2 unit change in 3–4 months with good cooperation. If need unilateral distal movement, extraction of 7 on that side can be considered (provided 8 in good position).

Headgear safety

There have been a number of cases where damage to the eye as a result of headgear has resulted in loss of vision. For this reason headgear should only be used by those who have received training and to avoid injury to the face, it should only be used in conjunction with safety mechanisms which prevent displacement &/or recoil of the facebow. If eye injury should occur immediate referral to an ophthalmologist is required.

Spacing

Uncommon in UK; crowding is the norm.

Generalized spacing is due either to hypodontia or small teeth &/or large jaws. Note that hypodontia is associated with small teeth p. 70. Rx of spacing is problematic, a purely orthodontic approach is liable to relapse and requires prolonged retention. In milder cases try and encourage the patient to accept the situation. In more severe cases a combined restorative/ orthodontic approach will be required. This may involve composite additions or veneers to increase the width of the teeth &/or orthodontics to localize the space for provision of a prosthesis.

Median diastema

Prevalence 6-yr-olds = 98%, 11-yr-olds = 49%, 12–18-yr-olds = 7%.

Aetiology Small teeth in large jaws; absent or peg-shaped 2|2; midline $; proclination of ULS; physiological (caused by pressure of developing teeth on upper incisor roots which resolves as 3 erupts), or due to a frenum.

The upper incisive frenum is attached to the incisive papilla at birth. As 1|1 erupt the frenum recedes, but this is less likely if the arch is spaced. A frenum contributes to a diastema in a small number of cases and is associated with the following features:

- Blanching of incisive papilla when frenum put under tension.
- Radiographically there is a V-shaped notch in the interdental bone between 1|1, indicating the attachment of the frenum.
- Anterior teeth may be crowded.

Management Always take a periapical X-ray to exclude presence of a $.
1 Before 3 erupted: if diastema <3 mm—review after eruption of canines as will probably ↓ unaided. If >3 mm—may need to approximate incisors to provide space for canines to erupt, but care is required not to resorb roots of 2|2 against crowns of 3|3. Usually requires FA and prolonged retention.
2 After 3 erupted: orthodontic closure will require prolonged retention as has high tendency to relapse. If frenum undoubtedly a major aetiological factor perform a frenectomy during closure, but retention still wise. Alternatively, measure width of 1 2, and if they are narrower than average (1 = 8.5 mm, 2 = 6.5 mm) consider composite additions or veneers to close space. If teeth of normal width and no other orthodontic Rx required, could try and talk patient into accepting their diastema.

Buccally displaced maxillary canines

▶ Width $\underline{3}$ > width $\underline{4}$ > width $\underline{C}$.

$\underline{3}$ is usually the last tooth to erupt anterior to $\underline{6}$. If the upper arch is crowded, $\underline{3}$ may be squeezed buccal to its normal position, in which case space needs to be created for its alignment. Usually $\underline{4}$ is the tooth of choice for extraction and, if so, this should be carried out just as $\underline{3}$ is about to erupt. If there is plenty of space it is sufficient to keep the patient under review, otherwise fit a space-maintainer.

Where $\underline{2}$ and $\underline{4}$ are in contact, extraction of $\underline{4}$ alone will not provide sufficient space to accommodate the canine and thought should be given to extracting $\underline{3}$.

Less commonly, a canine may develop well forward over the root of $\underline{2}$. In this case orthodontic Rx to align $\underline{3}$ will be prolonged. If the arch is crowded it may be simpler to extract $\underline{3}$ and align remaining teeth.

Alignment of mesially inclined, buccally displaced canines can, if they are the only Rx required, be accomplished by URA otherwise FA

Transposition almost exclusively involves a canine tooth. In the maxilla $\underline{3}$ is usually transposed with $\underline{4}$ and is the mandible the laceral incisor is more commonly involved. Rx options include alignment of teeth in transposed position, extraction of the most displaced tooth, or correction if transposition nor complete.

Palatally displaced maxillary canines

► Early detection is essential.

Width $\underline{3}$ > width $\underline{4}$ > width $\underline{C}$.

Prevalence Up to 2%. Occurs bilaterally in 17–25% of cases. F > M.

Aetiology In normal development the maxillary canine develops palatal to $\underline{C}$ and then migrates labially to erupt down the distal aspect of $\underline{2}$ root. The aetiology of palatal displacement is not fully understood, but some suggest a lack of guidance is the reason behind the association with missing or short-rooted $\underline{2}$.[1] Others argue that it is an inherited polygenic trait and that the link with missing or short-rooted $\underline{2}$ is part of association with other dental anomalies including microdontia and hypodontia[2].

Prevention Early detection may allow corrective interceptive Rx, ∴ when examining any child >9 yrs, palpate for unerupted $\underline{3}$. If there is a definite hollow &/or asymmetry between sides, further investigation is warranted. Extraction of $\underline{C}$ may result in improvement of a displaced $\underline{3}$[3], but this eliminates the possibility of maintaining $\underline{C}$ should sufficient improvement in the position of $\underline{3}$ not materialize; ∴ confine to those cases where the $\underline{3}$ is not too far displaced. More markedly displaced $\underline{3}$ should be referred to a specialist.

Assessment Clinically by palpation and from inclination of $\underline{2}$ and by X-rays. A DPT and an intra-oral view or two intra-oral views with tube shift can be used to assess the position of the canine by parallax (p. 21 remember your PAL goes with you!). Consider also position and prognosis of adjacent teeth (including $\underline{C}$), the malocclusion, and available space.

Management If the canine is only very slightly palatally displaced or impacted between $\underline{2}$ and $\underline{4}$, provision of space should result in eruption. The majority of palatally displaced canines, however, do not erupt spontaneously, so hopeful watching and waiting may only result in an older patient who is less willing to undergo the prolonged Rx required to align the displaced tooth. Rx alternatives available:

1 Interceptive extraction of $\underline{C}$ in mixed dentition (see above).
2 Maintain $\underline{C}$ and keep unerupted canine under radiographic review. Provided no evidence of cystic change or resorption, removal of $\underline{3}$ can be left until GA required, e.g. for extraction of 8s. Patient must understand that $\underline{C}$ will eventually be lost, necessitating a prosthesis.
3 No Rx, if $\underline{2}$ and $\underline{4}$ are in contact and appearance is satisfactory, or if patient refuses other options. Again, $\underline{3}$ will require removal in due course.
4 Exposure and orthodontic alignment only feasible if (a) canine in favourable position for orthodontic alignment; (b) sufficient space available for $\underline{3}$, or can be created; (c) patient willing to undergo surgery and prolonged orthodontic Rx (usually 2+ yrs). Sequence is to arrange exposure, and allow tooth to erupt for 3 months, and then commence orthodontic traction to move tooth towards arch. FAs are required.

1 A. Becker 1981 *Angle Orthodontist* **51** 24.
2 S. Peck 1994 *Angle Orthodontist* **64** 249.
3 S. Ericson 1988 *Eur J Orthod* **10** 283.

5 Transplantation is not an instant solution, as space is needed to accommodate <u>3</u>, which may involve appliances &/or extractions. Poor long-term results have been reported, e.g. only 1/3 still functional after 10 yrs.[4] However, shorter splinting times (1–2 weeks) and RCT for teeth with closed apices within 3 weeks of transplantation may ↑ prognosis.

Resorption Unerupted and impacted canines can cause resorption of incisor roots. For this to occur a 'head-on' collision between the two seems to be required. If detected on X-ray, a specialist opinion should be sought, quickly. Extraction of the canine may be necessary to limit resorption, but if extensive, removal of the affected incisor may be preferable, thus allowing the canine to erupt.

4 J. P. Moss 1975 *Br J Oral Surg* **12** 268.

Increased overjet

When is an o/j increased? This is really a matter of opinion, but provided the arches are well-aligned, an o/j <6mm is acceptable. If Rx is required for other reasons, consider reduction of o/j >4mm.

Aetiology

Skeletal pattern Increased o/j can occur in association with Class I, II, or even III skeletal patterns. If Class II, is often due to a normally sized mandible being positioned posteriorly on the cranial base. Be wary of patients with vertical proportions at either extreme of the range, as they are difficult to treat.

Soft tissues The effects of the soft tissues are usually determined by the skeletal pattern, as the greater the discrepancy the less likely it is that the patient will have competent lips. Where the lips are incompetent, the way an anterior oral seal is achieved will influence incisor position; e.g. if the lower lip is drawn up behind the upper incisors this may have contributed to the increased o/j, but if the incisors can be retracted within control of the lower lip at the end of Rx the prognosis for stable o/j reduction is good. This is less likely if the LFH is increased and the lower lip lies beneath the upper incisors, as it will be less likely to control their position following o/j reduction. The soft tissues can also help to compensate for the skeletal pattern by proclining the lower &/or retroclining the upper incisors.

Dental *Crowding* may contribute to an increased o/j, ∴ relief of crowding may aid stability. Digit-sucking can cause proclination of the upper and retroclination of the lower incisors, but in a growing child this will resolve once habit is stopped unless maintained by adverse soft-tissue activity.

In the majority of cases skeletal pattern will determine ease of Rx, but the soft tissues will influence the stability of the end result.

Stability of overjet reduction

Provided the inc have been retracted to a position of balance within the lower lip, this should not be a problem. Nevertheless, a period of retention is usually necessary to allow for periodontal fibre and soft-tissue adaption. However, prolonged retention will not make stable an inherently unstable position. A common mistake is to stop Rx before o/j reduction is complete and the lips competent. If the patient returns to retracting the lower lip behind the ULS to achieve an anterior oral seal, the o/j is likely to increase.

Management of increased overjet

(See also Functional appliances, p. 190.)

Principles

1 Provision of space for o/j reduction &/or relief of crowding.
2 Reduce o/b before o/j reduction (p. 170).
3 Appliance required to ↓ o/j.
4 Consider stability of treated result and plan retention.

Class I or mild Class II skeletal pattern

Stability of o/j reduction ↑ with age as the lips mature and are held together by the patient, ∴ early Rx is likely to require prolonged retention. Unless a functional appliance is indicated, it is advisable to await the 2° dentition before embarking on Rx to reduce an o/j. If the overjet is <6mm and orthodontic Rx not indicated for other reasons, consideration should be given to accepting the position of the incisors, particularly if the <u>inc</u> are not proclined, or stability following overjet reduction is questionable. In a small proportion of cases with proclined incisors, where space to retract the overjet is available or can be created by the extraction of first premolars, an URA can be used. However, the majority of patients in this category are managed using fixed &/or functional appliances. A functional appliance (p. 190) can be used to reduce an increased overjet in a growing child, either as the sole appliance if the arches are well aligned, or as the first phase of Rx to reduce the overjet before fixed appliances &/or extractions are used to complete alignment.

Moderate to severe Class II skeletal pattern

Approaches available:
1 Modification of growth—either by restraint of maxillary growth with headgear, or by encouraging mandibular growth with a functional appliance.
2 Orthodontic camouflage—by extractions in upper arch and bodily movement of <u>inc</u> and FA.
3 Surgical correction.

Because mandibular growth predominates during teens, a greater proportion of Class II than Class III skeletal problems are amenable to orthodontic correction. Research would suggest that the amount of growth modification that can be achieved is limited, but every little helps and in practice the majority of growing children in this category are treated by a combination of approaches **1** and **2**. This usually takes the form of an initial phase of functional appliance therapy, followed by FA &/or extractions. Adults whose skeletal pattern is not too severe may be treated by orthodontic camouflage, but in cases with a more severe skeletal problem &/or an ↑ o/b a surgical correction may be the only option.

Increased overbite

Normal o/b is between 1/3 and 1/2 overlap of the lower incisors. It is more practical to record o/b in terms of whether it is increased, decreased, or normal, rather than to try to measure it with a ruler. Increased o/b is associated with Class II/2 incisor relationship, where typically 1|1 are retroclined and 2|2 are proclined, reflecting their relationship to the lower lip. But the o/b can also be ↑ in Class III and II/1 malocclusions. Increased o/b per se is not an indication for Rx, unless it is traumatic and this is relatively rare, but ↓ of o/b may be necessary before correction of other anomalies. In Class III cases an ↑ o/b is advantageous as this will help to retain the corrected incisor position.

Aetiology ↑ o/b occurs because the incisors are able to erupt past each other due to a combination of some or all of the following interrelated factors: ↓ LFH, high lower lip line, retroclined incisors, ↑ inter-incisal angle. Normal inter-incisal angle is 135°. Highest acceptable angle is 145°. Above this value the tendency for the lower incisors to erupt may be inadequately resisted.

Approaches to reducing overbite
1 *Extrusion/eruption of molars.* Passive eruption of lower molars occurs when an URA incorporating a biteplane is worn. Active extrusion of molars in either arch is possible using FA. However, unless the patient grows vertically to accommodate this increased dimension, the molars will re-intrude under the forces of occlusion once appliances are withdrawn. This approach is of limited value in adults.
2 *Intrusion of incisors.* This is difficult, requires FA, and in most cases the major effect is extrusion of the buccal segments. More successful in growing patients.
3 *Proclination of lower incisors.* This will only be stable if the LLS has been trapped behind the ULS, in which case, provision of a removable biteplane may allow the lower incisors to spontaneously procline. Active proclination should only be attempted by the experienced orthodontist, who will be better able to judge those cases where this is indicated.
4 *Surgery.* Indicated in severe cases especially if associated with A–P skeletal discrepancy, and in adults.

Stability of overbite reduction depends upon eliminating or reducing the aetiological factors, but ↓ LFH and high lower lip line can only be altered if growth is favourable. Reduction of the inter-incisal angle is necessary to provide a 'stop' to the incisors re-erupting, but requires FA to move incisor apices lingually.

Management of increased overbite

Class II/2   It is often prudent to avoid extractions when the lower arch is mildly crowded in a Class II/2, as extractions may be followed by lingual tipping of the lower incisors resulting in a further ↑ of the o/b. Cases with sufficient crowding to warrant premolar extractions in the lower arch and moderately to severely increased overbite are best treated with FA to close space by forward movement of the buccal segments and to correct incisor relationship.

Where o/b ↓ is required, the inter-incisal angle will need to be reduced in order to achieve a stable result. Usually this necessitates FA, but in growing patients with a skeletal II pattern and no or mild crowding an alternative approach is to procline <u>inc</u> with an URA and then use a functional appliance to reduce the resultant overjet, or use a Twin Block functional as a spring can be added to the upper block to procline <u>inc</u>.

Class II/1   o/b ↓ is required before o/j ↓. If a functional appliance is indicated for A–P correction then some o/b reduction can often be achieved during this phase by trimming the appliance in the buccal segments. If headgear is being used then it may be helpful to commence o/b by using an URA clipped over the bands on the upper molars. Rx of most II/I will need FA either as the sole Rx or following a functional appliance or headgear. Including $\overline{7}$ in the FA will aid intrusion of the LLS, but inevitably some extrusion of the molars will occur.

Class III (p. 176)   Avoid reducing o/b as it will aid retention of the corrected incisor position.

Retention   Reducing the inter-incisal angle will aid stability. Following FA Rx incorporation of a flat anterior biteplane into the upper retainer may be helpful. Where the incisal relationship has been changed, retention ideally should be continued until growth is complete. In some patients this is not practicable.

Anterior open bite (AOB)

Vertical overlap of incisors (o/b)

←——→

↑ o/b   normal o/b   incomplete o/b   AOB

AOB can occur in Class I, II, and III malocclusions.

Aetiology Either *skeletal*—vertical > horizontal growth (↑LFH &/or ↑MMPA), or *environmental*—habits, tongue thrust, iatrogenic. Or a combination. If the distance between maxilla and mandible is sufficiently increased such that even if incisors develop to their full potential they do not meet, an AOB will result. This is often associated with incompetent lips and a lip-to-tongue anterior oral seal, which may exacerbate the AOB. Tongue thrusts are usually adaptive and can maintain an AOB due to a habit even after the habit has stopped. Localized failure of maxillary dento-alveolar development resulting in an open bite is seen in CLP.

Treatment is generally difficult except where due mainly to a habit, ∴ it is wise to refer patient to a specialist for advice.

  Skeletal In milder cases can align arches and accept, or try to restrain vertical development of the maxilla &/or upper molars with headgear &/or a functional appliance with posterior bite blocks. Extrusion of the incisors is unstable. For more severe cases the only alternative is surgery, but even this is not straight forward and liable to relapse.

  Habits Better to await natural cessation of habit, but not if that means deferring Rx for other aspects of malocclusion. Once habit stops o/b should re-establish within 3 yrs, unless perpetuated by soft tissues or because it is skeletal in origin.

  Tongue thrust None.

Hints for cases with ↑ vertical dimensions and ↓ o/b or AOB.
• Avoid extruding molars, e.g. cervical pull headgear to 6|6, URA with a biteplane.
• Avoid upper arch expansion as this will tip down the palatal cusps of buccal segment teeth, reducing o/b.
• Extraction of molars will not 'close down bite'.
• Space closure is said to occur more readily in patients with ↑ LFH and ↑ MMPA.

Reverse overjet

This will include only those cases with >2 teeth in linguo-occlusion, i.e. Class III cases. For management of one or two teeth in crossbite, see p. 178.

Aetiology

Skeletal Reverse overjets are usually associated with an underlying Class III skeletal pattern. This is most commonly due to either a large mandible &/or a retrusive maxilla. Class III malocclusions occur in association with the whole range of vertical patterns. Crossbites are a common feature, due either to a large mandible or the anterior position of the mandible relative to the maxilla.

Soft tissues A patient's efforts to achieve an anterior oral seal often result in dento-alveolar compensation, i.e. retroclination of the lower and proclination of the upper incisors. ∴ the incisor relationship is often less severe than underlying skeletal pattern.

Dental crowding This is usually greater in the upper than the lower arch.

Assessment (p. 140) Consider also the following:
- Patient's opinion about their facial appearance (be tactful!).
- Severity of skeletal discrepancy.
- Amount of dento-alveolar compensation. If upper incisors already markedly proclined, further proclination is undesirable.
- Amount of overbite. Remember that proclination of ULS will reduce o/b and retroclination of LLS will ↑ o/b.
- Can patient achieve an edge-to-edge contact of the incisors. If not, simple Rx C/I.

Rx planning, see p. 146.
▶ Class III malocclusions tend to become worse with growth.
▶ In severe cases seek a specialist opinion before embarking on Rx or extractions, as if surgery is necessary, decompensation (i.e. correcting the position of the incisors to their normal inclination) will probably involve the reverse of orthodontic camouflage.

Major factors determining Rx approach are skeletal discrepancy and overbite:

Skeletal pattern	Normal or ↑ o/b	↓ o/b
Mild to normal	Procline ULS	Accept
Moderate	FA to procline ULS and retrocline LLS	Accept or FA to retrocline LLS ± procline ULS
Severe	Surgery	Align and accept if possible, or surgery

If child on borderline between groups, assume more severe as growth will probably prove you right.

Management of reverse overjet

Relief of crowding Extractions in the upper arch alone may run the risk of worsening the incisor relationship, ∴ it is advisable to extract at least as far forward in lower arch as upper.

Moderate crowding responds best to extraction of premolars. Extraction of 5|5 will maintain 4|4 to support the ULS, but often crowding in the upper arch necessitates extraction of 4|4. Proclination of ULS, if indicated, will provide some space for relief of crowding. If using FA to retrocline LLS, space will be required in the lower arch to accomplish this. Distal movement of the upper buccal segments is C/I in Class III as restraint of maxillary growth is undesirable.

Practical Rx

Accept This may be the wisest option for those patients with increased LFH and reduced o/b, with Rx directed towards achieving alignment within the arches only.

Proclination of ULS only This is only suitable for milder well-aligned cases where ULS is not already proclined and where sufficient o/b will be present to retain the corrected incisor position. Best carried out in the mixed dentition, provided 3|3 are not sitting labial to the roots of 2|2. If extraction of C|C necessary for space, it is advisable to match this with loss of C|C to avoid compromising the incisor relationship. Provided there is sufficient o/b, stability is not usually a problem, but if URA has been used it is advisable to retain for 3 months nights-only wear. Often there is adequate o/b for the 1|1, but not 2|2; if so, a bonded retainer is advisable, but remember that further eruption will be limited.

Retroclination of LLS ± proclination of ULS requires FA. By interchanging the position of the incisors within the neutral zone, stability is not compromised. Class III elastic traction from the back of the upper arch to the 3 region helps to retrocline LLS. However, in addition to extruding the incisors, which is desirable, also results in extrusion of the upper molars, which reduces o/b. ∴ these cases should be managed by a skilled operator.

Orthodontics and orthognathic surgery, p. 194.

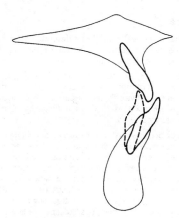

Correction of a Class III incisor relationship by retroclination of the lower incisors increases overbite

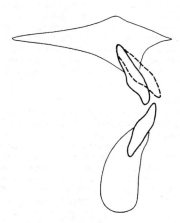

Correction of a Class III incisor relationship by proclination of the upper incisors alone reduces overbite

Crossbites

By convention the lower teeth should be described relative to the upper (p. 136). Crossbites can be anterior or posterior (unilateral/ bilateral), with displacement, or with no displacement.

Aetiology Xbites can be skeletal &/or dental in origin. For posterior Xbites, the skeletal component is usually the major factor. Antero-posterior discrepancies obviously play a part in anterior Xbites, but can also result in posterior Xbites in Class II (lingual Xbite) and Class III (buccal Xbite) skeletal patterns.

Displacement may occur when a premature or deflecting cuspal contact is encountered on closure and the mandible is postured either anteriorly or laterally to achieve better interdigitation. This new path of closure becomes learned and the patient closes straight into maximum interdigitation. To help detect displacement on closure, try to get the patient to close on a hinge axis by asking them to curl their tongue back to touch the back of the palate and then close together slowly, whilst guiding the mandible back via the chin. In addition, look for other clues like a centre-line shift (of lower in direction of displacement) in association with a posterior unilateral Xbite. Evidence suggests that displacing contacts may predispose to TMPDS.

Anterior crossbites

Class III malocclusions are considered on p. 174. Should be treated early, especially if associated with a displacement, provided sufficient o/b exists to retain the result. If not, probably best to defer until the 2° dentition and use FA. Correction of one or two teeth with reverse overjet and a +ve overbite can be accomplished using an URA; however, need to have space available to accommodate the tooth in the arch (or create with extractions). Application of a force to procline the ULS results in an URA being unseated anteriorly, ∴ good anterior retention is usually required. In the mixed dentition, the morphology of the primary teeth makes this difficult. A screw appliance has the advantage that the teeth to be moved can also be clasped. Buccal capping should be added to free the tooth to be moved from contact with lower arch. Upper lateral incisors that are displaced bodily and palatally due to lack of space are not amenable to simple proclination. Refer patient to a specialist.

Posterior crossbites[1]

Unilateral Generally, the greater the number of teeth involved the greater the skeletal contribution to the aetiology. If only one or two teeth, movement of opposing teeth in opposite directions for correction may be required. This can be achieved by cross-elastics attached to attachments on the affected teeth. 5s are often crowded palatally, but are easily aligned using a T-spring on an URA. Unilateral Xbite from the canine region distally is usually associated with a displacement, as true skeletal asymmetry is rare. If the arches are of a similar width, displacement to the right or left will give better interdigitation. In these cases Rx should be directed towards expanding the upper arch so that it fits around the lower, provided the upper teeth are not already buccally tilted.

Bilateral buccal crossbite This suggests a greater underlying transverse skeletal discrepancy. Less commonly, associated with displacement. Correction of a bilateral Xbite should be approached with caution, because partial relapse may result in the teeth occluding cusp to cusp and development of a unilateral Xbite with displacement.

Bilateral lingual crossbite (or scissor bite) occurs due to either a narrow mandible or a wide maxilla. In milder cases only 4|4 may be involved, and if these teeth are extracted to relieve crowding or for retraction of 3|3, so much the better. Where all of the buccal segments are involved, Rx will probably involve expansion of the lower &/or contraction of the upper; ∴ refer to a specialist.

Rapid maxillary expansion

Involves a screw appliance comprising bands attached to 64|64 and connected to a midline screw. The object is to expand the maxilla by opening the midline suture and is ∴ more successful in younger patients. Large forces are required to accomplish this, ∴ the screw is turned 0.2 mm twice a day for about 2 weeks. Over-expansion is necessary as the teeth relapse about 50% under soft-tissue pressure. Not to be attempted by the inexperienced!

Quad helix appliance

This is a very efficient fixed, slow expansion appliance. Suitable for mixed or 2° dentition. Attaches to upper teeth by bands on 6 and is W-shaped.

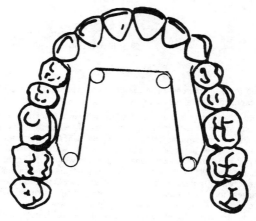

Quad helix appliance which is attached to bands, cemented onto the upper first molar teeth

Anchorage

Anchorage is defined as the source of resistance to the reaction from the active component(s) in an appliance. In practice, it is the balance between the applied force and the available space. E.g., in a case where 3|3 are being retracted following extraction of 4|4, an equal, but opposite force will also be acting on 65|56. The amount of forward movement of these anchor teeth will depend largely upon their root surface area and the force used.

Anchorage loss can be minimized by limiting the number of teeth being moved at any one time, applying the correct force for the movement required, and ↑ the resistance of the anchor teeth (e.g. by permitting only bodily movement). In some situations, movement of the anchor teeth is desirable, e.g. in a Class III where space is being opened up for an unerupted 5. However, it is important to assess the anchorage requirements of a particular malocclusion before embarking on treatment If no or little movement of the anchor teeth is desirable, then anchorage should be reinforced from the start.

Reinforcing anchorage

Intra-maxillary (teeth in same arch)   By including the maximum number of teeth in the anchorage unit. Applicable to both fixed and removable appliances.

Inter-maxillary (teeth in opposing arch)   This is achieved by running elastics from one arch to the other. It is mainly applicable to FA, as an URA will be dislodged. The direction of elastic pull is described according to the type of malocclusion to which it is applicable.

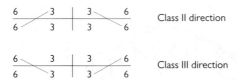

Increased mucosal coverage   By virtue of its palatal coverage an URA has more potential anchorage than an FA.

Extra-oral   Anchorage is transmitted to the appliance by elastic or spring force from a head or neck strap. This involves a face-bow, which engages tubes soldered on to molar cribs (URA) or bands (FA). The direction of pull can be selected according to the malocclusion with an overall direction of pull above the occlusal plane for patients with ↑ vertical proportions (hi-pull) and vice versa for ↓ vertical proportions (cervical pull). For EO anchorage, 250 g for 10 h/day should suffice. For EO traction (i.e. using the headgear force to achieve movement rather than just resist it) forces in the region of 500 g for 14–16 h/day are necessary.

Following reports of a number of cases where eye damage (including blindness) occurred due to headgear, the use of at least two safety mechanisms is imperative. Better still, avoid headgear if possible.

Anchorage loss

May occur because of **1** failure to appreciate fully anchorage requirements at Rx planning stage; **2** active force exceeding available anchorage (often due to over-activation or too many teeth being moved at a time); **3** poor patient compliance.

Removable appliances—scope and limitations

Removable appliances are single-arch appliances that can be taken out of the mouth by the patient. They are only capable of tilting movements of individual teeth, but can be used for moving blocks of teeth. In addition they can be used to allow differential eruption of teeth via biteplanes or buccal capping.

Advantages of removables	Disadvantages of removables
Easier to clean than FA	Patient can leave appliance out
Easy to adjust, ∴ ↓ chairside time	Only tipping movement possible
Contact with mucosa ↑ anchorage	Affects speech
Can be used for o/b ↓	Good technician required
Can transmit forces to blocks of teeth	Intermaxillary traction not possible
	Lower removable appliances are difficult to tolerate
	Inefficient for multiple tooth movements

Indications

Active

Where only require simple tipping movement of an individual tooth.
Movement of blocks of teeth, e.g. correction of a buccal crossbite by expansion of upper arch.
As an interceptive Rx in the mixed dentition, e.g. correction of an upper incisor in crossbite.
Overbite reduction.
In conjunction with other appliance, e.g. to facilitate distal movement of upper molar(s) with headgear; to free occlusion to allow movement of a tooth over the bite during fixed appliance Rx.

Passive

Space maintainer, e.g. following loss of an upper central incisor due to trauma.
Retaining appliance, e.g. following fixed appliance Rx.

Correction of unilateral posterior crossbites

Removable appliances are useful in the correction of unilateral posterior crossbites, particularly in the mixed dentition where mobile primary teeth may make placement of a fixed appliance problematic. Usually the design involves a midline screw which works by reciprocal anchorage, i.e. each side of the arch moves equally in opposite directions.

Interestingly, a recent Cochrane systematic review indicated that for cases with a posterior crossbite in the mixed dentition, active intervention was indicated to prevent perpetuation of the crossbite in the permanent dentition.[1] The most effective Rx was grinding of the primary teeth responsible for causing the premature contact, and if this was not successful then the use of an URA to expand the upper arch was also effective.

1 J. Harrison 2001 Cochrane Library, Issue 2, Oxford.

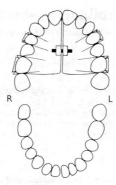

Upper removable appliance to expand upper arch with midline screw.
cribs <u>6|6</u> 0.7 mm SS
   <u>4|4</u> 0.6 mm SS
buccal capping or FABP

Removable appliances—design

Four components need to be considered for every appliance.

Active component

Exerts force required for desired movement.

Springs

Springs are the most commonly used active component because they are versatile and cheap to construct.

The relationship between the distance (d) that an orthodontic spring is deflected on activation, the length of the spring (l), the diameter or radius (r) of the wire it is composed of, and the force generated is:

$$F \propto \frac{dr^4}{l^3}$$

In practice this means that for two identical springs, one made in 0.5 mm wire and one in 0.7 mm wire, to deliver the same amount of force, the 0.5 mm spring would be activated about 3 mm, whereas the 0.7 mm spring requires only 1 mm activation.

Palatal finger springs are the most commonly used active components for mesial or distal movement along the arch. They are fabricated in 0.5 mm wire and are easy to adjust and activate. If boxed out from the acrylic and made with a guard wire they are more stable in the vertical plane than a buccal spring and ∴ should be used in preference.

For details of other types of spring the reader should consult a specialist text.

Elastics

Less commonly used nowadays, but are useful for aligning displaced teeth, e.g. palatal canine, using an attachment bonded onto the tooth surface, to which an elastic is applied by the patient to a hook soldered on to a labial bow or crib.

Screws

The Glenross type of screw design is used almost exclusively. This type of screw is opened (or closed) by means of a key, a quarter turn of which separates the two halves by 0.2 mm. A screw appliance is useful when the teeth to be moved need to be clasped for retention (e.g. expanding the upper arch in the mixed dentition). It is advisable to start patients turning the screw only once a week, progressing on to a maximum of two turns per week. If worn intermittently, a screw appliance will become progressively ill-fitting. Remember that these screws have about 18 activations and if considerable movement is necessary a second appliance may be required.

Retention

This is the means by which the appliance is retained in the mouth. The best retention posteriorly is provided by the Adams crib, which is made in SS in either 0.7 mm (for permanent molars) or 0.6 mm (for premolars and primary molars) wire. These clasps are very technician-sensitive and no amount of adjustment will compensate for a badly made crib. Should engage about 1 mm of undercut, which on a child's molar may be at, or just under, the gingival margin and in an adult may only be part-way down the clinical crown. The versatility of the crib can be increased by soldering tubes for EOT, labial bows, or buccal springs onto the bridge of the clasp.

Anterior retention can be gained by a labial bow or either an Adams or Southend Clasp. All these components are usually constructed in 0.7 mm wire.

Anchorage

Resists force generated by active component(s); see p. 180.

Baseplate

Not only holds other elements together, but may also itself be active. Heat-cure acrylic is more robust than self-cure.

• A flat anterior biteplane should only be prescribed if o/b ↓ is required. In case your technician isn't telepathic, it is wise to specify the height

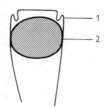

Adjustment of Adams crib
1 Arrowhead moves horizontally towards tooth
2 Arrowed moves towards tooth and also vertically towards gingival crevice

(e.g. half the height of <u>1/1</u>) and how far back the biteplane should extend (e.g. o/j = 3 mm). In order to ↑ the likelihood of the URA being worn the molars should only be separated by 1—2 mm by the biteplane, ∴ self-cure acrylic should be added during Rx in order to continue o/b ↓.

- Buccal capping frees the occlusion on the tooth being moved and allows further relative eruption of the incisors (∴ is C/l if o/b is already ↑). Should be trimmed so that the teeth to be moved are separated only by 1–2 mm.

▶ The easier it is for the patient to insert and wear their URA, the more likely it is that Rx will be successful, ∴ keep design simple.

Fixed appliances

▶ FA should only be used in cooperative patients with good OH, to minimize damage.

As the name implies, FA are attached to the teeth. They vary in complexity, from a single bracket used in conjunction with an URA, to attachments on all teeth. URA are limited to tilting movements, but FA can tilt, rotate, intrude, extrude, and move teeth bodily. Not surprisingly, FA have a greater propensity for things to go wrong, ∴ they should only be used by those with the necessary skills and training.

Principles

- Rx planning (p. 146), but with ↑ attention to anchorage requirements, especially if apical movement is planned.
- As FA are able to achieve bodily movement it is possible (within limits) to move teeth to compensate for a skeletal discrepancy.
- FA can be used in conjunction with other appliances &/or headgear.
- For initial alignment flexible archwires are used, but to minimize unwanted movements, progressively more rigid archwires are necessary.
- Archwires should be based on the pre-Rx lower arch-form for stability.
- Mesio-distal movement is achieved either by: **1** sliding the teeth along the archwire with elastic force (sliding mechanics), or **2** moving the teeth with the archwire.
- Intermaxillary traction is often used to aid antero-posterior correction and increase anchorage.

Components of fixed appliances

Bands Usually used on molar teeth so that the end of the arch wire is retained even if band becomes loose. Indicated for other teeth if bonds fail or lingual attachment is required for de-rotation. If tooth contacts are tight these will need to be separated prior to band placement using an elastic doughnut stretched around the contact point for 1–7 days. Use of GI cements helps to ↓decalcification.

Bonds are attached to enamel with (acid-etch) composite. There are three types: **1** metal (poor aesthetics); **2** plastic (become stained); **3** ceramic (prone to # and can cause enamel wear).

Archwires Flexible nickel titanium (NiTi) archwires are used in the intial stages of Rx and more rigid stainless steel wires for the planned tooth movements. Tungsten molybdenum, and cobalt chromium alloys are also popular.

Auxillaries Elastic rings or wire ligatures are used to tie the archwire to the brackets. Forces can be applied to the teeth by auxiliary springs or elastics.

Types of fixed appliance

Almost infinite variety, but most are based on:

Begg uses round wires which fit loosely into a vertical slot in the bracket, thus allowing the teeth to tip freely. Auxiliaries are required to achieve apical and rotational movements. Now superseded by Tip-Edge.

Edgewise uses rectangular brackets that are wide mesio-distally for rotational control. Round wires are used initially for alignment, but rectangular wires are necessary for apical control. Largely historical.

Pre-adjusted systems These 'pre-programmed' brackets allow ↑use of pre-formed archwires. As each tooth has its own individual bracket with a built-in prescription for that tooth, these systems are more expensive, but that is offset by savings in operator time. Numerous types - MBT prescription currently fashionable.

Tip edge is based on the Begg philosophy but the brackets also have pre-adjusted values incorporated to give the 'finish' produced by using a straight wire appliance.

Lingual appliances Popular with patients, but not with orthodontists as they are difficult to adjust !

Damon brackets have a clip mechanism to hold the archwire in place which ↓ friction, making space closure quicker.

More details can be found in specialist texts (sorry could not resist the opportunity to plug my book!).[1]

1 L. Mitchell 2001 *An Introduction to Orthodontics*, OUP.

Functional appliances—rationale and mode of action

Definition Functional appliances utilize, eliminate, or guide the forces of muscle function, tooth eruption, and growth to correct a malocclusion.

Philosophy The term functional appliance dates back to a belief that by eliminating abnormal muscle function normal growth and development would follow. Nowadays, the importance of both genetic and environmental factors in the aetiology of malocclusion is acknowledged, but functional appliances are still successfully used to correct Class II malocclusions by a combination of skeletal and dental effects. Functional appliances (or just 'functionals') can also be used in the Rx of AOB and Class III, but generally alternative approaches are more successful, ∴ we shall only consider Class II malocclusions.

Mode of action In the average child the face grows forward relative to the cranial base and mandibular growth predominates. Functional appliances help to harness this change to correct Class II malocclusions by a combination of force application and force elimination. The relative contributions of each depends upon the design of appliance. Force application usually takes the form of inter-maxillary traction, i.e. a restraining effect on the maxilla and maxillary teeth and a forward pressure on the mandible and mandibular teeth. A similar effect is produced with Class II elastics (p. 180). Functional appliances are ineffective for individual tooth movement.

Application

1 To achieve some antero-posterior correction for a Class II malocclusion prior to FA ± extractions. Ideally, for Class II/1 with mandibular retrusion, average or reduced LFH, or upright or retroclined LLS. A useful test is to examine the profile with patient postured forward to a Class I incisor relationship, and if not improved consider another appliance.

2 Can be used as sole appliance in milder cases with well-aligned arches.

Changes produced by functional appliances[1]

Skeletal

- Research would suggest that changes seen are 25% skeletal and 75% dental.
- Restraint or redirection of forward maxillary growth.
- Optimizing of mandibular growth. Some proponents of functional appliances have claimed increased mandibular growth. Others have replied that the changes seen are small and unsubstantiated long term. The debate continues! It is ∴ better to consider functional appliances as providing an environment for achieving an individual's best mandibular growth potential.
- Forward movement of the glenoid fossa.
- ↑ in LFH.

1 K.D. O'Brien *Am J Orthod Dentofac Orthop* **124** 234.

Dental
- Palatal tipping of the upper incisors.
- Labial tipping of the lower incisors (not a consistent finding).
- Inhibition of forward movement of the maxillary molars.
- Mesial and vertical eruption of the mandibular molars.

Keys to success with functional appliances
- Cooperative and keen patient. Remember that cooperation is finite.
- Favourable growth; ∴ coincide Rx with pubertal growth spurt (girls 11–13, boys 13–15).
- Confident operator, so that child believes appliance will work and will persevere with wearing it.

Types of functional appliance and practical tips

Choice of appliance

Except for those designed for cases with ↑ LFH, the effects produced by the different types of appliance are similar. It is wiser to become familiar with one particular design. For each appliance well-extended upper and lower impressions are required. A wax bite should be recorded with the mandible postured forwards 7–10 mm.

Some of the more popular types:

Twin Block Comprises a separate URA and a lower removable appliance which by means of sloping buccal blocks help to posture the mandible forward. They are well tolerated by patients and can be worn for meals. In addition, a screw can be incorporated in the upper twin block if expansion is required, as well as springs (e.g. to align 2). This design is the most commonly used type of functional appliance in the UK.

Frankel Advocated for cases with abnormal soft-tissue pattern, e.g. lower lip trap. Several subtypes, of which FRII is the most popular. Buccal shields allow expansion of the arches, but the long-term stability of this is unsubstantiated. Construction bite is forward 6 mm and open 3–4 mm in premolar region. Worn full-time. Difficult to repair or adjust, but can be re-activated by dividing buccal shields and advancing.

Medium opening activator A preliminary phase of upper arch expansion is required in most patients to co-ordinate arch widths. Construction bite as for Frankel. Worn full- time. Must be made in heat-cure acrylic as lower arch extensions prone to fracture.

Functionals in Class II/1 with ↑ LFH

Need appliance with molar capping to try and prevent molar eruption, encourage auto-rotation of the mandible, and thus ↓ LFH. ↑ the bite opening of an appliance, is thought to result in a more forward direction of mandibular growth.[1] Some designs include high-pull headgear to restrain vertical maxillary growth.

Practical tips

- Advise patient to wear appliance full-time. Only twin block appliance can be worn for eating. See every 2 months.
- Problems with appliances that fall out in bed at night are often cured by ↑ wear during the day.
- Expect at least 1 mm o/j ↓ per month.
- Wise to continue until o/j almost edge-to-edge.
- Retain by wearing nights only, for about 3 months before progressing on to FA.

---

1 S. E. Bishara 1989 *Am J Orthod Dentofac Orthop* **95** 250.

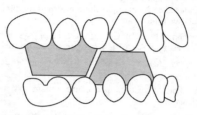

Diagram to show how the inclined bite blocks of the Twin Block appliance hold the mandible forward in a postured position.

Orthodontics and orthognathic surgery

Orthognathic surgery is the correction of skeletal discrepancies outwith the limits of orthodontic Rx, because of either their severity or a lack of growth. Usually deferred until growth complete.

Diagnosis and Rx planning

This is best undertaken jointly by orthodontist and maxillofacial surgeon. Require the following information:

Patient's perception of problem C/O appearance of jaws or teeth, speech, or problems with eating? Are patient's expectations realistic?

Clinical examination Assessment of the balance and proportions of full face and profile.[1]

Study models For bimaxillary procedure mount on semi- or fully adjustable articulator.

Radiographs require DPT and lateral skull, plus PA skull for asymmetries. It is helpful to compare patient's cephalometric tracing with the ideal (Bolton Standard) to visually assess areas of discrepancy. A number of computer programs are available to aid in Δ and planning, of varying complexity and cost. However, these should not supersede clinical assessment in planning.

Photographs Required as pre-Rx record and can also be manipulated with lateral skull for visual predictions.

It is important to correlate desired facial changes with patient's occlusion. Pre-surgical orthodontics will be required to decompensate teeth so that a full surgical correction is possible.

Include the patient in Rx planning so they understand what is involved. It is also helpful if the prospective patient can meet a previous (successful!) candidate.

Sequence of Rx

Pre-surgical orthodontics Aim of orthodontic Rx is to align and coordinate the arches so that the teeth will not interfere when the jaws are placed in their correct position. This usually involves decompensation, i.e. removal of any dento-alveolar compensation for the skeletal discrepancy so that the teeth are at their correct axial inclinations and a full surgical correction can be achieved. If a segmental procedure is planned space will be needed interdentally for surgical cuts. It is inefficient to carry out movements that can be accomplished more readily at surgery (e.g. expansion of upper arch if Le Fort 1 planned), or following surgery (e.g. levelling of lower arch in Class II/2). In addition, the FA provides a means of fixation at surgery.

Surgery, p. 508.

1 N. P. Hunt 1984 *Br J Orthod* **11** 126.

Post-surgical orthodontics Lighter round wires and inter-maxillary traction are used to detail occlusion. Then retention, usually with removable retainers.

Relapse Relapse This can be surgical or orthodontic or both. Relapse more likely in Rx of deficiencies as soft tissues are under greater tension post-operatively.

Cleft lip and palate

Prevalence CLP varies with racial group and geographically. Occurs in 1:750 Caucasian births, but prevalence ↑. M > F. If unilateral L > R. Family history in 40% of cases.

Isolated cleft palate occurs in 1:2000 births. F > M. Family history in 20%.

Aetiology Polygenic inheritance with a threshold. Environmental factors may precipitate susceptible individual towards threshold.

Classification Many exist, but best approach is to describe cleft: primary &/or secondary palate; complete or incomplete; unilateral or bilateral. Submucous cleft is often missed until poor speech noticed, as overlying mucosa is intact.

Problems

Embryological anomalies Tissue deficit, displacement of segments, abnormal muscle attachments.

Post-surgical distortions Unrepaired clefts show normal growth. In repaired clefts maxillary growth is ↓ antero posteriorly, transversely, and vertically. Mandibular growth also ↓.

Hearing and speech are impaired.

Other congenital anomalies occur in up to 20% of cases with CLP and are more likely in association with isolated clefts of palate than lip.

Dental anomalies In CLP ↑ prevalence of hypodontia and $ teeth (especially in region of cleft). Also ↑ incidence of hypoplasia and delayed eruption.

Management (of unilateral complete CLP)

Team usually includes cleft surgeon, secondary surgeon, ENT surgeon, health visitors, orthodontist, speech therapist, clinical psychologist, and central coordinator. Centralization of care and audit of outcome gives better results.

Birth Parents need explanation, reassurance, and help with feeding. Pre-surgical orthopaedics are now out of vogue as benefits not proven.

Lip closure The majority of centres do lip repair at about 3 months, but neonatal repair is carried out by some surgeons. Delaire or Millard &/or modifications are the most popular. Some surgeons do Vomer flap at same time. Bilateral lips are closed either in one or two operations.

Palatal closure Usually between 9 and 18 months. Delaire or Von Langenbeck ± modifications are the most popular. Deferring repair until patient older ↓ growth disturbance, but resultant poor speech has a greater psychological impact.

Primary dentition Lip revision may be carried out before patient starts school. Speech and hearing assessments are required.

Mixed dentition May be necessary to procline upper incisors if they erupt into linguo-occlusion, otherwise orthodontic Rx is better deferred until just prior to secondary bone grafting at 8–10 yrs.

Secondary bone grafting Involves grafting cancellous bone from the iliac crest into the cleft alveolus. Advantages:

1 Provides bone for $\underline{3}$ to erupt through (∴, ideally before eruption of $\underline{3}$).
2 Allows tooth movement into cleft site ∴ intact arch possible.
3 ↑ bony support for alar base.
4 Aids closure of oro-nasal fistulae.

Orthodontic expansion of collapsed arches and alignment of the upper incisors required prior to grafting to improve access. Closure is with local keratinized flaps; ∴, if any 1° extractions are planned these should be carried out in advance.

Permanent dentition Once permanent teeth have erupted, FA are usually required for alignment and space closure. Ideally, if $\underline{2}$ missing, Rx should aim to bring $\underline{3}$ forward to replace it, thus avoiding a prosthesis.

Growth complete A final nose revision is often performed at this stage. Orthognathic surgery to improve facial aesthetics (p. 508) may also be considered, in which case it is preferable to postpone the nose revision until bony surgery complete.

Periodontology

Principal sources J. Lindhe 2003 *Clinical Periodontology and Implant Dentistry* 4th edn, Munksgaard. *Journal of Clinical Periodontology*, Munksgaard.

Oral microbiology

The mouth is colonized by microorganisms a few hours after birth, mainly by aerobic and facultative anaerobic organisms. The eruption of teeth allows the development of a complex ecosystem of microorganisms (>300 species have been identified)[1] and the healthy mouth depends on maintaining an environment in which these organisms coexist without damaging oral structures.

Microorganisms worth noting

Streptococcus mutans group   Several species are recognized within this group, including *S. mutans* and *S. sobrinus*. Aerobic. Synthesizes dextrans. Colony density rises to >50% in presence of high dietary sucrose. Able to produce acid from most sugars. Most important organisms in the aetiology of caries.

Streptococcus oralis group includes *S. sanguis*, *S. mitis*, and *S. oralis*. Account for up to 50% of streptococci in plaque. Heavily implicated in 50% of cases of infective endocarditis.

Streptococcus salivarius group Accounts for about half the streptococci in saliva. Inconsistent producer of dextran.

S. intermedius, S. angiosus, S. constellatus (formerly *S. milleri* group) Common isolates from abscesses in the mouth and at distant sites.

Lactobacillus   Secondary colonizer in caries. Very acidogenic. Often found in dentine caries.

Porphyromonas gingivalis   Obligate anaerobe associated with chronic peri-odontitis and aggressive periodontitis.

Prevotella intermedia   Found in chronic periodontitis, localized aggressive periodontitis, (juvenile periodontitis), necrotizing periodontal disease, and areas of severe gingival inflammation without attachment loss.

Prevotella nigrescens   New, possibly more virulent.

Fusobacterium Obligate   anaerobes. Originally thought to be principal pathogens in necrotizing periodontal disease. Remain a significant periodontal pathogen.

Borrelia vincenti (refringens)   Large oral spirochaete; probably only a co-pathogen.

Actinobacillus actinomycetemcomitans   Microaerophilic, capnophilic, Gram –ve rod. Particular pathogen in juvenile periodontitis and rapidly progressive peri-odontitis.

Actinomyces israelii   Filamentous organism; major cause of actinomycosis. A persistent rare infection which occurs predominantly in the mouth and jaws and the female reproductive tract. Implicated in root caries.

---

1 J. Hardie 1992 *BDJ* **172** 271

Candida albicans Yeast-like fungus, famous as an opportunistic oral pathogen; probably carried as a commensal by most people.

Spirochaetes Obligate anaerobes implicated in periodontal disease; present in most adult mouths. *Borrelia, Treponema*, and *Leptospira* belong to this family.

Plaque

Dental plaque, which is a biofilm, is a firmly adherent mass of bacteria in a muco-polysaccharide matrix. It cannot be rinsed off but can be removed by brushing. It is the root of most dental evils.

Attachment   Although it is possible for plaque to collect on irregular surfaces in the mouth, to colonize smooth tooth surfaces it needs the presence of *acquired pellicle*. This is a thin layer of salivary glycoproteins, formed on the tooth surface within minutes of polishing. The pellicle has an ion-regulating function between tooth and saliva and contains immunoglobulins, complement, and lysozyme.

Development   Up to 10^6 viable bacteria per mm^2 of tooth surface can be recovered 1 h after cleaning;[1] these are selectively adsorbed streptococci. Bacteria recolonize the tooth surface in a predictable sequence. *Streptococcus mutans* synthesizes extracellular polysaccharides (glucan and fructan) specifically from sucrose and promotes its early colonization in this way. Cocci predominate in plaque for the first 2 days, following which rods and filamentous organisms become involved. This is associated with ↑ numbers of leucocytes at the gingival margin. Between 6 and 10 days, if no cleaning has taken place, vibrios and spirochaetes appear in plaque and this is associated with clinical gingivitis. It is generally felt that the move towards a more Gram –ve anaerobe-dense plaque is associated with the progression of gingivitis and periodontal disease.

Plaque in caries   (p. 28) As several oral streptococci, most notably mutans streptococci, secrete acids and the matrix component of plaque, there is a clear relationship between the two. However, various other factors complicate the picture, including saliva, other microorganisms, and the structure of the tooth surface.

Plaque in periodontal disease   There is a direct correlation between the amount of plaque at the cervical margin of teeth and the severity of gingivitis,[2] and experimental gingivitis can be produced and abolished by suspending and reintroducing oral hygiene.[3] It is commonly accepted that plaque accumulation causes gingivitis, the major variable being host susceptibility. While there are numerous interacting components which determine the progression of chronic gingivitis to periodontitis, particularly host susceptibility, the presence of plaque, particularly 'old' plaque with its high anaerobe content, is widely held to be crucial, and most Rx is based on the meticulous, regular removal of plaque.

1 R. Gibbons 1973 *J. Periodont* **44** 347.
2 M. Ash 1964 *J. Periodont* **35** 424.
3 H. Loe 1965 *J. Periodont* **36** 177.

Calculus

Calculus (tartar) is a calcified deposit found on teeth (and other solid oral structures) and is formed by mineralization of plaque deposits. It can be subdivided into:

Supragingival calculus, most often found opposite the openings of the salivary ducts, i.e. 76|67 opposite the parotid (Stensen's) duct and on the lingual surface of the lower anterior teeth opposite the submandibular/sublingual (Wharton's) duct. It is usually yellow, but can become stained a variety of colours.

Subgingival calculus is found, not surprisingly, underneath the gingival margin and is firmly attached to tooth roots. It tends to be brown or black, is extremely tenacious, and is most often found on interproximal and lingual surfaces. It may be identified visually, by touch using a WHO 621 probe, or on radiographs. With gingival recession it can become supragingival.

Composition Consists of up to 80% inorganic salts, mostly crystalline, the major components being calcium and phosphorus. The microscopic structure is basically that of a randomly orientated crystal formation.

Formation is always preceded by plaque deposition, the plaque serving as an organic matrix for subsequent mineralization. Initially, the matrix between organisms becomes calcified with, eventually, the organisms themselves becoming mineralized. Subgingival calculus usually takes many months to form, whereas friable supragingival calculus may form within 2 weeks.

Pathological effects Calculus (particularly, subgingival calculus), is associated with periodontal disease. This may be because it is invariably covered by a layer of plaque. Its principal detrimental effect is probably that it acts as a retention site for plaque and bacterial toxins. The presence of calculus makes it difficult to implement adequate oral hygiene.

Host

Local and systemic modifying factors influence progress of the disease.

Systemic factors include immune status, stress, endocrine function, (e.g. diabetes) smoking, drugs, age, and nutrition. There has been evidence reported suggesting a link between periodontal, ischaemic heart, and cerebrovascular disease. It is unclear if this is a cause and effect relationship. Watch this space.

Local factors are tooth position and morphology, calculus, overhangs and appliances, occlusal trauma, and mucogingival state.

Epidemiology of periodontal disease—1

Epidemiology is the study of the presence and effect of disease on a population. In order for this to be of value it is essential to be able to quantify the prevalence and degree of severity of any given disease, in a reproducible manner. The search for suitable **indices** in periodontology has left the literature replete with often confusing and redundant scoring systems.

The original purpose of periodontal indices was to study the extent of disease within population groups; however, the value of indices in the screening and management of individual patients soon became apparent. The following two indices fulfil both these criteria and are simple and easy to perform:

Debris or Oral Hygiene Index This can be modified for personal use by using disclosing agents.[1]

0 No debris or stain.
1 Soft debris covering not more than $\frac{1}{3}$ of the tooth surface.
2 Soft debris covering more than $\frac{1}{3}$ but less than $\frac{2}{3}$.
3 Soft debris covering over $\frac{2}{3}$ of tooth surface.

Basic Periodontal Examination (BPE) Also known as **Community Periodontal Index of Treatment Needs (CPITN)**.[2] This technique is used to screen for those patients requiring more detailed periodontal examination. It examines every tooth in the mouth (except third molars), thus taking into account the site-specific nature of periodontal disease. A World Health Organization (WHO) periodontal probe (ball-ended with a coloured band 3.5–5.5 mm from the tip) should be used. The mouth is divided into sextants, i.e. two buccal and one labial segment per arch. Six sites on each tooth are explored and the highest score per sextant recorded, usually in a simple six-box chart.

0 = No disease,
1 = Gingival bleeding but no pockets, no calculus, no overhanging restoration. Rx: OHI.
2 = No pockets >3 mm, subgingival calculus present or subgingival retention site, e.g. overhang. Rx: OHI, scaling, and correction of any iatrogenic problems.
3 = Deepest pocket 4 or 5 mm. Rx: OHI, scaling, and root planning.
4 = One or more tooth in sextant has a pocket >6 mm. Rx: scaling and root planing, &/or flap as required.
* = Furcation or total loss of attachment of 7 mm or more. Rx: full periodontal examination of the sextant regardless of CPITN score.

Individuals identified as having areas of advanced periodontal disease will require a full probing depth chart, together with recordings of mobility, recession and furcation involvement, and radiological examination. BPE cannot be used for close monitoring of the progress of Rx.

---

1 J. Greene 1960 *J Am Dent Assoc* **61** 172.
2 J. Ainamo 1988 *Int Dent J* **32** 281.

Epidemiology of periodontal disease—2

Other techniques for assessing the levels of periodontal disease include.

Marginal bleeding index (MBI)   Score 1 or 0 depending on whether or not bleeding occurs after a probe is gently run around the gingival sulcus. A percentage score is obtained by dividing by the number of teeth and multiplying the result by 100.

Plaque index (PlI)   This is based on the presence or absence of plaque on the mesial, distal, lingual, and buccal surfaces revealed by disclosing.

$$\text{Percentage score} = \frac{\text{number of surfaces with plaque} \times 100}{\text{total number of teeth} \times 4}$$

Both the MBI and PlI can be expressed as bleeding or plaque-**free** scores in this way obtaining a high score is a good thing, which may be both easier for the patient to understand and a more positive motivational approach.

Although periodontal diseases are very common, severe forms affect no more than about 10–15% of the population. Overall, periodontitis accounts for between 30 and 35% of all tooth extractions; caries and its consequences account for up to 50%.[1]

The direct association between the presence of tooth surface plaque and periodontal damage has been confirmed, but the rate of destruction has been shown to vary, not only between individuals but also between different sites in the same mouth, and at different times in the same individual.

---

1 P. Papapanou 1996 *Annals of Periodontology* **1** 1.

WHO probe for use in BPE/CPITN.

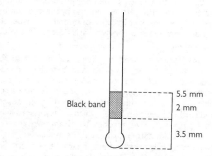

Black band

5.5 mm
2 mm

3.5 mm

If black band disappears on probing pocket, perform full periodontal examination in that sextant.

Chronic gingivitis

Chronic gingivitis is, as the name suggests, inflammation of the gingival tissues. It is **not** associated with alveolar bone resorption or apical migration of the junctional epithelium. Pockets > 2 mm can occur in chronic gingivitis due to an increase in gingival size because of oedema or hyperplasia (false pockets). Four different types of gingivitis are described; the commonest type is plaque induced.

Plaque-induced gingivitis   This is present in virtually all mouths to some extent. The classic triad of redness, swelling, and bleeding on gentle probing are diagnostic and are usually associated with a complaint by the patient that their 'gums bleed on brushing'. False pocketing may also be present. This gingivitis occurs as a result of low-grade infection caused by the presence of undisturbed dental plaque, which is associated with a change in the flora from Gram +ve aerobes to Gram −ve anaerobes (p. 202). This gives rise to inflammatory changes in the associated gingivae; these are detectable histologically prior to the appearance of overt clinical gingivitis, which is observed after about 7 days of undisturbed plaque accumulation. The inflammatory response seen comprises an alteration in the integrity of the gingival microcirculation, an ↑ in the numbers of inflammatory cells in the gingival connective tissue (i.e. plasma cells, lymphocytes, macrophages, and neutrophils), a ↓ in the number of fibroblasts, and a ↓ in collagen density. These inflammatory changes are easily reversible after institution of effective plaque control. While gingivitis is reversible, it should be remembered that calculus and other factors which promote plaque retention (e.g. overhanging restorations) will make adequate oral hygiene difficult. These factors should ∴ be corrected by scaling and appropriate restorative treatment in addition to OHI. Gingivitis may be a precursor to, or marker of, adult periodontitis, and this must be excluded by measuring probing attachment levels (looking for 'true' pockets) and excluding the presence of alveolar bone loss by radiographs, if indicated. Other forms of gingivitis include:

Gingivitis   modified by systemic factors. These would include puberty-associated gingivitis, menstual cycle-associated gingivitis, pregnancy-associated gingivitis, pyogenic granuloma, diabetes mellitus-associated gingivitis, and gingivitis associated with blood dyscrasias, e.g. leukaemia-associated gingivitis.

Gingivitis   modified by medications. These would include drug-influenced gingival enlargement and drug-induced gingivitis, e.g. oral contraceptive-associated gingivitis and drug-induced gingival overgrowth due to phenytoin or cyclosporin.

Gingival disease modified by malnutrition. These would include ascorbic acid-deficiency gingivitis (scurvy) and gingivitis due to protein deficiency.

Classification of periodontal disease

There appears to be a deep need among the 'labellers' to rename and reclassify microorganisms and diseases. Periodontitis has suffered more than most from this.

In truth, the only real benefit your patient receives from this exercise is if the classification has a bearing on Rx, and fortunately this is something that is starting to happen among periodontologists.

There are, of course, the usual caveats about patients being individuals and the real difficulty in making highly specific Δ in individual cases. Despite this, the current classification[1] may prove helpful in thinking your way through the different periodontal diseases:

I Chronic periodontitis.
II Aggressive periodontitis.
III Periodontitis as a manifestation of systemic disease.
IV Necrotizing periodontal diseases.
V Abscesses of the periodontium.
VI Periodontitis associated with endodontic lesions.
VII Development or acquired deformities and conditions.

1 G. C. Armitage *Ann Periodontol* 1999: **4** 1.

Chronic adult periodontitis

Chronic periodontitis (CP) can be regarded as a progression of the combination of infection and inflammation of gingivitis into the deep tissues of the periodontal membrane. It is characterized by breakdown of periodontal fibre bundles at the cervical margin, resorption of alveolar bone, and apical proliferation of junctional epithelium beyond the amelocemental junction. The progression of chronic gingivitis to periodontitis is by no means straightforward, as it varies in rate and progression not only between individuals, but also between sites within the same mouth, and with time. It is now thought that periodontal destruction occurs in acute bursts of disease activity, each followed by a quiescent phase. The active phase is characterized by a rapid loss of attachment. This lasts for a variable period of time and is probably induced by a change in the quantity &/or quality of the subgingival microflora in undisturbed plaque, although other parameters may be involved. These include host response due to systemic disease, and local factors such as occlusal trauma, iatrogenic damage, or an as yet undetermined variable in the inflammatory response. The quiescent phase is associated with no advance in disease on either clinical or radiographic grounds and may last for extended periods of time. However, complete healing of the lesion does **not** occur because plaque remains on the root surface, and inflammation ∴ persists in the connective tissues.

Microbiology In the majority of cases the microbial pathogens remain within the plaque in the periodontal pocket and do not invade the periodontal tissues. It has already been mentioned (p. 206) that sampling of pockets in cases of CP consistently recovers a greatly ↑ proportion of Gram −ve anaerobic rods and spirochaetes. Debate still continues between adherents of the specific (CP caused by specific organisms), and the non-specific plaque (CP caused by quantity rather than quality of plaque) theories. Nevertheless, certain Gram −ve anaerobes appear particularly prominently in active disease sites; namely *Prophyromonas gingivalis, Prevotella intermedia/nigrescens, Bacteroides forsythus, Campylobacter rectus,* and *Treponema denticola* (apologies to the reader, microbiologists appear to have a pathological need to rename organisms). Some of these organisms synthesize enzymes such as proteases which would exert a deleterious effect on the periodontal membrane, and all Gram −ve organisms release endotoxin (their cell wall) on death.

Diagnosis is based on:
- Probing to elicit bleeding (which is the single most useful indicator of disease activity), measuring pocket depth attachment levels, and detecting subgingival calculus.
- Testing teeth for mobility and vitality.
- Radiographic examination (vertical bitewings and periapicals). See radiological selection criteria.

Treatment pp. 228–52.
Generally aggressive periodontitis is a severe form of generalized periodontitis affecting young adults (20–35 yrs). Affects 1–2% of the Western population with an ↑ in Afro-Caribbeans. Microbiologically—round-up the usual

suspects plus *A. actinomycetemcomitans*. Immunologically there may be an associated neutrophil defect. Rx as for LAP.

Refractory periodontitis is characterized by low plaque scores and a poor response to appropriate periodontal therapy; 4–8% of patients with CP have refractory periodontitis. >90% are smokers.

Pocketing

Periodontal pockets can be divided into the following:

False pockets are due to gingival enlargement with the pocket epithelium at or above the amelocemental junction.

True pockets imply apical migration of the junctional epithelium beyond the amelocemental junction and can be divided into suprabony and infrabony pockets. Infrabony are described according to the number of bony walls: three-walled defect is the most favourable, as it is surrounded on three sides by cancellous bone and on one side by the cementum of the root surface. Two-walled defect may be either a crater between teeth having bone on two walls and cementum on the other two, or have two bony walls, the root cementum, and an open aspect to the overlying soft tissues. One-walled defects may be hemiseptal through-and-through defects, or one bony wall, two root cementum, and one soft tissue.

Pocket depths are measured from the gingival margin to the estimated base of the pocket. Attachment levels are measured from a fixed reference point: the cement–enamel junction or margin of a restoration to the base of the pocket. Pockets are ∴ dependent on the position of the gingival margin.

Periodontal probes are the key instruments in detecting pockets. Numerous designs exist, and while individual preference will influence choice, it is sensible to reduce variability by selecting a single type of probe and using that type of probe throughout any one individual's Rx. The use of the WHO probe for screening using the BPE index is described on p. 208. Patients who are identified as having advanced CP should then be investigated further, including probing around each tooth. The main other indicator of periodontal disease, bleeding, is also detected using a probe (gently), and again consistency with a single type of probe is necessary.

Probing variables The depth of penetration depends upon:
• Type of probe and its position.
• Amount of pressure used.
• Degree of inflammation.[1]

It is now apparent that the measurement obtained with a probe does not correspond to sulcus or pocket depth. In the presence of inflammation a probe tip can pass through the inflamed tissues until it reaches the most coronal dento-gingival fibres, about 0.5mm apical to the apical extent of the junctional epithelium, i.e. an overestimation of the problem. The amount of penetration into the tissues varies directly with the degree of inflammation, so that, following resolution of inflammation, an underestimate of attachment levels may be given. Formation of a tight, long junctional epithelium following Rx may also give a false sense of security if probing measurements are not interpreted with a degree of caution. For this reason the term 'probing pocket depth' is preferred to pocket depth.

1 M. A. Listgarten 1980 *J Clin Periodont* **7** 165.

Diagnostic tests and monitoring

It is widely accepted that disease active and inactive pockets exist. Progression is episodic and more likely in susceptible patients. Bleeding on probing has traditionally been the most useful indicator of disease activity; however, only 30% of sites which bleed will go on to lose attachment.[1]

With ↑ emphasis on specific periodontopathic bacteria (p. 200) and availability of assays for components of immunological response, chairside diagnostic tests using gingival crevicular fluid have been developed.

Three types exist:

1 Based on detection of antibodies to specific periodontopaths, e.g. Kodak Evalusite.
2 Based on components of immune response, e.g. elastase in Dentsply Prognostick.
3 Based on tissue breakdown by products, e.g. aspartate aminotransferase in Colgate-Palmolive's Periogard.

These aim to predict sites of future and actual disease progression, and the first may indicate need for specific antibiotic therapy (p. 232).

There is a huge amount of ongoing research into improving and refining these tests, but evidence is still required to demonstrate predictive ability and a higher level of accuracy than bleeding on probing.

Other peripheral techniques worthy of note are pocket temperature probes and computerized subtraction radiovisiography.

Radiographs are useful in comparing degree of bone loss and root surface deposits with pocket depth. Standardized sequential radio- graphs allow monitoring of disease.

• Horizontal bitewings provide a good view of interproximal bone, useful for relatively minor degrees of bone loss (pocketing <5 mm) and to detect calculus deposits. Vertical bitewings are recommed when pocketing is >5 mm.
• Full mouth periapicals (long cone technique), supplemented with vertical or horizontal bitewing, have been the radiological assessment of choice for patients with significant periodontal disease, i.e. irregular pocketing. They can clearly demonstrate root surface deposits, furcation involvement, extensive bone loss, infrabony pocketing, and perio-endo lesions. Radiation exposure is > OPG but it gives a more accurate representation of bone loss.

The results of a radiographic examination, clinical assessment, and assessment of pocket depth can all be marked on an updatable periodontal chart to monitor progress with Rx.

1 N. Lang 1986 *J Clin Periodont* **13** 590

Acute periodontal disease

Necrotising ulcerative gingivitis (NUG) is also known as, Vincent's gingivitis, Vincent's gingivostomatitis, ulceromembraneous gingivitis, or trench mouth. It should not be confused with Vincent's angina, which is also a fusospirochaetal infection but is typically localized over the tonsils.

NUG is characterized by painful papillary yellowish-white ulcers which bleed readily. Patients also often complain of a metallic taste and the sensation of their teeth being wedged apart. Regional lymphadenitis, fever, and malaise may occur in some cases. NUG is associated with poor oral hygiene, but stress and smoking act as co-factors. Inadequately treated NUG will lapse into a less symptomatic form which has become known as chronic ulcerative gingivitis, in which a slower rate of destruction occurs. NUG is usually a limited gingival condition, but a rare and more serious form known as cancrum oris or noma is found in patients who are malnourished, and in this form can lead to extensive destruction of the jaws and face.

Microbiology Originally *Borrelia vincenti* (*refringens*) and *Fusobacterium fusiformis* were held to be the major culprits in a mixed anaerobic infection. Further research has, however, served to confuse the picture, with *Porphyromonas* spp. being implicated, as well as *Treponema* spp. *Selenomonas* spp. and *Prevotella* spp. The crucial aspect of the microbiology of NUG is that it is a Gram −ve anaerobic infection which has been shown to actually invade the tissues but usually responds to local debridement. In recent years, the tendency for patients who are HIV +ve to develop severe NUG, sometimes with bone necrosis, has renewed interest in it. From the practical point of view it should be remembered that NUG presenting in an otherwise apparently healthy young adult may be a presenting sign of HIV infection. Practically, consider control of cross-infection, examining the mouth for other signs of infection (p. 476), and directing the patient to appropriate counselling &/or HIV testing.

Rx In most cases local measures, i.e. thorough debridement and adequate oral hygiene will suffice; however, if there is evidence of systemic upset (lymphadenopathy) metronidazole 200 mg tds for 3 days is indicated. It is wise to get the patient to rinse with chlorhexidine gluconate 0.2% prior to ultrasonic scaling to reduce aerosol spread. Chlorhexidine rinses may also be prescribed as an adjunct to brushing, which is painful initially. Later Rx, such as gingivectomy for persistent craters, is only rarely required.

Periodontal abscess is a localized collection of pus within a periodontal pocket. It occurs either due to the introduction of virulent organisms into an existing pocket or ↓ drainage potential. The latter classically occurs during Rx as reduction of inflammation in the coronal gingival tissues occludes drainage by a tighter adaptation to the tooth. May also occur due to impaction of a foreign body such as a fishbone in a pre-existing pocket or even in an otherwise healthy periodontal membrane.

Diagnosis   Need to distinguish from apical abscess.

Apical abscess	*Periodontal abscess*
Non-vital	Usually vital
TTP vertically	Pain on lateral movements
May be mobile	Usually mobile
Loss of lamina dura on radiograph	Loss of alveolar crest on radiograph

Insertion of a GP point into an associated sinus and a radiograph may be helpful.

Rx *Emergency*: Incision and drainage under LA; debridement of the pocket (e.g. ultrasonic scaler); systemic antibiotic, e.g. metronidazole 200–400 mg tds &/or amoxicillin 250–500 mg tds for 5 days if systemic involvement *Follow-up*: conventional Rx for periodontal pockets (p. 234), combined periodontal–endodontic lesion (p. 250).

Acute herpetic gingivostomatitis, p. 436.

Acute streptococcal gingivitis   Rare. Beefy, red, painful gingivae usually caused by a Lancefield A streptococcus. Rx: penicillin V 500 mg qds for 7 days and OHI.

Periodontitis in children

There are three main variants: localized aggressive periodontitis, generalized aggressive periodontitis, and prepubertal periodontitis. Originally termed 'periodontosis' (1942), they have become better defined in recent years.

Localized aggressive periodontitis (LAP)
Occurs in children and adolescents. Usually localized to upper and lower incisors and first molars. Retrospective studies have suggested it may affect primary dentition. The gingivae around affected teeth may appear entirely normal despite deep periodontal pockets. The degree of period-ontal destruction seems out of proportion to the deposits of plaque and calculus.

Prevalence is low (~0.2%). Afro-Caribbeans (2.5%) > Asians > Caucasians. F > M and often familial.

Microbiology A range of rare organisms have been cultured. *Actinobacillus actinomycetemcomitans (Aa)* is the major culprit. Others which may act in association include *Eubacterium-* and *Bacteroides*-like spp. *Aa* has been implicated because of high levels in LAP pockets, ↑ serum antibodies to *Aa* in LAP patients, and the ability of *Aa* to produce a range of periodonto-pathic mediators such as leucotoxin, chemotactic inhibition factor, fibro-blast growth inhibitor, and an endotoxic cell wall. These patients do show functional defects of neutrophils. There is some evidence that *Aa* invades local host tissue.

Rx Meticulous oral hygiene, conventional scaling, and root planing, often in conjunction with access flap surgery. Consider systemic tetracycline (oxytetracycline 250 mg qds or doxycycline 100 mg od for 2–3 weeks) or locally deposited (e.g. slow release) tetracycline. 3-monthly monitoring of subgingival microflora for *Aa* with targeted Rx is ideal.

Generalized aggressive periodontitis (GAP)
A disease of older children; often beginning around puberty. Unlike LAP, these patients have marked periodontal inflammation, and heavy plaque and calculus deposits.

Prevalence Figures from the USA suggest ~0.13% in adolescents.

Microbiology High levels of non-motile, Gram −ve facultative anaerobes, including *Porphyromonas gingivalis*. In common with LAP these patients have neutrophils with ↓ chemotaxis.

Rx As above optimal antibiotic not yet known.

Prepubertal periodontitis
Rare. Appears soon after eruption of 1° dentition. Characterized by severe gingival inflammation, and rapid bone and tooth loss.

Microbiology Usual periodontal pathogens.

Pathology Thought to be due to a defective leucocyte glycoprotein, preventing leucocyte migration and causing ↓ effective immune response.

Exclude hypophophatasia before making Δ, as cementopathia seen in this can mimic prepubertal periodontitis.

Rx As for LAP but avoid tetracycline. Use amoxicillin 125–250 mg tds instead.

Chediak–Higashi, p. 757.

Papillon–Lefevre, p. 759.

Prevention of periodontal disease

Following the comments on the pages covering the aetiology and epidemiology of periodontal disease, it is quite clear that dental plaque is the cause of the problem and its elimination will prevent gum disease. This is easier said than done—remember most of the world's population has gingivitis &/or periodontitis. The key to prevention is regular and thorough plaque removal, ∴ OHI is probably the most useful advice you can give to your patients. Smoking exacerbates periodontal disease and adversely affects Rx outcome. Patients should be advised of this.

OHI should include an explanation of the nature of the patient's disease and hence the reasons for good oral hygiene. Identify and demonstrate to the patient the disease (swollen gingivae, bleeding on probing) using a hand mirror, then demonstrate the cause (plaque), either directly, by scraping off a deposit, or by disclosing. Explain how plaque starts to grow immediately after toothbrushing, so that regular removal is necessary, and that it cannot be rinsed away. Then demonstrate how to remove it, avoiding overt criticism of the patient's present efforts, as this is often counter-productive.

Toothbrushing requires a brush, ideally with a small head and even nylon bristles (3–4 tufts across by 10–12 lengthways), which should be renewed at least monthly. Toothpaste makes the process more pleasant and is a useful medium for topical fluoride and other agents. Anticalculus pastes ↓ plaque formation by about 50%. Chlorhexidine-containing toothpastes are active against plaque microorganisms. Numerous methods can be described, based on the movement of the brush stroke: rolling, vibratory, circular, vertical, horizontal. The best is the one which works for that patient (as demonstrated by absence of plaque on disclosing after brushing) and does no harm to tooth or gingivae. The horizontal scrub is notorious for possibly exacerbating gingival recession. Modifications to toothbrushes and brushing technique are often required in children, the elderly, and those with disabling diseases.

Interdental cleaning Brushing alone is unlikely to clean the interdental spaces adequately; however, it must be mastered first by the patient, before interdental cleaning is taught. Flossing, mini interdental brushes (particularly good for concave root surfaces), and interspace brushes are available for cleaning interproximally. The use of dental floss is something of an art form and must be learned by demonstration.

Professional preventive techniques

Regular periodic examination for periodontal disease, which is largely asymptomatic, is essential. This requires a full oral examination, including probing for pockets as part of routine examination (p. 14). In patients who have been demonstrated to have periodontal disease, 3-monthly follow-ups are advisable. Routine scaling and polishing is of little value unless accompanied by intensive education and motivation of the patient (however tedious this may be), as it is the patient's efforts which will prevent the re-formation of plaque and initiation of periodontal disease. Employment of a hygienist has obvious benefits in this area. Elimination, avoidance, and Rx of iatrogenic problems such as overhanging margins on restorations, ill-fitting crown margins, poorly designed appliances, etc., are mandatory.

Principles of treatment

- Establish diagnosis.
- Periodontal disease is an infection due to the presence of plaque,
  ∴ control of plaque is the key to success. More complex Rxs will always
  fail in the absence of effective plaque control.
- The aims of corrective techniques such as scaling, root planing,
  periodontal surgery, restorative work, endodontics, and occlusal
  adjustment, etc. are:
  1 to eliminate pathological periodontal pockets, or to create
    a tight epithelial attachment where the pocket once existed;
  2 to arrest loss of, and in some cases improve, the alveolar bone
    support;
  3 to create an oral environment which is relatively simple for the
    patient to keep plaque-free.

The overall aim could be summarized as the creation of a healthy mouth
which the patient is both capable of, and willing to, maintain.

It is often convenient to divide the principles of periodontal therapy into
three phases:

1 The *initial* (cause–related) phase, where the aim is to control or
  eliminate gingivitis and arrest any further progression of periodontal
  disease by the removal of plaque and other contributory factors.
2 The *corrective* phase is designed principally to restore function and,
  where relevant, aesthetics.
3 The *maintenance* (supportive) phase aims to reinforce patient
  motivation so that their OH is adequate to prevent recurrence of
  disease. This phase is receiving ↑ attention due to the relative ease
  with which disease activity can be monitored by probing and chairside
  diagnostic assays (p. 220).

Non-surgical therapy—1

Non-surgical therapy in periodontal disease consists of debridement, restorative Rx (to correct coexisting or exacerbating factors, e.g. periapical infection, overhanging margins), and the use of antiseptics and antibiotics.

Scaling is the removal of plaque and calculus from the tooth surface, either with hand instruments (e.g. curettes, hoes, chisels, and jaquettes) or mechanically (e.g. Cavitron). Scaling can be sub-or supragingival depending upon the site of the deposits. LA is usually not necessary. It is customary to make use of an ultrasonic scaler for the bulk of the work and finish off, particularly subgingivally, with hand instruments. The precise use of hand instruments is largely a matter of personal preference; however, it is essential to use controlled force and a secure finger-rest. Ultrasonic instruments are quicker, but they can be uncomfortable and leave an uneven root surface (though the significance of the latter is controversial). Ultrasonic scaling employs a frequency of 25–40 000 cycles/sec. Another instrument, known as a sonic scaler and vibrating at 1600–1800 cycles/sec, has been shown to be equally effective at removing calculus and may result in smoother root surfaces. With both it is essential to use a copious coolant spray.

The teeth are usually polished after scaling, preferably using a rubber cup and a fluoride-containing paste (e.g. toothpaste). Patients can then appreciate the feeling of a clean mouth, which they must then maintain.

Local delivery of medicaments

Due to controversy over the efficacy and unwanted effects of systemic antibiotics, methods of direct delivery into the pocket have been explored. These have included using injected pastes or gels, or by impregnated fibre. This gives a high local dose, low systemic uptake, and prolonged exposure of the pathogens to the drug. The rate of crevicular fluid turnover is such that the substantivity of these agents is low. Examples: Blackwell Dentomycin (minocycline), Colgate-Palmolive Elyzol (metronidazole), and Periochip (chlorhexidine). However, only small ↑ in attachment levels have been reported and currently local adjunctive antibiotics are only indicated for the Rx of persistent local defects.

Antimetabolites

NSAIDs are the main group being investigated. Experimental gingivitis and alveolar bone loss in animals are ↓ by flurbiprofen. This is *not* only due to cyclo-oxygenase pathway inhibition. Evidence of significant long-term benefit in humans is awaited. A future possibility is inclusion of NSAIDs in topical form in a toothpaste.

Non-surgical therapy—2

Antiseptics and antibiotics

As the mechanical control of plaque is a tedious and time-consuming procedure, the use of chemicals either as antiseptics or antibiotics would be a significant aid. Problems with their use include the unwanted side-effects of such chemicals, development of resistance, mode of delivery, and most importantly, the fact that no single organism has been identified as the main pathogen in periodontal disease. Nevertheless, elimination of Gram −ve anaerobic bacteria has been demonstrated to result in improved periodontal health.

Antiseptics The antiseptic of greatest proven value is chlorhexidine gluconate. This is commonly used in a 0.2% mouthwash or gel, although 0.12% mouthwash is also available. A standard regimen is 10 ml of solution rinsed for 1 min bd. The gel can be used instead of toothpaste. **NB** An interaction between conventional toothpaste and chlorhexidine reduces the antiseptic's efficacy. Other proprietary antiseptic rinses have yet to meet this 'gold standard'.

Antibiotics A review of the use of antibiotics in periodontology recommended their use for patients with recent, or a high risk of, periodontal breakdown.[1] Antibiotics are generally used as an adjunct to mechanical non-surgical therapy in early onset periodontitis and some forms of adult periodontitis. Short-term, relatively high doses, or high locally delivered doses, are used. The two most useful drugs are:

Tetracycline. Can be administered either systemically or directly into the pocket via a slow release mechanism (Dentomycin gel). It is active against spirochaetes, *Actinobacillus actinomycetemcomitans*, and many other periodontal pathogens. Most useful in the Rx of LAP. Oxytetracycline and doxycycline are currently popular. In addition to being antibacterial, tetracyclines ↓ host neutrophil collagenases and ↓ bone loss. Crevicular fluid concentrations are high. Currently there is much interest in doxycycline (20 mg bd for 3/12). At this dose it has no detrimental effect on the periodontal microflora and its action is mainly to reduce collagenolytic metalloproteinases.

Metronidazole. Effective against protozoa and strict anaerobes and capable of eliminating all the strict anaerobes found in periodontal pockets. As it does not interfere with aerobes or facultative anaerobes it is highly unlikely to allow the development of opportunist pathogens. There is frequent mention of the mutagenicity and teratogenicity of this drug in animal studies but, despite widespread use in medicine, no clinical evidence has emerged to support this. It is, in fact, an extremely safe and useful drug. When combined with mechanical pocket therapy, significant improvements in terms of probing depth have been demonstrated.[2] There is an emetic interaction with alcohol.

There is a clear place for antibiotics/antiseptics as adjuncts in selected types of periodontal disease, e.g. aggressive periodontitis and acute or severe periodontal infections.

1 J. Slots 1990 *J Clin Periodont* **17** 479.
2 W. J. Loesche 1984 *J Clin Periodont* **55** 325.

Minimally invasive therapy—1

There has been a progressive move away from pocket elimination surgery, towards the creation of a healthy periodontium which gives access for both professional and home cleaning. Recognition that periodontal disease is a localized infection due to the presence of dental plaque, and that its arrest and prevention is dependent on the removal of plaque and plaque-retaining factors, has allowed a far more rational and conservative approach to therapy to develop. The prime aims of periodontal surgery are now to:

- remove deposits from root surfaces;
- create subgingival root surfaces which are accessible for cleaning, either by professionals or by the patient;
- maximize the potential for healing of damaged periodontal tissues.

Minimally invasive techniques include deep subgingival scaling/root planing and the modified Widman flap (open flap debridement). These are suitable for those patients who, despite good supragingival plaque control, still have true pockets but do not need recontouring of the gingival margins.

Scaling and root planing Deep subgingival scaling and root planing are best carried out under LA. Deep scaling is a procedure which removes plaque and calculus from the root surface; it differs from supragingival scaling simply in its thoroughness, and the discomfort it causes. Root planing is a technique whereby endotoxin-damaged cementum is removed from the root surface by scraping the root. The same instruments are used for both procedures (p. 230), and in practice it is probably impossible to differentiate between subgingival scaling and root planing, as in both techniques plaque, calculus, root cementum, and small amounts of dentine will be removed. These are the core procedures for **all** periodontal techniques; the only real difference with formal surgery is that it allows Rx under direct vision, osseous recontouring and sculpting if desired, and repositioning of the gingiva.

It is often most effective to treat one quadrant at a time under LA, partly because it is painful and partly because it is tedious when performed meticulously, which is the only worthwhile way to do it. It has been suggested, however, that full mouth root planning be done in two visits separated by only 24 h, with concurrent use of a chlorhexidine mouth-wash. The choice of instruments is less important than the end result, as effective debridement of the root surface is essential. It is **not** necessary to curette the epithelial lining of the pocket. Success will allow tight adaptation of the pocket epithelium to the root, creating a *long junctional epithelium.*

As smoking ↓ outcome of Rx, some periodontologists have limited Rx in those continuing to smoke. While periodontal surgery hardly has the public impact of cardiac surgery, the ethical problem is the same.

Practical tips for periodontal surgery

Local anaesthesia The infiltration, block &/or lingual/palatal injections required will be determined by the site of surgery. Both LA and haemostasis are improved by injecting directly into the gingival margin and interdental papillae until blanching is seen.

Suturing techniques Interrupted interproximal sutures are used when buccal and lingual flaps are being reapposed at the same level. When flaps are repositioned at different levels, a suspensory suture is used, where the suture only passes through the buccal flap and is suspended around the cervical margins of the teeth.

Periodontal packs These are essential after gingivectomy to ↓ post-operative discomfort. Many favour them after all periodontal surgery to help reappose the flap to bone.
Classified:

- Eugenol dressings, e.g. ZnO, have the advantage of being mildly analgesic but can cause sensitivity reactions.
- Eugenol-free dressings, e.g. Coe-pack, are more popular.

Minimally invasive therapy—2

The modified Widman flap

This is a technique which enables open debridement of the root surface, with a minimal amount of trauma. There is no attempt to excise the pocket, although a superficial collar of tissue is removed. This has the advantage of allowing close adaptation of the soft tissues to the root surface with minimal trauma, and exposure of, underlying bone and connective tissue, thus causing fewer problems with post-operative sensitivity and aesthetics.

Technique (after Ramfjord and Nissle 1974).[1] A scalloped incision is made parallel to the long axis of the teeth involved 1mm from the crevicular margin, except when pockets are <2mm deep when an intracrevicular incision is made. This incision is extended interproximally as far as possible, separating the pocket epithelium from the flap to be raised, and then extended mesially and distally, allowing the flap to be raised as an envelope without relieving incisions. The flap should be as conservative as possible and only a few millimetres of alveolar bone exposed by a second incision intercrevicularly to release the collar of pocket epithelium and granulation tissue. A third incision at 90 degrees to the tooth separates the pocket epithelium, and this is removed along with accompanying granulation tissue with curettes and hoes. The root surface is then thoroughly scaled and root planed. Although bony defects can be curetted **no** osseous surgery is carried out. The flaps are then repositioned to cover all exposed alveolar bone and sutured into position. Post-operatively chlorhexidine 0.2% 10ml rinsed bd is given, and most periodontologists prefer to use a periodontal pack to improve patient comfort post-operatively.

Notes There continues to be considerable confusion about nomenclature with this type of flap. The original Widman flap described in 1918 by Leonard Widman used relieving incisions and osseous surgery, and attempted to remove the pocket. The Neumann flap used an intracrevicular incision, again attempting to excise the pocket, but the 'modified flap operation' described by Kirkland in 1931 did not require sacrifice of inflamed tissues or apical displacement of the gingival margin. The latter was, of course, the precursor of the 'modified Widman flap'.

---

1 S. Ramfjord 1974 *J Periodont* **45** 601.

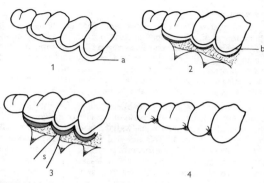

Modified Widman flap
1 Design of flap
  a Incision
2 Flap elevated
  b Gingival cuff to be discarded
3 Excision of supra-alveolar pocket
  s Scalpel blade
4 Flap repositioned and sutured in place

Periodontal surgery

Gingivectomy

Has ↓ in use over the last decade; its remaining indications are in cases with persistence of deep supra-alveolar pockets (e.g. gingival hypertrophy), to reshape severely damaged gingivae into an easily manageable contour to treat gingival overgrowth, and for crown lengthening prior to restorative procedures. It is **not** suitable for the management of deep 'true' pocketing as excision of the pocket will remove the entire thickness of keratinized gingivae. It is of no value in the Rx of infrabony lesions.

Technique Pockets are delineated by use of pocket marking forceps, e.g. Crane–Kaplan forceps. This marks out a line of incision, which may be either smooth or scalloped, made with the blade angled at 100–110° to the long axis of the tooth. This bevelled incision excises supragingival pockets and allows for gingival recontouring. Once the incision has been made the strip of gingiva remaining is released by an intercrevicular incision. The root surfaces are then curetted and an open area of freshly cut granulation tissue left to heal under a periodontal pack. Prescribe chlorhexidine mouthwash 10 ml bd. The pack is left in place for about 1 week.

Disadvantages Loss of attached gingiva, raw wound, exposed root surface (which ↑ likelihood of sensitivity and caries). Some remodelling of alveolar bone occurs, despite there being no operative interference.

Apically repositioned flap

This procedure is used to expose alveolar bone and includes the option for osseous surgery to correct infrabony defects. It allows excellent access to the root surface for debridement. The principal difference between this procedure and the modified Widman flap is the deliberate exposure of alveolar bone, and the apical repositioning of the flap with post-operative exposure of the root surfaces. This is primarily a buccal procedure, and although it can be performed on lingual pockets, it is obviously impossible on the palate where a conventional or reverse bevel gingivectomy approach has to be used.

Technique A reverse bevel incision is made in the attached gingiva angled to excise the periodontal pocket in a scalloped outline with vertical relieving incisions at either end. A split thickness flap is made down to bone and then converted to full thickness, leaving a residual collar of tissue around the root surfaces. This combination of pocket epithelium and granulation tissue is removed with a curette. If indicated the alveolar crest can be remodelled.

Advantages Include exposure of alveolar bone with controlled bone loss, exposure of furcation area, minimal post-operative pocket depth, ability to reposition the flap, and primary closure of the wound. In addition, keratinized gingiva is preserved.

Disadvantages Exposure of root surface (leading to ↑ susceptibility to caries and sensitivity) and ↑ loss of alveolar bone height, which accompanies full exposure of the bone at operation.

Osseous surgery

Bone recontouring has become less popular as it is always accompanied by some degree of alveolar resorption and ∴ ↓ support for the tooth. **Osteoplasty** is conservative recontouring of the bone margin (i.e. non-supporting bone).

Ostectomy is excision of bone aimed at eliminating infra-alveolar pocketing, but unfortunately it also ↓ alveolar support. The aim of osseous surgery should be to establish a more anatomically correct relationship between bone and tooth while maintaining as much alveolar support as possible.

Other flap procedures

These include simple replaced flaps which give ↑ bony access compared to the modified Widman flap. Also crown-lengthening procedures, which can range from a simple gingivectomy to an apically repositioned flap ± bone removal. In addition, many periodontologists have their own modification of the aforementioned techniques.

Apically repositioned flap
1 Design of flap
  a Reverse bevel incision
  b Relieving incisions
2 Elevating the flap. Tissue enclosing pocketing which is to be discarded is hatched
3 Flap elevated, pockets excised. Osseous surgery can be performed at this stage
4 Flap apically repositioned and sutured in position

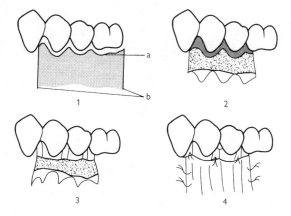

Regenerative techniques

Guided-tissue regeneration

The recognition that epithelium migrated along the root surface before any other cell type, after periodontal surgery, and created the *long junctional epithelium* which prevented new attachment, created the possibility that prevention of migration of epithelium would allow new connective tissue attachment. Guided-tissue regeneration (GTR) is essentially interposing a barrier to epithelial migration prior to completion of surgical or non-surgical therapy. Original barriers were Millipore and PTFE. Goretex membranes in a variety of shapes are now widely used and infrabony and furcation defects can be infilled using a combination of bone/hydroxyapatite/biocoral covered by the membrane. Goretex has to be removed at 4–6 weeks. Biocompatible resorbable materials, such as Vicryl and lyophilized collagen (Resolute) allow a one-operation technique. Tissue growth factor β-2 and bone morphogenetic protein may have a role in stimulating bone and connective tissue deposition. Main disadvantage is cost. Please note that a recent systematic review has also questioned the effectiveness of these techniques.

Endogain is a product containing enamel matrix derivative (EMD) proteins. These substances (e.g. amelogenin) are found in Hertwig's sheath and induce root formation in the developing tooth. Locally applied enamel matrix proteins may help form acellular cementum, the key tissue in the development of a functional periodontium.

Technique Access to the root surface is gained surgically, the cementum is mechanically cleaned, and EMD solution is applied to the root surfaces. The access flaps are then repositioned and sutured.

Outcome Regeneration of cementum, periodontal ligament, and alveolar bone appears to be possible experimentally; long-term clinical outcome awaits prospective RCCTs.

Peri-implantitis

Osseo-integrated implants are now well established (p. 428). Implants which have achieved full osseo-integration may fail by overloading, peri-implantitis (similar to periodontitis), or a combination of both, with failure rates being high in smokers. Implant salvage in the failing stage consists of ↓ overloading and the entire arsenal of periodontal therapies. Local antibiotics and bone-supplemented GTR may be particularly useful.

Tissue transformation using bone morphogenetic protein may also prove useful in the future.

Mucogingival surgery

Mucogingival surgery encompasses those techniques aimed at the correction of local gingival defects. The rationale for this type of surgery has been hotly debated over many years. Initially, it was felt that a margin of attached gingiva of around 3 mm was required to protect the periodontium during mastication and to dissipate the pull to the gingival margin from fraenal attachments. In fact, data from properly conducted experimental work have demonstrated that the width of attached gingiva and the presence or absence of an attached portion are **not** of decisive importance for the maintenance of gingival health.[1] As a result of this, the indications for mucogingival surgery have been rationalized:

1 where change in the morphology of the gingival margin would improve plaque control, e.g. presence of high fraenal attachments or deep areas of recession;

2 areas where recession creates root sensitivity or aesthetic problems;

3 a very thin layer of attached gingiva overlying a tooth which is to be moved orthodontically: the evidence for this is somewhat anecdotal.

Gingival recession

Gingival recession is one of the commonest reasons for carrying out mucogingival surgery. The two commonest causes are plaque-induced gingival inflammation and toothbrush trauma, revealing dehiscences in alveolar bone. ∴, basic periodontal care and correction of faulty toothbrushing technique are the first lines of Rx. While anatomical features may contribute, these and trauma from occlusion, high fraenal attachments, and impingement from restorations, etc., are a secondary consideration.

Mucogingival techniques

These can be divided into two main groups:

Vestibular extension procedures   essentially aim to ↑ the area of attached gingivae and deepen the buccal or labial sulcus. As they are always accompanied by a degree of bone resorption, these methods are not recommended as a therapeutic periodontal technique.

Grafting is subdivided into:

1 *Free grafts*, which are completely removed from their donor area. Free gingival grafts, commonly of palatal mucosa and connective tissue, are taken and grafted to donor sites prepared by incising between attached and alveolar mucosa. While this technique may successfully cover exposed root surfaces of around 2 mm square and will certainly ↑ the width of keratinized gingiva, long-term cross-over studies suggest that in the presence of meticulous OH there is no significant difference between attachment levels in grafted and non-grafted sites with similar degrees of recession.[2]

---

1 J. Wenstrom 1987 *J Clin Periodont* **14** 181.
2 H. S. Dorfmann 1980 *J Clin Periodont* **7** 316.

2 *Pedicle grafts* are not separated from their blood supply. Commonly used pedicle grafts are the laterally repositioned flap, coronally repositioned flap, and the double papilla flap. These techniques may be of some value in very narrow areas of isolated gingival recession. Technically, of course, these are flaps *not* grafts.

Reattachment/New attachment

Definitions[1]

Reattachment is defined as the reunion of connective tissue and root separated by incision or injury. *New attachment* is defined as the reunion of connective tissue with a root surface which has been pathologically exposed (i.e. due to periodontal disease). It is the ideal aim of periodontal therapy.

There are two ways in which new attachment may occur; these can be subdivided anatomically as those occurring within bony pockets and those occurring between the soft tissue of the previously existing periodontal pocket and the root surface. There have been numerous claims and counterclaims as to which of these may occur, following virtually all forms of periodontal intervention. However, there is very little satisfactory evidence to support the contention that new attachment takes place above the level of the alveolar crest. More recently, re-entry procedures in animals have suggested that new attachment formation is inhibited by the apical migration of dento-gingival epithelium forming a long, but apparently quite healthy, *long junctional epithelium*. Some newer procedures now describe methods to inhibit apical migration of dento-gingival junction epithelial cells in an attempt to obtain new attachment. However, animal experiments[2] suggested that granulation tissue originating from bone or gingival connective tissue was unable to establish new connective tissue attachment, even when the intervening dento-gingival epithelium was prevented from migrating into the treated area. In fact, when close apposition of connective tissue to root surface occurred, resorption and ankylosis often resulted, suggesting that the migration of dento-gingival epithelium into the Rx area may be a protective mechanism. Experiments to assess whether this behaviour also applied to the PDL have been carried out.[3] Interestingly, it would appear that PDL cells may develop new attachment if dento-gingival junction epithelial cells are prevented from migrating into the area, without the occurrence of resorption and ankylosis. This has been confirmed in clinical studies, using a variety of materials to form a barrier against ingress of epithelial cells by a process known as GTR (p. 240). This involves placement of a mechanical barrier (Goretex, Vicryl, Resolute) underneath the flap, extending from the outer surface of the alveolar process to the crown of the tooth above the gingival margin. This allows preferential colonization by PDL cells. Resorbable barriers avoid a retrieval operation.

EMD, p. 240.

Bony infill in osseous defects There are a number of studies which suggest that complete regeneration can occur in up to 70% of three-walled infrabony defects. This success rate, however, is not consistent, especially in combined and two-walled defects.

---

1 K. I. Kalkwarf 1974 *Perio Abstracts* 53.
2 S. Nyman 1980 *J Clin Periodont* **7** 394.
3 S. Nyman 1982 *J Clin Periodont* **9** 157.

Occlusion and splinting

All matters relating to occlusion seem to have developed a high degree of mysticism about them in the dental world; this is also true of the relationship between occlusion and periodontal therapy.

It used to be claimed that angular bony defects and ↑ mobility were directly attributable to trauma from the occlusion. This belief is less commonly held nowadays as angular defects can be found around both occlusally traumatized and non-traumatized teeth.[1] It is, however, self-evident that an already periodontally diseased tooth can change its relationship in the arch to become traumatized, or that a tooth which is already in traumatic occlusion can develop periodontal disease, and that the two factors can exacerbate one another.

Tooth mobility ↑ tooth mobility may simply be a result of loss of periodontal attachment and bony support. It may also result purely as a localized effect due to a heavy occlusal loading, causing a widening of the periodontal membrane space, though this is usually iatrogenic in origin. It is now felt that the Δ of occlusal trauma should only be made where progressive *increasing* tooth mobility is observed, but in order to do this it is necessary to have an objective method of measuring tooth mobility. This can be done using a Mobility Index:[2]

Grade 1 = Mobility <1 mm buccolingually
Grade 2 = Mobility 1–2 mm buccolingually
Grade 3 = Mobility of >2 mm buccolingually &/or vertical mobility.

Rx First priority should be to diagnose and treat any existing periodontal disease and correct any pre-existing iatrogenic causes, e.g. poor crowns or bridges, high restorations. If tooth mobility persists as a direct result of diagnosable occlusal trauma, occlusal adjustment is a sensible Rx modality. If the tooth is mobile as a result of lack of alveolar bone support, this is not automatically an indication for splinting (see below).

Splinting Indicated in the following situations:
- Tooth with healthy but ↓ periodontium where mobility is ↑.
- Tooth with ↑ mobility which patient finds uncomfortable during function.

It is very easy to design splints which are impossible for the patients to keep clean as all additions to the natural tooth surface will ↑ plaque retention. A wide range of different techniques and materials have been described, including orthodontic wire fastened to teeth by resin-composite, resin-composite alone, fixed bridges, partial prostheses, acid-etch retained splints, and, more recently, fibre-reinforced resin-composite splinting.

1 J. Waerhaug 1970 *J Periodont* **50** 355.
2 A. Grace 1989 *Periodontal Control: An Effective System for Diagnosis, Selection, Control and Rx Planning in General Practice*, p. 52, Quintessence.

Perio-endo lesions

▶ It is essential to vitality test any heavily restored tooth with periodontal involvement.

Given the relative frequency of both periodontal disease and periapical pathology, it is not surprising that both may occur together, which can result in diagnostic confusion. In fact, there is little evidence to support the popular notion that periodontitis leads to pulp necrosis. However, there is no doubt that pulp pathology can exacerbate periodontal problems.

Pulpal problems

Acute pulpitis, p. 260.

Non-vital pulp (p. 260) may cause asymptomatic periapical lesion or periapical abscess.

Lateral canal &/or non-vital pulp may mimic periodontal abscess, as can a root perforation following endodontic therapy.

Vertical root fracture &/or non-vital pulp can lead to periodontal inflammation and may mimic periodontal abscess.

Horizontal root fracture may mimic periodontal abscess.

Periodontal pathology and its effect on the pulp

Deep pocketing may encroach on lateral canals in the apical ⅓ of the root, but is otherwise unlikely to cause direct pulpal pathology.

Gingival recession is directly associated with hypersensitivity of root dentine.

Root planing and furcation procedures actively involve dentine, and can clearly lead to hypersensitivity and sometimes acute pulpal changes.

Differential △

	Primarily periodontal	*Primarily pulpal*
History	No preceding toothache	Often toothache
Percussion	TTP especially lateral	TTP especially vertical
Probing	Pocketing always	May be no pockets
Probing sinus	May lead to pocket	May lead to apex
Vitality test	Usually +ve	−ve
Radiographs	Vertical bone loss	Apical area

Combined perio-endo lesions

These may be either:

• Coexisting, but separate from each other, in which case standard endodontic and periodontal therapy are used as indicated.
• Interconnected, in which case probing both pocket and sinus will reach the apex. This can be confirmed by taking a periapical film with a GP point inserted into the pocket.

Rx of combined interconnected lesion First, resolve the acute infection and inflammation by drainage (&/or antibiotics), then treat with orthograde RCT (the greater the pulpal component the better the prognosis). The apparent periodontal lesion will often be seen to resolve to a substantial degree over a period of months,∴ the decision to carry out surgery should be deferred. Combined apicectomy and periodontal surgery is quite feasible but carries a poorer long-term prognosis. The worst prognosis applies to those teeth where the periapical/pulpal pathology has been due entirely to apical extension of the periodontal pocket. These are often diagnosed after the fact, when endodontics completely fails to resolve the lesion.

Furcation involvement

The extension of periodontal disease into the bi- or trifurcation of multirooted teeth is known as furcation involvement.

Diagnosis is established by probing into the furcation and by radiographs. The possibility of pulpal pathology is ↑ in teeth with furcation involvement and vitality testing is essential. Radiographs give a guide to the degree of alveolar bone loss both mesially and distally, and in the furcation area.

Classification

1st degree: horizontal loss of support not exceeding 1/3 tooth width. Requires scaling and root planing, possibly with furcation plasty.

2nd degree: horizontal loss of support exceeding 1/3 but not encompassing the total width of the furcation area. May require furcation plasty, &/or tunnel preparation, &/or root resection, &/or extraction.

3rd degree: horizontal through-and-through destruction in the furcation area. May require tunnel preparation, &/or root resection, &/or extraction.

Rx techniques

Scaling and root planing (p. 230) Unless the post-Rx morphology can be kept clean by the patient it will not be successful.

Furcation plasty An open procedure involving a muco-periosteal flap to allow root planing and scaling, followed by the removal of tooth structure in the furcation area to achieve a widened entrance to give access for cleaning. Osseous recontouring may be used if indicated. The flap is repositioned and sutured to ↑ access post-operatively. There is an obvious risk of pulpal damage and post-operative dentine sensitivity.

Tunnel preparation is a similar procedure to furcation plasty using buccal and lingual flaps, the main difference being that the entire furcation area is exposed and the flaps are sutured together intra-radicularly to leave a large exposed furcation. There is a high risk of post-operative caries, dentine sensitivity, and pulpal exposure, making this a method to be used with caution. It is of most value for mandibular molars in patients with optimal OH. In many cases considered for furcation plasty or tunnelling, it may be more sensible to proceed to a more radical approach such as root resection.

Root resection Involves amputation of one (or even two) of the roots of a multirooted tooth, leaving the crown and the root stump. It is important to ensure that the root to be retained can be treated endodontically, is in sound periodontal state with good bony support, is restorable, and will be a viable tooth in the long term. At operation it is wise to raise a flap to enable direct visualization of the root surface. Resection of the root with a high-speed bur is followed by smoothing, recontouring, and restoration of any residual pulp cavity. It is sometimes not possible to proceed with root resection, despite apparently favourable radiographs, especially in maxillary molars, so warn patient pre-operatively.

Hemisection Involves dividing a two-rooted tooth in half to give two smaller units each with a single root. Again, RCT is necessary pre-operatively and restoration of the divided crown is required post-operatively.

Extraction   Ensures removal of periodontal disease but carries its own problems.

Guided tissue regeneration,[1]   p. 240.

Enamel matrix derivatives EMD,   p. 240.

It is important to note that the techniques described above are of less significance to long-term outcome than the degree of plaque control that can be achieved and maintained by the patient. Mini interproximal brushes are a valuable aid in cleaning furcation defects and are available in a variety of sizes and shapes.

1 R. Ponteriero 1989 *J Clin Periodont* **16** 170.

Restorative dentistry

Relevant pages in other chapters 　Caries diagnosis, p. 30; amalgam, p. 664; resin composite, p. 666; the acid-etch technique, p. 670; dentine adhesive systems, p. 672; glass ionomers, p. 674; cermets, p. 678; cements, p. 682; impression materials, p. 686; casting alloys, p. 688; acid-etch tip, p. 110.

Principal sources and further reading 　Operative Dentistry. Dental Update. The British Dental Journal. B. G. N. Smith 1997 *Planning and Making Crowns and Bridges*, Dunitz. P. A. Brunton 2002

Decision Making in Operative Dentistry, Quintessence. J. L. Gutmann *et al.* 1997 *Problem Solving in Endodontics*, 3rd edn, Mosby. E. A. M. Kidd *et al.* 2003 Pickard's *Manual of Operative Dentistry*, 8th edn, OUP. S. J. Davies and R. J. Gray 2002 *A Clinical Guide to Occlusion*, British Dental Association. J. M. Whitworth 2002 *Rational Root Canal Treatment in Practice*, Quintessence.

To attempt to resolve the problem of caries by preparing and restoring teeth is comparable to trying to resolve the problem of poliomyelitis by manufacturing more attractive and better quality crutches, more quickly and more cheaply.

Treatment planning

A proper treatment plan can only result from a thorough patient assessment, which must include a history, an examination, relevant special tests, and ultimately, a diagnosis.

Under ideal circumstances an integrated treatment plan is formulated for each patient at the start of every course of treatment. Very often, however, the treatment plan will need to be revised in the light of clinical findings as the treatment progresses, e.g. patient cooperation, response to periodontal therapy, investigation of teeth of doubtful prognosis, etc. When dealing with patients with a range of problems it is therefore wise to formulate a treatment plan which has a number of achievable goals, and then on completion of this to reassess the patient to decide on what further treatment is necessary.

Sequence of treatment

This list is obviously an oversimplification but should serve as a general guide to the order in which treatment should be carried out.

1 Relief of pain.
2 Control of active disease and achievement of stability:
   – OHI, dietary advice, topical fluoride, and initial periodontal therapy;
   – extraction of unsaveable teeth;
   – treatment of large and active carious lesions;
   – consideration of definitive denture design;
   – remaining simple restorations;
   – RCT.
3 Reassessment of success of initial treatment, OH, periodontal condition, and prognosis of teeth.
4 Definitive treatment: crowns, bridgework, and dentures.
5 Maintenance and review.

Practical points

- The priority of items of treatment must be taken into account when formulating a treatment plan, which may lead to deviations from the scheme described above. For example, in an apprehensive patient it would be more appropriate to complete small restorations before dealing with the large ones.
- Explain what the treatment plan involves to the patient and the role they will have to play in controlling their dental disease. Success is dependent upon patient compliance, ∴ time spent discussing their expectations, treatment options, time involved, cost implications present and future, and their role in maintenance is never wasted. Equally without such a discussion consent is not by definition informed
- If need to check a medical history with patient's GMP or refer patient to a specialist, allow sufficient time to elapse before arranging to carry out any treatment that is dependent upon the outcome.
- It is important to bear in mind subsequent items on a treatment plan, e.g. the design of a P/- may influence the choice of material and contour of restorations.
- For complex cases, several short treatment plans, each ending with a reassessment, are more logical and efficient than one long one that keeps changing.

- When formulating a treatment plan group items together into appointments to form a visit plan. Decide how long you will need for each visit.
- Although it is usually advantageous to complete as much work as possible at each visit, in a proportion of patients (or if carried to an extreme, in any patient) this can be counter-productive. If in doubt about how much treatment to do at a visit, discuss this with the patient.
- Regularly reinforce the OH throughout the treatment (e.g. whilst waiting for LA to take).
- Record-keeping is very important. At the end of each visit carefully note what has been done and the materials used (including sizes and shades). Cross that item off the treatment plan and adjust the patient's chart. Note what is to be done next visit: this will save time.
- It is important to recognize your own limitations, and where appropriate refer a patient for advice or treatment.

Stabilization or caries control In patients with multiple carious lesions it may take several weeks/months to complete the permanent restorations necessary to secure OH. In these cases it may be advisable to prevent any symptomless large lesions increasing in size by placing temporary dressings. The cavities should be rendered caries-free at the margins, and temporarily restored with a strong cement, e.g. traditional or resin-modified GI cement.

Dental pain

When a patient attends the surgery and complains of toothache, pain may be arising from a variety of different structures and may be classified as follows:

- Pulpal pain
- Periapical/periradicular pain.
- Non-dental pain.

Dental pain can be very difficult to diagnose, and the clinician must first gather as much information as possible from the history, clinical and radiographic examinations, and other special tests (see Chapter 1).

Pulpal pain

The pulp may be subject to a wide variety of insults, e.g. bacterial, thermal, chemical, traumatic, the effects of which are cumulative and can ultimately lead to inflammation in the pulp (pulpitis) and pain. The dental pulp does not contain any proprioceptive nerve endings, ∴ a characteristic of pulpal pain is that the patient is unable to localize the affected tooth. The ability of the pulp to recover from injury depends upon its blood supply, not the nerve supply, which must be borne in mind when vitality (sensibility) testing is carried out (p. 18).[1] It is impossible to reliably achieve an accurate Δ of the state of the pulp on clinical grounds alone; the only 100% accurate method is histological section.

Although numerous classifications of pulpal disease exist, only a limited number of clinical diagnostic situations require identification before effective treatment can be given.

Reversible pulpitis

Symptoms Fleeting sensitivity/pain to hot, cold or sweet with immediate onset. Pain is usually sharp and may be difficult to locate. Quickly subsides after removal of the stimulus.

Signs Exaggerated response to pulp testing. Carious cavity/leaking restoration.

Rx Remove any caries present and place a sedative dressing (e.g. ZOE) or permanent restoration with suitable pulp protection.

Irreversible pulpitis

Symptoms Spontaneous pain which may last several hours, be worse at night, and is often pulsatile in nature. Pain is elicited by hot and cold at first, but in later stages heat is more significant and cold may actually ease symptoms. A characteristic feature is that the pain remains after the removal of the stimulus. Localization of pain may be difficult initially, but as the inflammation spreads to the periapical tissues the tooth will become more sensitive to pressure.

Signs Application of heat (e.g. warm GP) elicits pain. Affected tooth may give no or a reduced response to electric pulp tester. In later stages may become TTP.

1 A. H. R. Rowe 1990 *Int Endo J* **23** 77.

Rx Extirpation of the pulp and RCT is the treatment of choice (assuming the tooth is to be saved). If time is short or if anaesthesia proves elusive then removal of the coronal pulp and a Ledermix dressing can often control the symptoms until the remaining pulp can be extirpated under LA at the next appointment.

Dentine hypersensitivity

This is pain arising from exposed dentine in response to a thermal, tactile, or osmotic stimulus (but not all exposed dentine gives rise to symptoms). It is thought to be due to dentinal fluid movement stimulating pulpal pain receptors. Prevalence is ~ 1:7 adults with a peak in young adults, then ↓ with age.[1] Δ is by elimination of other possible causes and by evoking symptoms.

Rx Involves ↓ aetiological factors (i.e. OHI, possibly including tooth-brushing technique and intrinsic and extrinsic dental erosion) and by ↓ permeability of dentinal tubules (e.g. by toothpaste containing strontium, formalin, &/or fluoride; placement of varnishes, dentine desensitizers, dentine adhesive systems, or, if indicated, a restoration).

Cracked tooth syndrome

Symptoms　Sharp pain on biting—short duration.

Signs　Often relatively few, ∴ Δ difficult. Tooth often has a large restoration. Crack may not be apparent at first but transillumination and possibly removal of the restoration may aid visualization. Positive response to vitality (sensibility) testing and pain can normally be elicited by getting the patient to bite with the affected tooth on a cotton-wool roll or a tooth sleuth. May be associated with bruxing habit.

Rx　An adhesive resin composite restoration may be appropriate in teeth which are minimally restored, but some cases a cast restoration with full occlusal coverage will be needed. Occasionally RCT may be required.

Periapical/periradicular pain

Progression of irreversible pulpitis ultimately leads to death of the pulp (pulpal necrosis). At this stage the patient may experience relief from pain and thus may not seek attention. If neglected, however, the bacteria and pulpal breakdown products leave the root canal system via the apical foramen or lateral canals and lead to inflammatory changes and possibly pain. Characteristically the patient can precisely identify the affected tooth, as the periodontal ligament, which is well supplied with proprioceptive nerve endings, is inflamed.

Pulpal necrosis with periapical periodontitis

Symptoms　Variable, but patients generally describe a dull ache exacerbated by biting on the tooth.

Signs　Usually no response to vitality testing, unless one canal of a multi-rooted tooth is still vital. The tooth will be TTP. Radiographically the apical PDL may be widened or there may be a periapical radiolucency (granuloma or cyst).

1 P. Dowell 1985 *BDJ* **158** 92.

Rx RCT or extraction.

Acute periapical abscess

Symptoms Severe pain which will disturb sleep. Tooth is exquisitely tender to touch.

Signs Affected tooth is usually extruded, mobile, and TTP. May be associated with a localized or diffuse swelling. Vitality (sensibility) testing may be misleading as pus may conduct stimulus to apical tissues. Radiographic changes can range from a widening of the apical PDL space to an obvious radiolucency. It is important to differentiate this condition from a periodontal abscess.

Rx Drain pus and relieve occlusion, if indicated. Drainage of pus can often be achieved by entering the pulp chamber with a high-speed diamond bur. The tooth should be steadied with a finger to prevent excessive vibration. After drainage has been achieved it is preferable to prepare the canal and place a temporary dressing. Leaving the tooth on 'open drainage' should be avoided if possible, but if absolutely necessary for <24 h, as after this time further contamination of the root canal by anaerobic bacteria makes subsequent RCT very difficult. If a fluctuant swelling is present in the soft tissues, this should be incised to achieve drainage. Antibiotics should be prescribed if there is systemic involvement (pyrexia, lymphadenopathy) or if the infection is spreading significantly along tissue planes. When the acute symptoms have subsided, RCT must be performed or the tooth extracted.

Chronic periapical abscess

Often symptomless. Possibly associated with persistent sinus. Presentation may be: coincidental or acute exacerbation.

Lateral periodontal abscess

Symptoms Similar to periapical abscess with acute pain and tenderness, and often an associated bad taste.

Signs Tooth is usually mobile and TTP, with associated localized or diffuse swelling of the adjacent periodontium. A deep periodontal pocket is usually associated, which will exude pus on probing. Radiographs normally show vertical or horizontal bone loss, and vitality (sensibility) testing is usually positive, unless there is an associated endodontic problem (perio-endo lesion).

Rx Debride the pocket and achieve drainage of pus. Irrigate with a chlorhexidine solution. If there is systemic involvement or it is a recurrent problem, prescribe antibiotics (metronidazole or amoxicillin).

Non-dental pain

When no signs of dental or periradicular pathology can be detected then non-dental causes must be considered. Other causes of pain that can present as toothache include:

- TMPDS (p. 482);
- sinusitis (p. 422);
- psychological disorders (atypical odontalgia) (p. 462);
- tumours (pp. 420 and 452).

Isolation and moisture control

Isolation is required to aid visibility, prevent contamination during moisture-sensitive techniques, maintain a relatively aseptic environment, and protect the patient from caustic materials or aspiration of foreign material.

High-volume suction, e.g. an aspirator.

Low-volume suction, e.g. a saliva ejector. Many designs available—most useful are (a) fianged metal type to keep tongue at bay when working in the lower arch, and (b) disposable plastic type for working on upper teeth.

Compressed air This tends to redistribute the moisture to somewhere else (e.g. your eye) rather than remove it. Should be used with care in deep preparations as prolonged use can cause pulpal damage, let alone displace adhesive materials when the solvent is being evaporated prior to curing.

Absorbents
- Cotton-wool rolls. Insert with a rolling action away from the alveolus. Moisten before removal to prevent tearing mucosa.
- Paper pads.
- Carboxymethylcellulose pads (Dry Tips). Very effective if inserted the correct way round with the impermeable plastic against the tooth.

Rubber dam This provides effective isolation and also improves access to operating site. It is indicated where moisture control and airway protection are essential, e.g. RCT (RCT without rubber dam is considered negligent), acid-etch technique. With practice, rubber dam can be applied quickly and often saves time in the long run. The dam must be secured to the teeth; several methods are available:
- Rubber dam clamps. These consist of two metal jaws linked by one or more bows. Commonly used for posterior teeth.
- Floss ligatures.
- Wedges.
- Proprietary rubber bands (Wedjets) or pieces of dam, worked through contact points.
- By pinching dam between a tight contact point.

Types of dam **1** Sheet grade, 6-inch square (15 cm), which is supported with a frame. Moderate to thicker gauges are preferable. **2** Mask type, which is supported by a paper margin and looped over ears with elastic. Increasingly, latex-free rubber dam is available and arguably should be used routinely.

Placement Several regimens have been described; the following is popular:
- Place cotton-wool roll in sulcus beside tooth for treatment.
- Mark position of centre of each tooth to be included with a ball pen while dam held stretched. Or preferably, use an ink stamp to indicate tooth position.
- Punch holes cleanly in the rubber dam, which correspond to tooth size.
- Try-in clamp (with floss tied to it).
- Fit clamp into appropriate hole, with bridge distally, and using forceps place clamp and dam on to tooth.
- Position dam on other teeth, using fioss to ease through contact points.

- Secure dam anteriorly using one of the methods above.
- If frame required, position.
- Put napkin on patient's chin under dam. A saliva ejector will add to the patient's comfort.

If using caustic materials, a rubber dam sealer (e.g. Oraseal) should be used.

Removal

- Take away clamps/ligatures, etc.
- Stretch dam, carefully cut interdental septa with scissors, and remove.

Protection of the airway Mandatory when fitting crowns, bridges, inlays, and carrying out RCT. Best provided by rubber dam, but if this is not possible a butterfly sponge or gauze can be used.

Gingival retraction ↓ gingival exudate and exposes subgingival preparations prior to impression-taking. Some retraction cords are impregnated with substances such as adrenalin to ↓ bleeding. The cord should be gently placed into the gingival crevice with a flat plastic instrument (leaving no tag hanging out) prior to impression-taking and temporization. Braided cords are better than twisted. Bleeding from the gingival margin can be ↓ by applying an astringent. A new paste (Expasyl) which contains aluminium chloride provides for retraction and haemorrhage control. Expasyl is useful for preparations finished within or just below the level of the gingival crevice, otherwise retraction cord is more appropriate.

Electrosurgery May be indicated where a margin extends subgingivally and gingival overgrowth is hampering restoration placement or impression-taking. Also for crown-lengthening procedures, although bone removal is required too.

Principles of tooth preparation

Why restore?
- To restore function.
- To prevent further spread of an active lesion which is not amenable to preventive measures.
- To preserve pulp vitality.
- To restore aesthetics.

However, these reasons need to be evaluated with regard to the patient and the rest of the dentition. For example, there is little point in attempting restoration of a non-functional 8.

Preparation design With caries prevalence declining, emphasis has changed from extension for prevention, to minimizing removal of tooth tissue. Tooth preparation should be based on the morphology of the carious lesion and the requirements of the restorative material being used.

General principles of tooth preparation
- Gain access to caries.
- Remove all caries at ADJ (to prevent spread laterally).
- Cut away all significantly unsupported enamel.
- Extend margins so that they are accessible for instrumentation and cleaning.
- Shape preparation so that remaining tooth tissue and restorative material will be able to withstand functional forces.
- Shape preparation so that restoration will be retained, i.e. undercut for amalgam, none required for resin composite or bonded amalgams.
- Check preparation margins are appropriate for the restorative material. Small areas of unsupported enamel may be left if a resin composite restoration is being placed
- Remove remaining caries unless indirect pulp cap to be carried out.
- Wash and dry preparation.

Helpful hints
- While care must be exercised not to overcut a preparation, do not skimp on access so that caries removal is compromised by poor visibility.
- Mark centric stops with articulating paper prior to tooth preparation and try to preserve if possible, or place the preparation margins past the occlusal contact areas.
- Avoid crossing marginal ridges.
- In removing caries a tactile appreciation of the hardness of dentine is important, ∴ use slow-speed instruments or excavators.
- The base of the preparation should not be flattened as this runs the risk of pulp exposure.
- Unless caries dictates, margins should be supragingival.
- All internal line angles should be rounded to ↓ internal stresses. Removing caries with a large diameter round bur automatically produces the desired shape.
- In a proximal box, the margin should extend below the contact point because this is where the caries is!

Amalgam[1] (see also p. 664)

- Amalgam is brittle, ∴ an amalgam cavo-surface margin of at least 70°, preferably 90°, is required to prevent ditching. Also avoid leaving amalgam overlying cavity margins and overcarving.
- Accepted minimal dimensions for amalgam are 2 mm occlusally and 1 mm elsewhere.
- In deep preparations, sealers &/or liners are required to seal the dentine and prevent ingress of bacteria.

Resin composite, p. 666

Glass ionomer, p. 674

- Wear precludes their use in load-bearing situations except for 1° teeth, management of root caries, temporary restorations, and the atraumatic restorative technique.

Gold

- Relies on minimally divergent walls and cement lute for retention.
- A preparation margin of >135° is advisable to give good marginal fit to restoration and to allow burnishing.

It would be foolish to think that experience in tooth preparation can be adequately assimilated from the written text. The purpose of the following pages is to give the reader some practical tips on how to do the procedures considered, as well as to describe recent innovations and techniques.

Nomenclature

Black's classification of cavities is now not widely used. It has been replaced by the following:

Occlusal (Class I)	Cavity in pits and fissures
Proximal (Class II or III)	Cavity in proximal surface(s) of any tooth
Incisal (Class IV)	Proximal in an anterior tooth, but including incisal edge
Cervical (Class V)	Cavity in cervical third of buccal or lingual surface of any tooth.

1 P. B. Robinson 1985 *Dental Update* **12** 357.

Occlusal (Class I)

Amalgam

Amalgam is still the most widely used material for occlusal cavities, probably because it is more forgiving of technique than some of the newer materials. It is now widely accepted, however, that resin composite placed in conjunction with minimal preparation techniques has a role in initial lesion management. If enamel margins are cut to an angle of 90° (or, if cusps steeply inclined, >70°) the resultant preparation will be adequately retentive.

Lining Recently, emphasis has changed, with linings being used to seal the underlying dentine for moderate to deep cavities. Light-cured GIs (e.g. Vitrebond) are now recommended. A preparation sealer (Gluma Densensitizer) can be used in minimal preparations.

Resin composite

The controversy surrounding posterior resin composites is dealt with on pp. 270 and 668. A technique which has gained more widespread acceptance is:

Preventive resin restoration Introduced by Simonsen (then by others as the minimal resin composite restoration!). Preparation is limited to caries removal and the resultant preparation restored using fissure sealant alone if small, or resin composite followed by sealant if larger. Alternatively, GI can be used instead of resin composite. The rationale of this approach is that adjacent fissures are sealed for prevention. It is particularly useful for investigating any suspect areas of a fissure, a technique that is often referred to as an enamel biopsy (obviously coined by an academic). This involves exploring the area with a small bur, and if no caries is found further preparation can be aborted and sealant placed. If carious, a PRR can be carried out. It is often possible to complete preparation of a PRR without LA; however, if the cavity appears larger than originally thought, LA can then be given. If the preparation extends significantly into load-bearing areas, conventional tooth preparation should be carried out and the tooth restored with resin composite.

Technique **for medium-sized cavities**
- Assess whether LA required. If not, ask patient to signal if tooth becomes sensitive.
- Isolate tooth (preferably with rubber dam).
- Gain access to caries with a small bur at high speed.
- Use a small round bur run at slow speed to remove caries. Only remove as much enamel as required for access.
- Etch preparation margins and occlusal surface. Wash and dry.
- Apply a dentine adhesive system.
- Restore preparation with resin composite placed and cured in increments, but don't overfill.
- Paint sealant over whole of occlusal surface and cure.
- Check occlusion.

Where possible a related sealant and resin composite should be used to ensure a good bond.

Hints for resin composite restorations

- Use etchant gel in a syringe to aid placement. Many newer adhesive systems do not have a separate etch stage, however, and rely on the use of acidic primers often used in conjunction with bonding resins or as a separate stage.
- Additions are generally easy as new resin composite will bond to old.
- Avoid eugenol-containing cements with resin composite restorations.
- Resin composite must be cured incrementally, with increments being no deeper than 2 mm.

Proximal (Class II)

▶ Avoid the creation of an overhang at the cervical margin and ensure a good contact point with adjacent tooth with a well-contoured matrix band and wedges.

Amalgam   In practice, preparation size is determined by the size of the carious lesion and extension beyond this should be minimal. Proximal preparations comprise an approximal box with vertical grooves. The preparation should only extend occlusally if there is evidence of caries in the occlusal fissures. Retention from occlusal forces is derived from a 2–5° divergence of the walls towards the floor in both parts of the preparation. The margins of the box should extend just outwith the contact area unless caries dictates a wider position. Amalgam restorations are prone to # at the isthmus in restorations extended occlusally, ∴ sufficient depth must be provided in this area. The width of the isthmus should not be overcut (ideally 1/4 to 1/5 intercusp width). If the cusps are extensively undermined or missing they should be replaced with a bonded restoration (p. 314). A chisel can be used to plane away unsupported enamel from the margins of the completed preparation to produce a 90° butt joint. In molar teeth with mesial and distal caries it is preferable to try and cut two separate cavities, but often a confluent MOD preparation is unavoidable. Increasingly the use of resin composite placed in conjunction with a dentine adhesive system is advocated for the restoration of small to moderate proximal preparations in premolar and molar teeth.

Tunnel preparations   A 'tunnel' approach to interproximal caries has been described.[1] Access to the caries is made through either the occlusal or buccal surfaces, leaving the marginal ridge intact. This approach is only suitable for small lesions, as when preparation is completed at least 2 mm of marginal ridge must remain. The access cavity may need to be widened buccolingually to complete caries removal. Carisolv may have a place here to ensure complete caries removal. A piece of mylar strip wedged into place will act as a matrix. A RMGIC is used to fill the bulk of the preparation and the occlusal access cavity restored with a posterior resin composite. In view of the difficulty of accurately removing all the caries, let alone the incidence of marginal fracture, this technique is rarely used.

Resin composite   Posterior resin composites should be used predominately to restore posterior teeth, but the technique is more demanding, taking ~50% longer. In addition, it is difficult to establish adequate contact points and occlusal stops. Polymerization shrinkage can cause cuspal flexure, post-operative pain, and marginal gaps. Posterior resin composites are best avoided in the following situations:
- Cusp replacements.
- Poor moisture control.
- Restorations with deep gingival extensions, although a bonded base approach can be adopted.
- Bruxism or heavy occlusion.

1 J. W. McLean 1988 *BDJ* **164** 293.

If a resin composite is to be used then a hybrid material with >75% filler is advisable. Pre-wedging one but not both proximal contacts aids creation of a contact point. Resin composite should be placed, and cured, incrementally. If possible, centric stops should be preserved on sound tooth tissue or the restorative material, but never on the marginal interface of the restoration.[1]

1 R. W. Bryant 1992 *Aust Dent J* **37** 81.

Proximal (Class II)—resin composite and inlays

Resin composite and porcelain inlays   These inlay techniques appear to overcome some of the problems associated with direct resin composite restorations. When used in conjunction with an acid-etch technique existing tooth tissue can be reinforced. Curing resin composite outside the mouth with the addition of heat (110° for 5 mins) or pressure overcomes polymerization shrinkage and possibly ↑ strength. As the inlays are bonded to the tooth with an adhesive, parallel walls are less important, but undercuts must be removed or blocked out with an RMGI cement. In general porcelain inlays offer improved aesthetics, surface finish, and bond in comparison to resin composite inlays; however, placement and adjustment can be more difficult.

Technique: preparation
- The preparation should have slightly divergent walls, rounded line angles, and a slight bevel of the enamel margins, but not occlusally. For onlays, a minimum 1.5 mm reduction of cusps is necessary.
- Block out any undercuts with RMGIC.
- Take an impression of the preparation and opposing arch, and if necessary make an inter-occlusal record.
- Choose shade.
- Make and place temporary with a proprietary resin-based temporary material (e.g. Fermit).

Technique: cementation
- Place rubber dam.
- Remove temporary and clean tooth.
- Try-in inlay, and carefully check marginal fit and adjust as necessary. Do not adjust the occlusion at this stage.
- Polish any adjusted areas.
- Remove inlay and clean with alcohol. For porcelain only, place layer of silane coupling agent on fitting surface.
- Etch enamel and dentine (total etch concept). Wash and remove excess moisture, but do not dry.
- Place dentine-adhesive system to moist surface.
- Apply dual-cure resin composite luting cement to prep and inlay and carefully seat.
- Cure for 10 sec and then remove any excess resin composite.
- Complete light-curing (dual-cure resin composite will finish setting chemically under inlay in ~6 mins).
- Trim any excess cement and polish.
- Check occlusion and adjust.

Proximal (Class III), incisal (Class IV), cervical (Class V), and root surface caries

Anterior proximal

Resin composite is the most widely used material for anterior proximal restorations.

Access should be gained from either the buccal or lingual aspect, depending on the position of the lesion. As resin composite is adhesive the preparation is just extended sufficiently to remove all peripheral caries. Some unsupported enamel can be retained labially, but the margins should be planed with chisels to remove any grossly weakened tooth structure. Tooth preparation can be almost entirely completed with slow-speed burs and hand instruments. Ideally the margins are bevelled. A slight excess of material should be moulded into the preparation with a mylar strip, wedged cervically. Once the material is set, the excess can be removed. After checking the occlusion the restoration can be polished using one of the proprietary products (e.g. Soflex discs, Enhance).

Incisal

The restoration of choice is resin composite, the so-called 'acid-etch tip' (p. 110); however, for large incisal cavities in the adult patient, a dentine-bonded crown or porcelain veneer may give better retention and aesthetics.

Cervical

Although cervical cavities are seen less frequently in younger patients, they are an ↑ problem in older age-groups with gingival recession. Resin composite, compomer, or RMGIC are the preferred materials in this situation. Amalgam should be avoided in this situation due to the possibility of a lichenoid reaction.

Once caries has been removed the occlusal margin should be bevelled. The cervical margin should not be bevelled as it has been shown to ↑ microleakage. The materials are ideally placed incrementally under rubber dam isolation.

Root surface caries

As gingival recession is a prerequisite to root caries, it occurs predominantly in the >40 age group. Dentine, which has a critical pH below that of enamel, is thus directly exposed to carious attack. It is sometimes seen secondary to ↓ saliva flow (which reduces buffering capacity and may alter dietary habits) caused by salivary gland disease, drugs, or radiation. Long-term sugar-based medication may also be a factor. Rx requires, first, control of the aetiological factor, and for most patients this involves dietary advice and OHI. Topical fluoride varnishes and mouthrinses may aid remineralization and prevent new lesions developing. However, active lesions require restoration, typically with a traditional or resin-modified GI cement. See also rampant caries (severe early childhood caries), p. 94.

Management of the deep carious lesion

Assessment
- Is the tooth restorable and is restoration preferable to extraction?
- Is the tooth symptomless? If not what is the character and duration of the pain?
- Test vitality and percuss the tooth (before LA!).
- Take radiographs to check extent of lesion and if apical pathology.

Management depends upon a guesstimate of pulpal condition (p. 260). Irreversible pulpitis/necrotic pulp—Rx: RCT (p. 318) or extraction. Reversible pulpitis/healthy pulp—aim to maintain pulp vitality by selective removal of carious dentine without pulp exposure. If in doubt Rx as reversible pulpitis. Can always institute RCT later.

Indirect pulp cap   Ideally, tooth preparation should involve the elimination of all caries, but where this would risk pulp exposure and the tooth is vital it may be more prudent to carry out an indirect pulp cap. This involves leaving a small amount of softened (affected but uninfected) dentine at the base of a deep cavity with the aim of arresting further bacterial spread and maintaining pulpal health.

Rationale
- Softening of dentine precedes bacterial invasion.
- Pulpitis does not occur until bacteria are within 0.5–1 mm of the pulp, ∴ if a vital tooth is asymptomatic the softened dentine closest to the pulp is unlikely to contain bacteria.
- Prognosis for continuing vitality of healthy pulp is better if exposure avoided.
- Materials with antibacterial properties help ↓ bacterial activity.
- Bacteria sealed under a restoration are denied substrate, ∴ lesion arrests.

Sequence of treatment for vital pulp
1 LA.
2 Apply rubber dam to ↓ risk of further bacterial contamination.
3 Prepare the tooth, removing caries from ADJ and cut back unsupported enamel.
4 Cautiously remove softened dentine from floor. If possible complete removal, but if likely to result in exposure and dentine only slightly softened, stop.
5 Apply hard-setting calcium hydroxide to floor.
6 Cover with traditional or resin-modified GI cement (Vitrebond).
7 Adjust margins and restore.
8 Warn patient that some sensitivity should be expected initially, but to return if symptoms occur after that.
9 Follow-up for at least 1 yr.

If it is necessary to leave dentine that is probably infected, place hard-setting calcium hydroxide and a traditional GI cement dressing. Leave tooth for 3 months before re-entering to complete caries removal. If the tooth is asymptomatic it would be prudent to cut back the GI cement dressing and place a resin composite restoration as it is likely that the caries has burnt out.

Exposure

- If traumatic, small, and uncontaminated, perform direct pulp cap with hard-setting calcium hydroxide and restore.
- If carious exposure, and continued pulp vitality is doubtful, RCT will be required. If time short, can dress tooth with Ledermix and a traditional GI cement, and extirpate pulp at next visit.

Pulpotomy is removal of coronal part of pulp in order to eliminate damaged or contaminated tissue. It is indicated for teeth with immature apices, as continued vitality of apical pulp will allow root formation to proceed. Once the apex has closed, conventional RCT can be carried out. The pulp is amputated to the cervical constriction, dressed with non-setting or hard-setting calcium hydroxide or MTA (mineral trioxide aggregate) and the tooth temporarily restored.

Materials used in the management of pulp vitality

Calcium hydroxide has a pH of 11, which makes it bacteriostatic and promotes the formation of a calcific barrier. When calcium hydroxide comes into contact with the pulp a zone of pulpal necrosis is formed. This is subsequently mineralized with calcium ions from the pulp. It is the material of choice for direct pulp caps, particularly the hard-setting type.

Ledermix is a mixture of triamcinolone acetonide (a steroid) and demethylchlortetracycline in a water-soluble base. It has anti-inflammatory and bacteriostatic properties, but also suppresses pulpal defences, ∴ resulting in the rapid spread of any bacteria not affected by the antibiotic it contains. It is a useful compromise for the management of irreversibly inflamed pulps where anaesthesia may be a problem, or when pulp extirpation has to be delayed.

Survival and failure of restorations

Survival of restorations

The results of Elderton's study into the durability of routine restorations placed in the General Dental Services in Scotland provided both a shock and a stimulus to the profession, as he found that 50% lasted for less than 5 yrs.[1] This led to debate over both clinical technique and the profession's readiness to replace restorations. It has been reported that 60% of practitioners' time is spent replacing restorations. It is also interesting to note that those patients who change dentists frequently are more at risk of replacement restorations than those who are loyal to the same GDP.[2] In order to ↑ longevity we need to consider the reasons for the failure of restorations and Δ of secondary caries.

Reasons for failure of restorations

- Incorrect Δ and treatment planning; e.g. pulpal pathology; caries of another surface; extraction of tooth for another reason.
- Poor understanding of the occlusion.
- Incorrect preparation; e.g. caries left at ADJ; incorrect margin preparation; inadequate retention; preparation too shallow; weakened tooth tissue left unprotected.
- Incorrect choice of restorative material; e.g. inadequate strength or resistance to wear for situation.
- Incorrect manipulation of material, e.g. inadequate moisture control; over- or under-contouring.

Before replacing a failed restoration it is important to identify the cause of failure and decide whether this can be dealt with by replacement or repair. When making this decision bear in mind that cavity size is ↑ on average by 0.6 mm each time a restoration is removed.[3]

Secondary caries

Unfortunately, placement of a restoration does not confer caries immunity upon a tooth. When caries occurs adjacent to a restoration it is called secondary or recurrent caries. More correctly it is defined as a new lesion which just happens to be adjacent to an existing restoration, and it should be managed in its own right. While secondary caries is an accepted phenomenon, we as a profession have perhaps been a little too ready in the past to diagnose and treat it. Ditched amalgam margins are not a reason for replacement per se, and active intervention is only required if caries can definitely be demonstrated as active. Secondary caries is difficult to diagnose, but careful observation (clinically and radiographically) rather than intervention, is now advocated. Intervention is only indicated when the lesion is in dentine, and there is evidence of progression &/or cavitation is present.

To prevent secondary caries it is important not only to educate the patient to reduce their caries rate, but also to examine our restorative technique, to ensure good long term-restorations.

1 R. J. Elderton 1983 *BDJ* **155** 91.
2 J. A. Davies 1984 *BDJ* **157** 322.
3 R. J. Elderton 1979 *Proc Br Paedodont Soc* **9** 25.

Occlusion—1

In a book of this size it is (thankfully) not possible to consider all aspects of occlusion; therefore we will try to concentrate on the practical aspects and leave the more esoteric considerations to other texts. We also suggest that significant occlusal adjustment is rarely indicated and should only be attempted by a specialist.

Definitions

Ideal occlusion   Anatomically perfect occlusion—rare.

Functional occlusion   An occlusion that is free of interferences to smooth gliding movements of the mandible, with absence of pathology.

Balanced occlusion   Balancing contacts in all excursions of the mandible to provide ∴ ↑ stability of F/F dentures; not applicable to natural dentition (except rarely in full-mouth reconstruction).

Group function   Multiple tooth contacts on working side during lateral excursions, but no contact on non-working side.

Canine-guided occlusion   During lateral excursions there is disclusion of all the teeth on the working side except for the canine, and no contacts on non-working side.

Hinge axis   The axis of rotation of the condyles during the first few millimetres of mandibular opening.

Terminal hinge axis   The axis or rotation of the mandible when the condyles are in their most superior position in the glenoid fossa.

Retruded arc of closure   The arc of closure of the mandible with the condyles rotating about the terminal hinge axis.

Intercuspal position (ICP) or centric occlusion   Position of maximum interdigitation.

Retruded contact position (RCP) or centric relation   Position of the mandible where initial tooth contact occurs on the retruded arc of closure. Occurs when condyles are fully seated in the glenoid fossa. In ~20% of patients RCP and ICP are coincident; the remainder have forward slide from RCP to ICP.

Rest position   The habitual postural position of the mandible when the patient is relaxed with the condyles in a neutral position.

Freeway space   The difference between the rest and intercuspal positions.

Centric stops   The points on the occlusal surface which meet with the opposing tooth in ICP. Normally the cusp tips, marginal ridges and central fossae.

Supporting or functional cusps   The cusps that occlude with the centric stops on the opposing tooth. Usually palatal on upper and buccal on lower.

Non-supporting cusps   The cusps that do not occlude with the opposing teeth. Usually buccal on upper and lingual on lower.

Deflective contacts   Deflect mandible from natural path of closure.

Interferences Contacts that hinder smooth excursive movements of mandible.

Occlusal vertical dimension (OVD) Relationship between maxilla and mandible in ICP, i.e. face height.

Do occlusal factors play a role in TMJ dysfunction?

TMPDS is recognized as being of multifactorial aetiology (p. 482). The evidence would suggest that occlusal interferences usually cause either subclinical or no dysfunction because they lie within the adaptive capacity of the patient's neuromusculature. However, this may be lowered by stress and emotional problems so that in susceptible patients occlusal interferences can result in muscle hyperactivity at certain times. It is important ∴ to ensure that iatrogenic interferences are not introduced during restorative procedures.

Occlusion—2

Occlusal examination

Prior to carrying out restorative treatment the dentist should examine the patient's occlusion. Occlusal contacts can be identified with a 10 μm metal foil (Shimstock) and marked using thin articulating paper (20 μm). Important features to look for are:

- Number and distribution of occluding teeth.
- Over-eruption, tilting, rotation, etc.
- Presence or absence of centric stops.
- The RCP and any slide between RCP and ICP.
- Anterior guidance—look for disclusion of posterior teeth on protrusion.
- Lateral excursions—?group function, ?canine guidance—check for non-working interferences.
- TMJs and muscles of mastication.

The clinical examination can only reveal a limited amount of information and in some circumstances (such as prior to crown and bridgework or in patients with TMPDS) a more detailed occlusal examination is required. This is called an **occlusal analysis** or a **diagnostic mounting**, and is done by mounting study models on an adjustable articulator (see below) to facilitate the examination of the features above.

Occlusal considerations for restorative procedures

In most situations restorations are made to conform to the patient's existing occlusion and the main consideration is to prevent the introduction of iatrogenic occlusal interferences. This approach to treatment is known as the **conformative approach**. In some circumstances the conformative approach is not appropriate and a new occlusal scheme must be planned. This is often the case when extensive crown and bridgework is required, such that the patient's existing occlusion will be effectively destroyed by the preparations. A new occlusion is established, free of interferences and with the patient occluding in centric relation, which is the only reproducible position. This approach to treatment is called the **reorganized approach** and further consideration of this line of treatment is beyond the scope of this book.

For simple intracoronal restorations there is generally no need to employ any complex methods, but care must be taken to ensure the correct occlusal scheme is reproduced. Before preparing a tooth it is worthwhile marking the centric stops with articulating paper and trying to preserve them if possible. On completion of the restoration it must be checked in centric occlusion to ensure that it is not high, but also to ensure that it has recreated the centric stops, as if it is out of occlusion then over-eruption will occur (which may produce interferences). The restoration should then be checked in all mandibular excursions to ensure that no interferences have been introduced.

One or two units of extracoronal restorations can again be constructed in a relatively simple manner. This is usually done in the laboratory using hand-held models to reproduce the occlusion. Again, great care must be taken at the try-in stage to check the occlusion as above. This technique should be used with care when restoring the most distal tooth in the arch as it is very easy to introduce errors in this situation; it may be more appropriate to use an occlusal record (transfer coping technique—see later) and mount the models on an articulator.

More complex laboratory-made restorations need to be constructed with the models mounted on an articulator. This allows the restorations to be constructed in harmony with the patient's occlusion in all mandibular positions, which should minimize the amount of time spent adjusting the restoration at the try-in stage. Also, if any changes to the patient's occlusion are planned, then they can be made on the articulator in a controlled fashion. An articulator is a device which holds the models in a particular relationship and simulates jaw movements. Numerous types of articulators are available but only certain types are appropriate for use in crown and bridgework, e.g. the Denar mark 2, which is a semi-adjustable articulator. The articulator must accurately reproduce mandibular movements and to do this the casts must be mounted in the correct relationship to the TMJs; this is achieved by taking a facebow record. In a conformative approach casts should be related in ICP for restoration.

Occlusal records

Occlusal records are required to mount the models on an articulator in a particular position. Two positions are commonly used for the mounting, the ICP and the RCP. A wax 'squash bite' has commonly been used to record ICP; however, it is inaccurate as the mandible can be deviated as the teeth 'bite' through the wax. It is far better not to use any record and to mount the models to the position of 'best fit'. After the preparations have been carried out it can be difficult to locate the working model to this position of best fit; in this situation the **transfer coping technique** can be used. In this technique Duralay copings are constructed on the working dies, which are taken to the clinic and seated in place on the preparations; they are then adjusted to ensure they are clear of the occlusion. A further mix of Duralay is applied to the occlusal surface of the coping and the patient asked to close together; this produces an indent of the opposing tooth in the resin and provides a very accurate occlusal registration.

When the models are to be mounted in RCP, this is achieved by recording the position of the mandible on the retruded arc of closure just before tooth contact occurs. This is termed a **pre-centric record** and is generally registered with a relatively hard wax (Moyco Dental Wax). The record is constructed on the maxillary model and trimmed flush with the buccal surfaces of the teeth. It is then softened and seated on the maxillary teeth and the mandible manipulated onto the retruded arc of closure to indent the wax, without allowing tooth contact to take place. The registration can be refined by using a low viscosity material (e.g. Temp Bond) in the wax record.

Alternatively, a proprietary inter-occlusal registration material (e.g. Jet Bite, Blu-mousse) may be used to record the space between prepared teeth and their opponents.

Anterior crowns for vital teeth—1

▶ Defer preparation of any crowns until the patient can attain good OH. Not only will this help to ↑ their motivation, but also healthy gingivae are necessary for correct placement of preparation margins and accurate impressions.

Preliminary treatment

- Check vitality; if any doubt, institute RCT first.
- Take a periapical radiograph to check for apical pathology, health of supporting tissues, and anatomy of pulp.
- Get study models. A trial preparation and diagnostic wax-up on a duplicate model can be helpful (especially for the less confident operator). This helps to anticipate any complications and can also be used for fabrication of a temporary crown.
- Record the shade, so that it can be checked at subsequent visits.
- Examine the occlusion.

Porcelain jacket crown (PJC)

This was previously the first choice for aesthetics in cases where occlusal loading was not a problem. Now being superseded by newer ceramic systems.

All-ceramic crown

Provides better aesthetics and ↑ strength compared with PJC (e.g. Inceram, Empress, Procera).

Principles

- Sufficient tooth reduction to permit adequate thickness of crown for strength.
- Reduction should follow tooth contours. **NB** two-plane reduction on labial face, of incisor teeth.
- Chamfer preparation: 1.0 mm labial (just into gingival crevice) and palatal (supragingival).
- 5° taper of opposing walls for retention.

Preparation

Check shade in natural and artificial light with help of dental nurse and patient.

Interproximal   Use a long, tapered chamfer bur. Walls should have 5° taper and converge lingually.

Labial   With the same bur, first place three depth grooves and remove intervening tooth tissue. Extend 0.5 mm subgingivally.

Lingual   If possible carry out under direct vision. Continue interproximal shoulder round to form cingulum wall, supra-gingivally. Remainder of palatal surface should be prepared with a flame-shaped bur to give 0.8–1.0 mm clearance from opposing teeth.

Incisal   A reduction of 1.5–2 mm is required.

Finishing   Finishing burs should be used to round off line angles.

Fabricate temporary crown (p. 312) next, as if time runs out impressions can be deferred, but a temporary crown cannot.

Impressions (p. 686) Opposing arch can be recorded in alginate (cheaper), inter-occlusal record, and facebow if required. Fit temporary and arrange next appointment.

Fitting crown Protect airway. Remove temporary crown. Check marginal fit, contact points, and occlusion. If any adjustments are required polish with porcelain polishing wheels. Make sure patient is happy before you cement crown.

Anterior crowns for vital teeth—2

Porcelain fused to metal (PFM) crown ↑ strength, but ↑ labial reduction (Note, some ceramic crowns can be more destructive than PFMs) and ↓ aesthetics. Preparation requires 0.5 mm reduction of lingual surface with chamfered margin and labial reduction of 1.2–1.5 mm, with shoulder. Transition from shoulder to chamfer is on proximal surface. The junction between porcelain and metal must not be in an area of contact with the opposing teeth. Ideally, all occlusal surfaces in contact with opposing teeth should be finished in metal.

Common problems with anterior crowns

- *Preparation likely to expose pulp* Consider veneer as interim measure.
- *Completed crown does not seat* Check: **1** no temporary cement left on preparation; **2** approximal contacts with floss, and if too tight, adjust; **3** ? distorted impression; check no undercuts on preparation and repeat impressions; **4** die over-trimmed leading to over-extension of margin, cut-back crown margin.
- *Core material showing through crown* Need to reduce preparation so that suficient bulk of enamel and dentine porcelain can be built up over core, and remake.
- *Colour not right* If technician handy can see if surface stains will give sufficient improvement. If not, re-choose shade and remake.

Removing old crowns **(Protect airway)**

  A crown-removing instrument can be used to try and remove a crown without destroying it. If crown is to be replaced:

  Cut a longitudinal groove in labial surface of crown. Insert a flat plastic and twist.

Anterior post and core crowns

In root-filled anterior teeth it may be necessary to insert a post and core prior to the placement of a crown. Post and cores provide support and retention; however, as the placement of a post makes further orthograde endodontics difficult, it is important to check first that the root-filling and apical condition are satisfactory. If in doubt, repeat RCT.

Preliminary preparation The first step is to prepare the crown of the tooth to receive the appropriate coronal restoration. The appropriate reductions and margin preparations are carried out with the intention of retaining as much coronal dentine as possible. Grossly weakened tooth substance is removed, but the root face should *not* be flattened off. The retention of a core of tooth substance is important as it effectively ↑ the length of the subsequent post; obviously in some cases this will not be possible, e.g. if the tooth has fractured at gingival level. The coronal GP is removed with a heated instrument or Gates–Glidden bur, taking care not to disturb apical seal. The root canal is then prepared according to the particular technique being used. As a general guide the post should be at least equal to the anticipated crown height, but a minimum of 4 mm of well-condensed GP should be left. A periodontal probe is helpful to check prepared canal length.

Types of post and core system

Many different types of post system are available and they can be classified in numerous ways:

Prefabricated or custom-made Prefabricated posts obviously have the advantage of being cheap and quick, however, they lack versatility and many of the systems require all coronal dentine to be removed. Custom-made techniques are preferred as they are more versatile, but they are also more expensive and require an additional laboratory stage.

Parallel-sided or tapered Parallel-sided posts are generally preferred to tapered as they provide greater retention and do not generate as much stress within the root canal. Tapered posts, however, are less likely to perforate in the apical region and are better for small tapered roots, e.g. lateral incisors.

Threaded, smooth, or serrated Threaded posts provide greater retention than smooth-sided; however, they will ↑ stress within the root canal and are ∴ C/I. Serrated posts do not concentrate stress but simply ↑ the surface area for retention. Other design features include antirotational components and cementation vents.

Examples

Custom-made The cast post and core is a popular choice. First of all the root canal is prepared using parallel-sided twist drills, and an antirotation groove is placed in the coronal dentine. The post and core can then be constructed either by a *direct technique* or by an *indirect technique*. In the direct technique a pattern is fabricated in the mouth using either inlay wax or a burn out resin (e.g. Duralay) which is then sent to the laboratory for casting. For the indirect technique, which is more widely used, an impression is taken using a matched plastic impression post placed in the prepared post hole. When using this technique it is generally inadvisable to have the post and subsequent crown constructed on the same impression.

Preformed   These are available in various different forms:

Parallel, serrated—e.g. Parapost.

Parallel, threaded—e.g. Radix, Kurer.

Tapered, threaded—e.g. Dentatus screw. These are the poorest design in terms of stress production and, in the authors' opinion, should not be used. If they are used in small tapered roots they should be cemented 'passively'.

Some of these systems have a prefabricated core on the post whilst with others it must be built up around the neck using resin composite. For the majority of crowns choice is one of personal preference. However, no one system will be versatile enough to cover every eventuality, so it is wise to be familiar with more than one method. Tooth-coloured posts based on ceramic or fibre-reinforced resins (Lightposts, Paraposts, Fibrewhite, and Snowposts) are increasingly available and the results are promising.

Anterior post and core crowns—practical tips

Some problems and possible solutions

- *Subgingival tooth loss* Either extrude tooth orthodontically or use cast post and core method, extending post into defect in the form of a diaphragm.
- *Insufficient space for separate core and PJC* Construct post crown in one piece with porcelain bonded to labial face.
- *Extensive tooth loss and calcified canal* (e.g. dentinogenesis imperfecta, severe toothwear) Use dentine pins (plus dentine adhesive system) to retain pinned resin composite core for porcelain bonded crown or consider crown lengthening surgery.
- *Perforation of root by post* Apical 2/3—if the post can be removed it is worth trying to encourage the laying down of a calcific barrier by dressing with calcium hydroxide. If successful re-prepare post hole to correct alignment. Alternatively, need surgical approach to cut back excess post and seal perforation with GI or MTA. Coronal 1/3—incorporate perforation into diaphragm preparation and make new cast post and core.
- *Loss of post* Check: **1** Length adequate? If not, remake with ↑ length. **2** Loose fit or too much taper? Can try sandblasting post and re-cementing with adhesive cement, e.g. Panavia 21. Alternatively, correct and remake. **3** Perforation? Take radiographs in parallax to check, and see above. **4** Root # ? Extract.
- *Apical pathology* If post and core crown satisfactory, arrange apicectomy. If not, remove and carry out revision endodontic therapy and place new post and crown.

Causes of failure in post and core crowns A survey of failed posts showed that most failed within 1 yr, but that a post crown that has survived satisfactorily for 3 yrs has a good chance of lasting for 10 yrs. Common causes of failure were caries, root #, and mechanical failure of the post.[1]

Removing old posts and cores Unretentive posts may be removed by grasping with Spencer–Wells forceps and twisting. Post removers are available (but C/I for threaded posts) that work by drawing out post using root face as anchorage, e.g. the Eggler post remover. Some proprietary kits, e.g. Masseran, can be used to cut a channel around the post to facilitate removal. In some cases an ultrasonic scaler tip can be used to vibrate the post loose, but heat generation can be a problem.

1 R. Lewis 1988 *BDJ* **165** 95.

Veneers

Indications Mild discoloration (can ↑ success by bleaching first), hypoplasia, fractured teeth, toothwear lesions, closing space, or modifying shape (within limits). Veneers are particularly useful in adolescents, where more extensive tooth preparation may risk exposure.

Contraindications Large existing restorations, severe discoloration, insufficient tooth substance to bond restoration to, and parafunction. Overlapping teeth, pencil-chewing, or nail-biting are relative C/I.

Types

Acrylic laminate veneers No longer used.

Resin composite resin Useful for the treatment of adolescent patients. Can be made directly or, more commonly, indirectly. Problems are shrinkage, staining, and wear. Average life-span ~4 yrs.[1]

Porcelain Better performance and aesthetics than resin composite and long-term follow-up now available.[2] In addition, porcelain is less plaque retentive. They are made indirectly in the laboratory and roughened on their fitting surface by etching or sandblasting. This surface is treated with a silane coupling agent prior to bonding to the etched tooth enamel with resin composite luting cement.

Technique for porcelain veneers

Tooth preparation The veneers are usually 0.5–0.7 mm thick, ∴ unless deliberate overbuilding is required, the tooth needs to be reduced labially. To guide reduction depth cuts of 0.5 mm are advisable. A definite chamfered finishing line will make the technician's job considerably easier and this should be established first. If the tooth is discoloured the margin should be sub-gingival (but still in enamel), otherwise keep slightly supra-gingival. The finishing line is extended into the embrasures, but kept short of the contact points. Incisally, the veneer can be finished to a chamfer at the incisal edge or wrapped over onto the palatal surface (see opposite).

An impression of the preparation is taken using an elastomeric impression material in a stock tray and the shade taken with a porcelain shade-guide. Temporary coverage is not usually required (see p. 312).

Try-in Careful handling is necessary so as not to contaminate the fitting surface of the veneer. Do not check the fit of the veneer on the stone cast. The prepared tooth should be cleaned and isolated and then the veneer tried in wet (to ↑ translucency). Minor adjustments are best deferred until after cementation to ↓ risk of #. The effect of different shades of resin composite &/or opaquers and tints can be tried prior to etching to get the best colour match. If several veneers are to be fitted, check them individually and then together to work out the order of placement.

Placement The fitting surface of the veneer is cleaned with alcohol, dried, and then coated with a thin layer of silane coupling agent followed

1 J. S. Clyde 1988 *BDJ* **164** 9.
2 F. J. Shaini 1997 *J Oral Rehabil* **27** 553.

by bonding resin. The tooth is re-isolated and cellulose acetate strips used to separate from adjacent teeth. After etching, washing, and flash drying, a dentine adhesive system is used. Numerous cementation systems are available, e.g. Calibra, Nexus, Variolink. The resin composite luting cement is placed thinly on the fitting surface of the veneer and the veneer carefully positioned. Excess luting cement should be removed with a brush dipped in bonding resin before curing. Adjustments are made with flame-shaped diamond or multi-blade tungsten carbide bur before polishing. The patient should be instructed in the use of floss.

Porcelain slips are veneered corners or edges used to restore # incisors or close spaces by building out the tooth mesially or distally. Now rarely used as direct placement of resin composite is preferred.

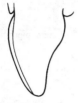 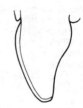

Incisal edge chamfer   Wrap around incisal edge

Porcelain veneer preparations.

Posterior crowns

Posterior crowns are indicated as bridge abutments, to restore endodontically treated teeth, for repair of tooth substance lost due to caries, wear, or #. Tooth loss due to these causes should first be restored using a suitable plastic restorative material. Prior to preparation any doubtful restorations should be replaced, let alone the vitality of the tooth checked and a pre-operative radiograph taken.

Full veneer gold crown

Principles
- Remove enough tooth substance to allow adequate thickness of gold, i.e. 1.5 mm on functional cusp, 1 mm elsewhere, following original tooth contours.
- Wide bevel on the functional cusp (normally buccal—lowers, palatal—upper) for structural durability.
- Convergence of opposing walls <10°.
- Height of axial walls as great as possible (without compromising occlusal reduction).
- Chamfer finishing line.
- Where possible, margins should be supragingival and on sound tooth substance.

Preparation
Occlusal Using a short diamond fissure bur reduce the cusp height, maintaining the original anatomy.

Bucco-lingual With a torpedo-shaped bur eliminate undercuts, retaining 5° taper in cervical 2/3, but usually remaining 1/3 will converge occlusally.

Approximal Using a fine tapered diamond bur within the confines of the tooth, eliminate undercuts at an angle of 5°.

Finishing Round axial line angles and cusps. Check no undercuts and smooth preparation with fine diamonds.
Impressions, p. 686, and temporary coverage, p. 312.

Porcelain fused to metal crown

This is used where a combination of strength and aesthetics is important. The preparation is similar to the full veneer gold crown except that where porcelain coverage is required more tooth substance must be removed. The amount of porcelain coverage must be decided before the preparation is commenced, and the patient consulted at this stage to make sure that they are happy.

Occlusal reduction If it is acceptable to the patient, it is better to provide an all-metal occlusal surface, as less tooth substance needs to be removed. If the patient is adamant that an all-porcelain occlusal surface is necessary, 2 mm will need to be removed from the supporting cusps and 1.5 mm from the non-supporting cusps, which will clearly compromise retention in teeth with short clinical crowns, let alone the vitality of the tooth.[1] Porcelain occlusals can also introduce occlusal interferences.

1 W. P. Saunders 1988 *BDJ* **185** 137.

Buccal reduction 1.2–1.5mm should be removed to provide enough room for the metal and porcelain.

Margins If it is acceptable to the patient, it is better to produce a metal to tooth margin, which will necessitate a narrow collar of metal around the gingival margin. In this case, the finishing line prepared should be a deep chamfer or a bevelled shoulder. If the patient insists on a porcelain to tooth margin then a 1.2–1.5 mm shoulder must be produced. Where no porcelain coverage is needed a chamfer finishing line is produced, as for the full veneer gold crown.

Three-quarter gold crown

The preparation is as for full veneer gold crown except:
- Buccal surface is left unprepared.
- Retention grooves are placed on the mesial and distal surfaces—these must both be parallel to the line of withdrawal of the preparation.
- A groove or 'occlusal offset' is prepared along the occlusal surface between the two retention grooves, just inside the tips of the buccal cusps. This serves to ↑ structural durability of the restoration, which can be quite weak in this region.
- For maxillary teeth a minimal buccal overlay is prepared. In mandibular arch the buccal cusps are the supporting cusps, ∴ an off-cut bevel is cut to ↑ strength of casting.

Crowning root-filled posterior teeth

Single-rooted posterior teeth can be treated as anterior teeth (p. 288). In multirooted teeth the major problem is the divergence of the root canals. The two most commonly used methods of solving this problem are:

Direct method Pre-formed posts are cemented into one or more canals. Amalgam may also be packed into the coronal aspect of the root canals (Nayyar core technique) and an amalgam core built up, which is the preferred technique. Resin modified GI or resin composite may also be used. These materials have the advantage that the preparation can be completed at the same visit. A dentine adhesive system should be used with resin composite to enhance retention.

Indirect method A sprue is placed in the least divergent canal and a lubricated post (e.g. SS wire) positioned in the more divergent. A wax pattern (or Duralay) is then built up to form a core. The lubricated post is removed before the pattern is sent to the lab for casting. The cast post (for the least divergent canal) and core is cemented in position, then either Wiptam or SS wire is cemented through the hole in the casting into the more divergent canal.

With either technique a gold shell or porcelain-bonded crown can be used for the final restoration.

All ceramic crowns

These new systems (e.g. Inceram, Empress I and II, Procera, Techceram) are built on high-strength alumina cores and may be used for posterior crowns. However, few long-term clinical studies of these crowns have been completed; although 5 yr data for Procera is good.[1]

1 P. A. Brunton 1999 *BDJ* **186** 430.

Problems with post and core crowns in multi-rooted teeth

- Short or very curved canals: use a sandblasted metal post in conjunction with a metal adhesive system, e.g. Panavia 21.
- Subgingival tooth loss: use pre-formed post (s) with amalgam core which is well-condensed into region of defect. Some corrosion between the dissimilar metals may be preferable to extending preparation and impressions below level of amalgam.

Bridges

Definitions

Bridge (fixed partial denture) A prosthetic appliance that is permanently attached to remaining teeth and replaces a missing tooth or teeth.

Abutment A tooth which provides attachment and support for a bridge.

Retainer The component that is cemented to the abutments to provide retention for the prosthesis.

Pontic The artificial tooth that is suspended from the abutments.

Connector The component that joins the pontic to the retainer. May be rigid or non-rigid.

Saddle The area of edentulous ridge over which the pontic will lie.

Units Number of units = number of pontics + number of retainers.

Retention Prevents removal of the restoration along the path of insertion or long axis of the preparation.

Support The ability of the abutment teeth to bear the occlusal load on the restoration.

Resistance Prevents dislodgement of the restoration by forces directed in an apical or oblique direction and prevents movement of the restoration under occlusal forces.

Types of bridge

Fixed–fixed The pontic is anchored to the retainers with rigid connectors at either end of the edentulous span. Both abutments provide retention and support. Both preparations must have a single line of draw.

Fixed–movable The pontic is anchored rigidly to the major retainer at one end of the span and via a movable joint to the minor retainer at the other end. The major abutment provides retention and support whilst the minor abutment provides support only. This design allows some independent movement of the minor abutment and has the advantage that the preparations need not be parallel.

Direct–cantilever Pontic is anchored at one end of the edentulous span only.

Spring cantilever A tooth-retained, mucosal-supported bridge. The retainer and pontic are remote from each other and connected by a metal bar which runs along the palate. Usually an upper incisor is replaced from the premolars or a molar. It is useful where there is an anterior diastema or if the posterior teeth are heavily restored; however, they are often poorly tolerated.

Resin-bonded Retained by resin composite (p. 308).

Compound Combination of more than one of above types.

Removable Can be removed by dentist for maintenance.

Types of retainers

- Full coverage crown.
- Three-quarter crown.
- Post-retained crown.
- Onlay.
- Inlay.

All of the above restorations have been used as retainers in conventional bridgework. They are listed in order from most retentive to least retentive. Wherever possible one of the first two should be used, as the failure rate of the last three is much higher. Post crowns should be avoided if possible, and onlays or inlays should only ever be used as minor retainers in fixed–movable bridges.

Selection of abutment teeth

When selecting abutment teeth general factors must be taken into account, such as caries status and existing restorations, but there are two other considerations which specifically relate to bridgework. These are **retention** and **support**.

Assessment of retention

The factors that affect the amount of retention offered by a potential abutment tooth are the clinical crown height and the available surface area. Obviously, the larger teeth offer more retention and should be chosen in preference to the smaller ones. The teeth of both arches are listed below in order of the amount of retention offered (if a full coverage restoration is used).

	Greatest	→	→	→	→	→	Poorest
Maxilla	6	7	4	5	3	1	2
Mandible	6	7	5	4	3	2	1

Assessment of support

Three factors are important:

Crown-root ratio Ideally should be 2:3 but 1:1 is acceptable. As bone is lost so the lever effect on the supporting tissues is ↑.

Root configuration Widely splayed roots provide more support than fused ones.

Periodontal surface area The more of the root that is attached to the bone via the PDL the greater the support offered. At one time great significance was applied to this factor and it formed the basis of Ante's law (1926) which states that '*the combined periodontal area of the abutment teeth must be at least as great as that of the teeth being replaced*,' Ante's law has no scientific basis and no longer has a place in contemporary bridgework design. It does not take into account that we are dealing with a biological system—as the load is ↑ on the abutment teeth a biofeedback mechanism operates to cause a reduction in this load.

The teeth of both arches are listed below in order of the amount of support offered, assuming that the periodontal tissues are intact.

	Greatest	→	→	→	→	→	Poorest
Maxilla	6	7	3	4	5	1	2
Mandible	6	7	3	5	4	2	1

Taper and parallelism
- Opposing walls of abutments should have 5° taper.
- For most designs abutments should be prepared with a common line of draw.
- Checking parallelism: direct vision, with one eye; survey mirror with parallel lines inscribed.
- Management of tilted abutments, p. 303.

Types of pontic
Ridge lap   As name suggests, this type of pontic should make (minimal) contact with buccal aspect of ridge. Gives good aesthetics and is the most popular type.

Hygienic   Does not contact saddle, ∴ easy to clean. Unaesthetic, ∴ limited to molar replacement.

Bullet   Makes point contact with tip of ridge.

Saddle   Extends over ridge buccally and lingually, ∴ difficult to clean. Should not be used.

Bridges—treatment planning and design

Treatment planning

First consider whether benefits of replacing missing teeth (improved aesthetics, occlusal stability, mastication, and speech) outweigh disadvantages (↑ oral stagnation, tooth preparation, cost). Do not forget to consider implants or shortened dental arch therapy. If replacement is indicated ? fixed or removable prosthesis. A number of factors affect this decision:

General	**Local**
Patient's motivation condition	OH and periodontal health
Age	Number of missing teeth
Health	Position of missing teeth
Occupation	Occlusion
Cost	Condition of abutments
	Length of span
	Degree of resorption

These factors need to be favourable if expensive and complex bridge-work is required. Removable prostheses are indicated if general or local factors are less than ideal (p. 336). Remember that removable prostheses can be more harmful than fixed partial dentures.[1]

Designing bridges

- Assess prognosis of all teeth in vicinity to reduce risk of another tooth requiring extraction in near future.
- Assess possible abutment teeth (check restorations, vitality, periodontal condition, mobility, and take periapical radiographs).
- Select design of retainers, e.g. full or partial crown. Full coverage is to be preferred.
- Consider pontics and connectors.
- With this information compile a list of possible designs for bridge.
- Consideration of the advantages and disadvantages of each design combined perhaps with a diagnostic wax-up should help to narrow down the choice. Where possible try the least destructive alternative first.

Specific design problems

Periodontally involved abutments First control periodontal disease. Then ? bridge indicated. Fixed–fixed type of design preferable to splint teeth together. Consider fibre-reinforced resin composite fixed partial dentures for this specific indication.

Pier abutments This is the central abutment in a complex bridge that supports pontics on either side, which are in turn anchored to the terminal abutments. In this situation the pier abutment can act as a fulcrum and when one part of the bridge is loaded the retainer at the other end experiences an unseating force which can lead to cementation failure. To overcome this a stress-breaking element must be introduced, e.g. fixed–movable joint, or avoid pier abutments by simplifying the design.

1 Budtz-Jorgensen 1990 *J Prosthet Dent* **64** 42.

Tilted abutments This occurs most commonly following loss of a molar. There are several approaches:

- Orthodontic treatment to upright abutments.
- Two-part bridge, e.g. fixed–movable.
- Telescopic crowns—placement of individual gold shell crowns on abutments, over which telescopic sleeves of bridge fit.
- Partial veneer preparations in which pins or slots are prepared to compensate for slight malalignment of abutments (least satisfactory).
- Precision attachments—a precision screw and screw tube can be incorporated into a two-part bridge. After cementation the screw is inserted, which effectively converts the bridge to a fixed–fixed design.

Canines The canine is often the keystone of the arch, and a very difficult tooth to replace. The adjacent teeth are poor in terms of the amount of retention and support that they offer and the canine is often subject to enormous stresses in lateral excursion (in a canine-guided occlusion). If a canine is to be replaced with a bridge the occlusal scheme should be designed to provide group function in lateral excursion—never canine guidance.

Bridges—practical stages

1 Take a **history**—Why is a bridge necessary? When and why was tooth lost? Remember the dental history, social history, and medical history.

2 Carry out a **clinical examination**—*extra-oral* and *intra-oral*. Extra-orally look for signs of TMJ dysfunction. Intra-orally look at the general condition of the mouth, the length of edentulous span, the condition and position of the potential abutment teeth. Carefully examine the occlusion and try to formulate some initial ideas on possible bridge designs.

3 Special tests- Radiographs of the potential abutments are mandatory along with vitality (sensibility) tests, accepting their limitations.

4 Diagnostic mounting- Take accurate impressions of both arches, a facebow record and have the models mounted on an adjustable articulator. The mounting can be carried out either in ICP (best fit) or in RCP, for which a precentric record will be necessary. If a reorganized approach to reconstruction is being considered, or if the clinical examination has revealed significant occlusal interferences, an RCP mounting should be performed. Carefully examine the occlusion and consider what occlusal consequences the proposed restoration will have.

5 Diagnostic waxing- In effect, this is a mock up of the final restoration on the mounted models. Wax can be added to the teeth to simulate the effect that the restoration will have on the final occlusion and aesthetic result. In the anterior part of the mouth a denture tooth can be used. In addition to assessing aesthetics and occlusion the diagnostic wax-up can serve as a template from which the temporary bridge can be constructed. An impression is taken of the wax-up in a silicone putty and saved for later. At this stage the design of the prosthesis must be finalized.

6 Preparations- Before the preparations are carried out any suspect restorations in the abutment teeth are replaced. Preparations are carried out in accordance with basic principles (p. 266) and care is taken to ensure that a single path of insertion is established. When checking for parallelism one eye should be kept closed and the use of a large mouth mirror is very helpful. Custom-made paralleling devices can be used but they are very cumbersome.

7 Temporary bridge- This is normally constructed using the matrix which has been formed from the diagnostic wax-up; in this way the temporary bridge should reproduce the aesthetics and occlusion of the final bridge (if the wax-up was done properly!). The matrix is filled with one of the proprietary temporary crown and bridge resins (e.g. Protemp) and seated over the preparations. After it has set it is removed, trimmed, polished, and cemented with a temporary cement (e.g. Temp bond).

8 Impressions- An impression is taken using an elastomeric material. Ideally all of the preparations should be captured on one impression, but this can be very difficult if multiple preparations are involved. If difficulties are encountered in this respect they can often be overcome by using the transfer coping technique. In this technique acrylic (Duralay) copings are made on dies of the preparations for

which a successful impression has been achieved. These are then taken to the mouth and seated on the appropriate tooth, and the impression repeated to capture the other preparations. On removal, the coping will be removed in the impression and the dies can be reseated in the copings and a new model poured around them.

9 Occlusal registration- Under most circumstances the models will be mounted in ICP in the position of best fit, and therefore an occlusal registration will not be necessary. Where numerous preparations have been carried out and it is difficult to locate this position, some form of inter-occlusal record will be necessary. A popular technique involves the use of transfer copings, and is described in the section on occlusion (p. 283).

10 Metal work try-in- If a porcelain fused to metal bridge is being constructed it is advisable to try in the metal work before the porcelain is added. At this stage the fit of the framework can be evaluated and the occlusion adjusted. On occasions it will be found that one retainer seats fully whilst the other does not. This can occur if there has been some minor movement of the abutments since the impression was taken. If this is the case the bridge should be sectioned, and hopefully both retainers will then seat. The two parts are then secured in their new position with acrylic resin (Duralay) and sent back to the lab for soldering.

11 Trial cementation- The finished bridge is tried in and any necessary adjustments made. The bridge should then be temporarily cemented (with modified Temp bond) for a period of a month or so. The advantage of a trial cementation period is that if any further adjustments are necessary they can be carried out outside the mouth and the restoration repolished and reglazed. The patient is instructed in how to clean the bridge (use of Superfloss).

12 Permanent cementation- After the period of trial cementation the bridge is re-evaluated and the patient questioned to check that they are happy with it. If all is well the bridge is removed and cemented with a permanent cement (usually traditional or resin-modified GI cement).

13 Follow-up- Arrangements are made to recall the patient to check that the bridge is still functioning satisfactorily.

Bridge failures

Most common reasons

- Loss of retention.
- Mechanical failure, e.g. # of casting.
- Problems with abutment teeth, e.g. secondary caries, periodontal disease, loss of vitality.

Management of failures

Depending upon type and extent of problem:
- Keep under review.
- Adjust or repair *in situ*.
- Replace.

Replacement

Before replacement of a bridge is embarked upon, a careful analysis of the reasons for failure is necessary. Minor problems in an otherwise satisfactory bridge should be repaired if at all possible. Fractured porcelain can be repaired with one of the specialized repair kits available (e.g. Cojet). Secondary caries or marginal deficiencies, if small, can be restored with traditional GI cement.

A survey of bridges placed by GDPs in Sweden found that 93.3% were still in service after 10 yrs.[1] The most common reason for failure was loss of vitality. This is not necessarily an indication for removal of the bridge because RCT can often be carried out through the retainer of the abutment.

Removing old bridges

To remove intact, try a sharp tap at cervical margin with a chisel or preferably a slide hammer. Orthodontic band-removing pliers can also be used but these require a small hole to be cut in the occlusal surface. If only one retainer is loose, support bridge in position while trying to remove it so that it does not bind.

Retainers can be cut through (p. 286), but this will destroy bridge.

1 S. Karlsson 1986 *J Oral Rehab* **13** 423.

Resin-bonded bridges

This technique involves bonding a cast metal framework, carrying the pontic tooth, to abutment teeth using an adhesive resin. This type of bridge is almost exclusively used for cantilever adhesive bridgework, i.e. one abutment and one pontic. Fixed–fixed designs have been problematic, with one retainer debonding being a common clinical finding. The resin bonds to the abutment tooth using the acid-etch technique and to the metal framework by either mechanical or chemical means.

Classification by:
1. Position: anterior or posterior.
2. Retention: Macromechanical: (a) perforated (Rochette);
                                    (b) mesh (Klettobond);
                                    (c) particular (Crystalbond).
                Micromechanical: (a) electrolytically etched (Maryland);
                                    (b) chemically etched.
                Chemical: (a) sandblasted;
                                    (b) tin-plated.

Chemical retention to a sandblasted metal surface is now used virtually exclusively. A dual-affinity cement (Panavia 21) is used, which chemically bonds to both enamel and non-precious alloys.

Indications	**Advantages**
Short span	Cheaper than conventional bridge
Sound abutment teeth	Minimal tooth reduction
Favourable occlusion	No LA required
	Disadvantages
	Tendency to debond especially if tooth preparation is poor
	Metal may show through abutments

Treatment planning   as for conventional bridgework. If orthodontic treatment is needed to localize space or upright adjacent teeth, it is advisable to retain with a removable retainer for at least 3 months prior to bridge placement.

Tooth preparation   is required to:
- Give a single path of insertion. Provide near parallel guiding planes eliminating undercuts, which allows coverage of maximal surface area for bonding.
- Provide space in occlusion to accommodate bridge. Need at least 0.5 mm for wings.
- ↑ retention, e.g. using a wrap-around design (covering >180° of tooth circumference) to resist lateral displacement.
- Mesial and distal grooves enhance resistance form.
- To prevent gingival displacement. A minimal chamfer is recommended.
- Provide axial loading of the abutments—prepare cingulum or occlusal rests.

NB Tooth preparation should usually be confined to enamel, and the framework should be designed with maximal coverage (to ↑ surface area available for bonding).

Technique (chemical method using Panavia 21) Following tooth preparation an elastomeric impression of the abutment teeth is taken plus an alginate impression of the opposing arch. At the try-in stage the bridge should be assessed for fit, aesthetics, occlusion, etc., and then the fitting surface thoroughly cleaned with alcohol. Contamination of the fitting surface with saliva must be avoided and cementation is best done under rubber dam. Following etching and washing of the abutment(s), and placement of a dentine adhesive system, the wings of the bridge are coated with Panavia 21 and the bridge seated into place and held firmly until set. Use of acetate strips and Superfloss at this stage will clear most of the excess cement and prevent it adhering to the adjacent teeth. The cement must then be covered with a substance known as Oxyguard, which prevents O_2 inhibition of the surface layer. After 5 min or so the rubber dam is removed and any excess cement removed.

Problems

- *Dentine exposed during preparation* Use a dentine adhesive system.
- *Metal shining through abutments* Cut wings away incisally before cementation or use a more opaque cement. May have to consider conventional bridge or placing veneer on labial surface.
- *Debonds* If one flange only, can usually detach other by a sharp tap with a chisel or by using ultrasonic scaler tips. If persistent problem, consider conventional bridge. The trend is for these bridges to be used for cantilevered bridgework and it is not usual for fixed–fixed adhesive bridgework to be prescribed due to problems with unilateral debonding.
- *Caries occurring under debonded wings* Remove bridge and repair.

Attrition, abrasion, and erosion

As these rarely occur individually, the term 'toothwear' is preferred. Also called 'non-carious tooth tissue loss' or 'tooth surface loss', but this is often an understatement!

▶ Some toothwear during life is inevitable, but where it has resulted in an unsatisfactory appearance, sensitivity or mechanical problems, the condition warrants investigation and treatment.

Abrasion is physical wear of a tooth caused by an external agent. Classically, toothbrushes are blamed for the characteristic cervical notches, but it is now believed that other factors may also be operating.[1] Abfraction lesions are now typically thought to be due to flexure of teeth under excursive occlusal loading, possibly coupled with some form of stress corrosion.

Attrition is physical wear caused by movement of one tooth against another. It affects interproximal and occlusal surfaces. ↑ in more abrasive diets and in bruxism. It is often assumed that attrition is greater in patients with reduced posterior support, but no evidence exists to support this.[2] Bruxism ↓ with ↑ age.

Erosion is loss of tooth substance from non-bacterial chemical attack. The incidence of erosion appears to be ↑, but this may be the result of an ↑ awareness of the problem. As the presence of acid results only in demineralization, for loss of tooth substance to occur erosion must act in conjunction with attrition, abrasion, or both. Erosion will be enhanced if the buffering capacity of the saliva is ↓, e.g. in dehydration secondary to alcoholism. Classically, one sees smooth plaque-free surfaces with proud restorations whether the acid is industrial (rare), dietary, or gastrointestinal in origin. The latter may be caused either by gastric reflux, which can be asymptomatic, vomiting (e.g. bulimia, p. 557, or pregnancy). Such conditions warrant referral.

Diagnosis From the clinical picture and history. As toothwear may be due to a factor which no longer operates, it may be necessary (tactfully) to delve into the patient's past. In a proportion of cases, the aetiology will remain obscure and this will complicate prevention. It is important to establish whether the toothwear is ongoing. If teeth are sensitive, probably yes; however, sequential study models will provide definitive evidence.

Toothwear indices are only of value if reproducible, i.e. used regularly. If interested, see paper by Smith.[3]

Management[4]

- Prevention requires an understanding of the aetiology. However, an explanation of possible exacerbating factors to the patient may help to limit loss even if the exact aetiology is unknown.

1 B. G. N. Smith 1989 *Dental Update* **16** 204.
2 A. F. Kayser 1985 *Community Dental Health* **2** 285.
3 B. G. N. Smith 1984 *BDJ* **156** 435.
4 E. A. M. Kidd 1993 *Dental Update* **20** 174.

- Monitoring. Take study models and photos to allow rate of wear to be monitored. Intervention is indicated in cases with an unsatisfactory appearance, sensitivity, or functional problems.
- GI or resin composite restorations may help improve appearance and ↓ sensitivity, but if toothwear is progressive full-coverage crowns are preferable.
- If toothwear is excessive it may not be possible to provide aesthetic crowns without ↑ OVD. The patient's tolerance to this should normally be tested first with an acrylic splint. The majority of patients seem to cope with an ↑ of <5 mm.
- Overdentures may be indicated in cases of excessive toothwear, but are aesthetically less satisfactory.
- Referral to a physician (gastrointestinal problems), psychiatrist (bulimic patient), or restorative specialist (complicated restorative problem).

Temporary restorations

Indications
- Protection of pulp and palliation of pulpal pain.
- Restoration of function.
- Stabilization of active caries prior to permanent restoration.
- Aesthetics.
- Maintenance of position of prepared and adjacent teeth.
- To prevent over-eruption of opposing teeth.
- To prevent gingival overgrowth.

Temporary dressings　Choice of material depends upon the main purpose of the dressing, i.e. therapeutic or structural, but the dressing must also be capable of promoting a good seal and being readily removed. For palliation of pulpal pain ZOE is indicated. For caries control, a calcium hydroxide liner and traditional GI cement. If the remaining tooth tissue requires support this can be gained using a copper ring or an orthodontic band. The interim seal during RCT is very important, ∴ a relatively strong material which prevents microleakage (e.g. GI) should be used.

Temporary crowns　Three main types.

Pre-formed　1 Polycarbonate crown (e.g. Directa), which is trimmed to correct shape and customized by lining with a bis-acryl material (e.g. Protemp). **NB** roughen the inside of the crown to facilitate retention. **2** Soft metal alloy crowns (e.g. Ion).

Laboratory made　Advisable if preparing multiple crowns or if temporary crown needs to last for several months while other aspects of treatment are completed. Preferred method for temporary bridges.

Chairside　This is a versatile technique. Crowns are custom-made using an alginate impression of the tooth taken prior to preparation as a mould. When the preparation is completed, any undercuts should be blocked out with carding wax to prevent the temporary crown material locking in the mouth. The material for the crown is then syringed into the impression around the preparation and re-seated in the mouth. When the initial set has been reached the impression is removed and the temporary left to finish curing before being polished. Suitable materials are Pro-temp (a bis-acryl resin) and Trim (poly-**n**-butyl methacrylate). Care must be taken when using the latter due to high exotherm on curing. An alternative technique is to make a duplicate model of the diagnostic waxing. This approach is useful for multiple crowns or where changes are being made to occlusion/aesthetics. Applicable to both anterior and posterior crowns.

If preparing several adjacent teeth, consider linking temporary crowns to aid retention.

Temporary post and core crowns　Some systems (e.g. Para post) come complete with temporary posts, otherwise they can be made at the chairside with a suitably sized piece of wire. The length of the post should be adjusted so that it protrudes 2–3 mm out of the canal without interfering with the occlusion. A one-piece temporary post and crown is made either by the chairside method described above or with a polycarbonate crown-former and acrylic.

Temporary bridges   The best type is made in the laboratory in acrylic and re-lined at the chairside. Alternatively, make a chairside bridge using the diagnostic waxing.

Veneers   Temporary coverage is usually not necessary, but if the patient complains of sensitivity tack a temporary composite veneer to the prepared surface by etching two small areas of enamel.

Temporary inlays   A light-cured temporary material (e.g. Fermit) has been introduced for this situation.

Temporary cements   The preferred material is Temp bond or similar. Fears about eugenol containing cements and subsequent use of resin composite materials are unfounded as the etching stage removes residual eugenol from the dentinal tubules.

Pinned restorations

Extensive loss of the crown of a tooth leads to problems with retention of subsequent restorations. In posterior (and occasionally anterior) teeth these can be alleviated by the use of dentine pins although their use is ↓. Pin retention may also be necessary to support the cores of full coverage crowns. Pins ↓ the compressive and tensile strength of amalgam and ∴ should not be over-prescribed. A rule of thumb is one pin per missing cusp. Now virtually all pins used are of the self-threading variety, where the pin is carried to the prepared channel in a handpiece. They are usually self-shearing when the correct depth (usually 2 mm) is reached. Pins have largely been replaced by bonding of amalgam coupled with the use of auxiliary forms of retention such as boxes and slots, circumferential grooves, and the use of Nayyar cores in the treatment of non-vital teeth.
Retention can be ranked: self-threading >> friction lock > cemented.

▶ Care is required to avoid perforation into the pulp or PDL.

Technique (**self-shearing threaded pin system**)
• Complete tooth preparation and place lining.
• Choose pin site: 1 mm away from amelo-dentinal junction and clear of bi-or trifurcation areas. A radiograph may be helpful.
• Use a small round bur to indent chosen site.
• Pin channel is then cut parallel to root surface and bur removed whilst still running, then reintroduced to full depth and removed.
• Line up pin with channel and insert. Pins usually shear off when base of channel is reached. If not, move handpiece to and fro until it does.
• Check occlusion and if necessary bend pin inwards. An old chisel with a groove cut in it is a suitable instrument.
• Fit matrix band or copper ring and condense amalgam (or resin composite).

Problems and their management
• Pin perforates into pulp: isolate to prevent contamination with saliva; place hard-setting calcium hydroxide and seal with resin-modified GI cement (e.g. Vitrebond). Monitor vitality of pulp.
• Pin perforates into PDL: can monitor; extend preparation margin to include defect and carefully re-site pin (!); or try to smooth off if accessible in gingival crevice.

Pin retention in anterior teeth Following the introduction of the acid-etch technique pins are rarely required in anterior teeth. Pins used to retain resin composite restorations may show through, detracting from the aesthetics, and are rarely indicated. Gold veneer pinledge preparations are occasionally used as bridge abutments. They rely on pins (which are an integral part of the gold casting) for retention and avoid proximal involvement necessary for 3/4 crown.

Bleaching

Bleaching provides a conservative solution for mild to moderately dis-coloured vital or root-filled teeth. Take photos as a pre-operative record or alternatively note shade of tooth, using a porcelain shade-guide.

Vital bleaching

Two methods have been described.

In-surgery or in-office bleaching This uses carbamide or hydrogen peroxide (30–35%) as the bleaching agent. It is caustic, ∴ protective eyewear and care is required. Dental curing lights are commonly used to activate the bleaching agent.[1] It is likely, however, that no activation is required.

Home bleaching A gel of 10–15% carbamide peroxide in a soft splint has also been advocated for 'home bleaching'. This is worn for a few hours, typically 8 h each day for several weeks, usually two, and is the preferred technique.

'In-office' bleaching technique

- Apply Orabase to gingivae prior to placing rubber dam over teeth to be treated.
- Polish teeth with pumice.
- Etch enamel, wash, and dry, although the need to etch has been ques-tioned.
- Apply the bleaching agent according to the manufacturer's instructions.
- Wash teeth with copious amounts of water.
- Remove rubber dam and polish teeth.
- Advise patient to avoid tea, coffee, red wine, cigarettes, etc., for 1 week and that some sensitivity may occur.
- Can repeat as required.

Home bleaching technique

- Take an alginate impression.
- Ask the laboratory to make a bleaching splint.
- Fit the splint, dispense the carbamide peroxide (10%), and give instructions.
- Advise 6–8 h treatment per day.
- Review weekly.

Non-vital bleaching

This provides a conservative alternative to a post-retained crown for the discoloured root-filled tooth. However, it usually only achieves an improvement in shade. There is a tendency for the discoloration to recur over time, ∴ warn the patient and over-bleach. Interestingly, it has been shown that the degree and duration of discoloration and the age of the patient do not affect the prognosis for a successful result.[1]

Walking bleach technique

- Place Orabase around gingivae of tooth to be treated and isolate with rubber dam.

---

1 R. A. Howell 1980 *BDJ* **148** 159.

- Open access cavity and remove root filling to 2 mm below gingival margin (a period probe is a useful guide).
- Place thin layer of GI cement over root filling to prevent root resorption.
- Remove any stained dentine within pulp chamber.
- Clean access cavity with etchant on a pledget of cotton wool and then repeat with alcohol. Wash and dry.
- Mix together sodium perborate (Bocasan) with water to a paste and place in the access cavity.
- Seal with a pledget of cotton wool and GI.
- Review patient after 1–2 weeks and repeat (up to two times) if necessary.
- Seal access cavity permanently with a light shade of resin composite.

Thermocatalytic techniques, where the hydrogen peroxide is heated within the pulp chamber, should no longer be used, as they are associated with the development of cervical resorption lesions.

Root canal therapy

RCT involves the removal of pulpal remnants, and cleaning and obturation of the resultant space, in order to prevent bacterial proliferation within the canal system. Resolution of apical pathology is dependent upon separation of invading microorganisms and their products from host's defence reactions.[1]

Indications

- Pulp irreversibly damaged &/or evidence of periapical disease.
- Crown of tooth requires extensive modification, e.g. overdenture.
- ▶ Those patients at risk from bacteraemia should be protected with antibiotic cover (p. 598) prior to endodontic treatment and for acute periapical conditions. Cover should be given for initial stages of RCT, but once working length has been determined (and all instrumentation confined within canals) it should not be necessary.

Anatomy

The apical foramina are usually sited 0.5–0.7 mm away from the anatomical and radiographic apex. The apical constriction usually occurs 0.5–0.7 mm short of the foramina. These distances ↑ with age due to deposition of secondary cementum. Root-filling to the constriction provides a natural stop to instrumentation, thus the working length should be established 1–2 mm from the radiographic apex.

Average working lengths (in mm):

	1	2	3	4/5	6	7
Maxilla	21	20	25	19	19	18.5
Mandible	19	19.5	24	20	19.5	18.5

Most canals are flattened mesio-distally, but become more rounded in the apical 1/3. Lateral canals are branches of the main canal and occur in 17–30% of teeth.

Remember:

Maxillary
4   74% have >1 canal with > 1 foramina.
5   75% have 1 canal with 1 foramina.
6,7 Assume these teeth have 4 canals (2 MB; 1P; 1DB) until second MB canal cannot be found.

Mandibular
1,2   >40% have 2 canals, but separate foramina are seen in only 1%.
4,5   May have 2 canals, but these usually rejoin to give 1 foramina.
6,7   Generally have 3 canals (MB; ML; D); but 1/3 have 4 canals (2 in D root).

Some endodontists are using a technique involving maintenance of apical patency, but at present there is little research evidence to support this approach.

1 European Society of Endodontology 1994 *Int Endodont J* **27** 115.

Assessment
- Check there is no doubt about which tooth requires treatment.
- Is tooth restorable following RCT?
- Good radiographs are essential. Minimum requirements are (1) pre-op assessment; (2) check working length; (3) check obturation and provide baseline for follow-up. In addition, a radiograph of the master-point prior to obturation is taken if indicated.

Root canal therapy—instruments

It is helpful to make up RCT kits containing the commonly used instruments, e.g. front surface mirror, extra-long probe, endo-locking tweezers, long-shanked excavator, flat plastic, root-canal spreaders and condensers, and a metal ruler. The whole kit can then be sterilized.

Broaches These are either smooth for exploring or barbed for pulp extirpation.

Reamers Rarely used or indicated. Disadvantages of reamers include their inflexibility with ↑ size, which can result in a wider channel being cut apically. Have now been replaced by files.

Files These are used either with a longitudinal rasping or a rotary action (e.g. wrist-watch action[1]). The main types of file available are:

K-type-file Made by twisting a square metal blank.

Hedstroem file Made by machining a continuous groove into a metal blank. More aggressive than K-file. Must never be used with a rotary action as liable to #.

K-flex file Similar to K-file but made by twisting a rhomboid shape blank→ alternating blades with acute and obtuse angles. More flexible than K-file but becomes blunt more quickly.

Flex-o-file Looks similar to a K-type-file but is made from a triangular blank of a more flexible steel. The file also has a blunt tip, which means that it is unlikely to create a false channel. This file is more flexible than K-types and is now becoming a popular replacement.

Gretaer taper (GT) Hand files made from nickel titanium (NiTi). They have increasing tapers (0.06–0.12) with matched GP cones.

Files have traditionally been made from steel, but newer varieties made of NiTi are gaining popularity as they are much more flexible. Larger-sized files can be sterilized and re-used more than the smaller sizes. All instruments should be examined regularly, and discarded if there are any signs of damage. It is good practice to dispose of smaller files after one use. In future files may all be single use (disposable). NiTi rotary instruments (Profile) reduce creation of blocks, ledges, transportations and perforations by remaining centred within the natural path of the canal. Useful for curved canals but ↑ risk of #. Prior to use check for patency/ glide-path up to the full working length with a size 10 file.

Spiral root fillers May be used to deposit paste materials within the canal, but are liable to #, ∴ the inexperienced operator should use them by hand. A preferred alternative is to coat a file with the paste and spin it by hand in an anticlockwise direction to deposit the paste in the canal.

Gates–Glidden burs These are bud-shaped with a blunt end and are used, at slow speed, for preparing the coronal 2/3 of the canal. A new instrument called (with some charm!) 'Orifice opener' works in the same fashion.

---

1 W. P. Saunders 1997 *Dental Update* **24** 241.

Rubber stops These indicate the working length on RCT instruments. Some have a notch to indicate the direction of a curvature.

Finger spreaders These are used to condense the cones of GP during canal obturation. They are sized to match the GP accessory cones.

Other equipment Sterile cotton-wool pledgets and paper points will be required for drying canals, and a syringe and needle for irrigating them.

Root canal therapy—materials

Irrigants These are required to flush out debris and lubricate instruments. Dilute sodium hypochlorite is generally considered to be the best irrigant as it is bacteriocidal and dissolves organic debris. The normal concentration is 2.5% available chlorine. Chelating agents which soften dentine by their demineralizing action are particularly helpful when trying to negotiate sclerosed or blocked canals (e.g. EDTA paste, File Eze, RC Prep).

Canal medication The emphasis in RCT should be placed on thorough mechanical debridement rather than trying to sterilize their contents (which is impossible!). Canal medicaments therefore play a secondary role in RCT. Strong antiseptics, such as phenolic compounds, have been used in RCT, but they are potentially toxic and their effects appear short-lived—so their use is not recommended. For routine cases it is normal practice to leave the root canal empty but in certain situations a medicament is helpful. Two types are worthy of consideration:

1 *Non-setting calcium hydroxide paste* (see below). It can be very effective in treating an infected canal where there is a persistent inflammatory exudate from the periapical tissues. Other sealers based on resin (AH Plus) and GI (Ketac Endo) are available.
2 *Antibiotic/steroid paste* (Ledermix) is useful if you are unable to achieve anaesthesia of a hyperaemic pulp. Dressing with Ledermix ↓ inflammation and may allow pulp extirpation under LA next visit.
3 *Iodine-containing pastes* are useful in retreatment cases as certain organisms are resistant to calcium hydroxide.

Filling materials GP, a form of latex extracted from tropical trees, comes the nearest to meeting the requirements of an ideal filling material. It is supplied in cones which come in two forms: *master cones*, sized according to ISO standards; *accessory cones*, sized to match the finger spreaders.

Sealers A wide variety are available. The calcium hydroxide materials (e.g. Sealapex) or the eugenol-based sealers (e.g. Tubliseal) are perhaps the safest choice. Some would advocate the routine use of non-setting calcium hydroxide paste (Hypocal) as an inter-appointment medicament.

Calcium hydroxide This is considered separately, because it has a wide range of applications in endodontics due to its antibacterial properties and an ability to promote the formation of a calcific barrier. The former is thought to be due to a high pH and also to the absorption of carbon dioxide, upon which the metabolic activities of many root-canal pathogens depend. It is also proteolytic. Indications for the use of calcium hydroxide include:

- To promote apical closure in immature teeth.
- In the management of perforations.
- In the treatment of resorption.
- As a temporary dressing for canals where filling has to be delayed. In the management of recurrent infections during RCT.

In RCT, a suspension of calcium hydroxide in carboxy-methyl cellulose (e.g. Hypo-cal) is useful. Alternatively, a suspension of (powder) calcium hydroxide and sterile water can be made up 'in-house'. Although, more difficult to handle, is clinically often more effective than proprietary brands.

Canal preparation—1

Aims of preparation   These are twofold, and generally described as *cleaning* and *shaping*.

Cleaning   Aims to remove bacteria and organic debris from the root canal.

Shaping   Aims to produce the ideal shape for the reception of the root filling material. As the filling material of choice is normally GP the shape should be a continuously tapering cone with its narrowest diameter at the apical constriction and its widest diameter in the coronal region.

Preparation of tooth   Prior to starting RCT all caries must be removed from the crown of the tooth and an interim restoration placed. Grossly weakened posterior teeth may need to be temporarily restored, ideally with amalgam. Large temporary dressings of, e.g., modified ZOE, in the posterior part of the mouth are not satisfactory. This initial preparation aids placement of rubber dam, prevents ingress of bacteria from the mouth, and provides a stable reference point for measurement of working length.

Isolation   Required to maintain an aseptic environment, protect the patient from toxic materials, and prevent inhalation of small RCT instruments. Use of rubber dam is mandatory.

Access   Should be designed to reduce the curvature required to nego-tiate the apical 1/3 of the canal and will involve removal of the entire roof of the pulp chamber, including the pulp horns. The access cavity in ante-rior teeth is midway between incisal edge and the cingulum, and in posterior teeth will vary according to the anatomy of the pulp chamber. Lining up a bur with the pre-operative radiograph will help to gauge the depth of preparation. The turbine handpiece should be used to gain initial access, reverting to slow speed for removal of the roof of the pulp chamber and subsequent preparation. When completed the access cavity should have a smooth funnel shape. Long-shanked burs are helpful, as are safe-ended (Batt) burs.

Extirpation of the pulp   Achieved using a barbed broach or fine files. Often the pulp remnants are necrotic and copious irrigation is required for complete removal.

Working length[1]   Definable as the distance from a fixed reference posi-tion on the crown of the tooth to the apical constriction of the root canal. Remember that the apical constriction is normally 1–2 mm short of the radiographic apex of the tooth. There are two methods of establishing the working length: (a) involves the use of radiography; (b) uses an electronic device known as an apex locator. The radiographic technique is the most commonly used and is described below. Apex locators work by measuring electrical impedance with an electrode in the root canal; when the elec-trode reaches the apical foramen it emits an audible or visible signal. Arguably the use of an apex locator reduces the number of radiographs taken for RCT.

---

1 C. J. R. Stock 1994 *BDJ* **176** 329.

Common errors in canal preparation

- *Incomplete debridement*: working length short, missed canals.
- *Lateral perforation*: often occurs as a result of poor access.
- *Apical perforation*: makes filling difficult.
- *Ledge formation*: can be very difficult to bypass.

Apical transportation (zipping) A file will tend to straighten out when used in a curved canal and straightening can transport the apical part of the preparation away from the curvature. The use of flexible files reduces the likelihood of this happening.

Elbow formation When apical zipping happens, a narrowing often occurs coronal to this in the canal such that the canal is hourglass in shape. This narrowing is termed an elbow.

Strip perforation A perforation occurring in the inner or furcal wall of a curved root canal, usually towards the coronal end.

Techniques of canal preparation

Numerous techniques have been described :

Stepback technique The apical part of the root canal is prepared first and the canal is then flared from apex to crown. Blockage of canals may occur using this technique, and irrigation can be difficult.

Stepdown technique This (along with several others) prepares the coronal part of the canal before the apical part. This has advantages (see later) and is the preferred technique.

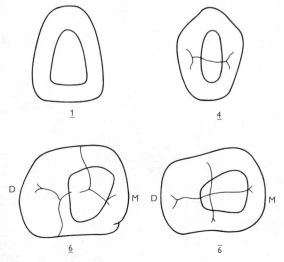

Access cavity preparations

Balanced force technique This involves using blunt-tipped files with an anticlockwise rotation whilst applying an apically directed force. It requires practise to master but is particularly useful when preparing the apical part of severely curved canals.

Anticurvature filing This was developed to minimize the possibility of creating a 'strip' perforation on the inner walls of curved root canals. It is used in conjunction with other techniques or preparation, and the essential principle is the direction of most force away from the curvature. Filing ratio 3:1 Outer wall: Inner wall.

To avoid confusion we have tried to provide a simplified guide to preparation of root canals. The recommended techniques are described on p. 328.

Canal preparation—2

Technique for the preparation of large, relatively straight root canals (modified crown-down technique)

1 Obtain a good-quality pre-operative radiograph. Identify the root canal.
2 Place a rubber dam and prepare the access cavity. Prepare the outline first (remembering your pulpal anatomy) with a high-speed bur and then change to a slow-speed rosehead. Remove the roof of the pulp chamber in its entirety leaving no ledges or overhangs.
3 Irrigate the pulp chamber, and identify the root canal with an explorer or fine file.
4 Estimate 2/3 length of canal from pre-operative X-ray. Check for patency with a size 15 file. Widen to form gradual coronal flare with Gates–Glidden bur 2, then 3, then 4 at successively shorter lengths.
5 Take diagnostic radiograph to confirm working length. Prepare apical region to three sizes larger than the size of the first file which binds at the working length. Irrigate well between each file.
6 The remainder of the canal is now flared by 'stepping back'. Take a file one size larger than the master apical file and insert it to a length 1 mm short of the working length. Work this file with a circumferential filing motion. Continue this enlarging procedure with successively larger size files, each 1 mm shorter than the previous, to complete the preparation. After each file is used it is important to reinsert the master apical file to the full working length (recapitulation) and irrigate thoroughly to ensure that the canal does not become blocked.

Technique for the preparation of fine and curved root canals

1 As above.
2 As above.
3 Irrigate the pulp chamber and identify the root canals using a fine file. Use the grooves in the floor of the pulp chamber as a guide to their location. Pass a fine instrument down the canals to ensure their patency.
4 Go back to your pre-operative radiograph and, for each canal, estimate the distance (in millimetres) from an occlusal reference position to the beginning of the canal curvature. This will vary depending upon the tooth in question. Widen to form gradual coronal flare with Gates–Glidden bur 2, then 3, then 4 at successively shorter lengths. Copious irrigation must be used to prevent the canal from becoming blocked.
5 The working length is now determined for each canal. It is important that this is not done before orifice enlargement, as the reference point on the crown will move as the coronal part of the canal is straightened. Remember to use the pre-operative radiograph to estimate the working length prior to taking the radiograph.
6 The next step is to prepare the apical stop. This is done with files using a longitudinal filing motion and copious irrigation. It is permissible to use a quarter turn with the finer files at this stage to help engage the dentine. As a general guide the apical stop should be prepared three sizes larger

than the first file that binds at the full working length, but it must also be at least a size 25 (preferably a 30). Remember that when using this technique in curved canals the larger files (generally 25 and above) will need to be precurved; this is done by bending around a mirror handle. When using precurved files try to use very short cutting strokes—long ones will produce an incorrect canal shape. The *balanced force* or modified double-flared techniques[1] can be very effective at this stage in curved canals, providing the operator is experienced in the technique.

7 The rest of the root canal is now flared by 'stepping back' in the conventional manner. This procedure is made much easier as the coronal part of the root has already been enlarged.

Advantages of orifice enlargement

- Effectively, ↓ the curvature in the coronal part of the root canal, allowing straighter access for files to the apical region. It therefore reduces the likelihood of apical transportation (zipping).
- It allows improved access for the flow of irrigant solution within the canal.
- It reduces the likelihood of apical extrusion of infected material as most of the canal debris is removed before apical instrumentation takes place. This is particularly important because the majority of bacteria in an infected root canal are located in the coronal region.

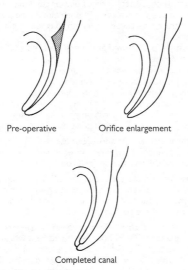

Pre-operative   Orifice enlargement

Completed canal

Diagram of stages of canal preparation

1 C. J. R. Stock 1995 *Color Atlas of Endodontics* 95.

Canal obturation

Purpose To provide a three-dimensional hermetic seal to the root canal that will prevent the ingress of bacteria or tissue fluids which might act as a culture medium for any bacteria that remain in the root canal system. In the past, the critical factor was considered to be the achievement of an apical seal, but now it is realized that coronal seal is also important. For this reason the whole of the root canal must be filled, and techniques that only seal the apical region (e.g. silver points) have fallen from favour.

Techniques

Numerous techniques have been described; all of those mentioned here use GP.

Cold lateral condensation This is a commonly taught method of obturation and is the gold standard by which others are judged. The technique involves placement of a master point chosen to fit the apical section of the canal. Obturation of the remainder is achieved by condensation of smaller accessory points. The steps involved are:

1 Select a GP master point to correspond with the master apical file instrument. This should fit the apical region snugly at the working length so that on removal a degree of resistance or 'tug-back' is felt. If there is no tug-back select a larger point or cut 1 mm at a time off the tip of the point until a good fit is obtained. The point should be notched at the correct working length to guide its placement to the apical constriction.
2 Take a radiograph to confirm that the point is in correct position if you are in any doubt.
3 Coat walls of canal with sealer using a small file.
4 Insert the master point, covered in cement.
5 Condense the GP laterally with a finger spreader to provide space into which accessory points can be inserted until the canal is full.
6 Excess GP is cut off with a hot instrument and the remainder packed vertically into the canal with a cold plugger.

Warm lateral condensation As above, but uses a warm spreader after the initial cold lateral condensation. Finger spreaders can be heated in a flame or a special electronically heated device (Touch of heat) can be used.

Vertical condensation In this technique the GP is warmed using a heated instrument and then packed vertically. A good apical stop is necessary to prevent apical extrusion of the filling, but with practice a very dense root filling can result. Time consuming.

Thermomechanical compaction This involves a reverse turning (e.g. McSpadden compactor or GP condenser) instrument which, like a reverse Hedstroem file, softens the GP, forcing it ahead of, and lateral to the compactor shaft. This is a very effective technique, particularly if used in conjunction with lateral condensation in the apical region, but requires much practice to perfect.

Thermoplasticized injectable GP (e.g. Obtura, Ultrafil) These commercial machines extrude heated GP (70–160°C) into the canal. It is difficult to control the apical extent of the root filling, and some contraction of the GP occurs on cooling. Useful for irregular canal defects, e.g. following internal root resorption.

Coated carriers (e.g. Thermafil) These are cores of metal or plastic coated with GP. They are heated in an oven and then simply pushed into the root canal to the correct length. The core is then severed with a bur. A dense filling results, but again apical control is poor and extrusions common. They are expensive and difficult to remove.

Once the filling is in place the tooth will need to be permanently restored, provided the follow-up radiograph is satisfactory. Fillings that appear inadequate radiographically may be reviewed regularly, or replaced, depending upon the clinical circumstances.

Follow-up The tooth should be reviewed radiographically after 6 months and thereafter annually for up to 4 yrs. Failure of endodontic treatment may present as pain, swelling, discharge, or radiographically as an enlargement of a periapical radiolucency. Following effective RCT most radiolucent periapical lesions show signs of resolution within 2 yrs.

Coronal seal This is now recognized as very important for success in endodontics. Too often good endodontic therapy is jeopardized by a poor restoration that does not provide a good coronal seal.[1]

1 W. P. Saunders 1994 *Endodontics and Traumatology* **10** 105.

Some endodontic problems and their management

Acute periapical abscess Relief of symptoms requires drainage of the abscess and where possible this should be obtained through the tooth. Open the pulp with a diamond bur in a turbine handpiece whilst supporting the tooth to ↓ vibration. Regional anaesthesia and occasionally sedation may be required. Once opened the canal is irrigated with sodium hypochlorite and, if at all possible, resealed. It may be necessary to see the patient again in 24 h, but this is more labour-saving long term than leaving the tooth on open drainage. Relieve any traumatic occlusion.

If a fluctuant abscess is associated with the tooth this should be incised. If drainage can be obtained through the tooth and there is no evidence of a cellulitis then antibiotics are not required (p. 408).

Pain following instrumentation This is usually due to instruments or irrigants, or to debris being forced into the apical tissues. Placement of a small amount of Ledermix in the canal may provide symptomatic relief, but care is required not to breach the apex. Occasionally, an acute flare-up of a previously asymptomatic tooth occurs following initial instrumentation—this is called a phoenix abscess. Loss of face is saved by warning patients that this can happen. Affected teeth should be opened and irrigated and if possible resealed. This may need to be repeated after 24–48 h.

Recurrent symptoms/intractable infection If thorough cleaning and repeated dressing of the canal with calcium hydroxide are unsuccessful, it may be necessary to do an apicectomy (p. 402). Do not routinely turn to surgery for failed cases—consider retreatment in the first instance.

Sclerosed canals As the incidence of pulp necrosis following canal obliteration is only 13–16%, elective RCT is not warranted.[1] However, where pulp death has occurred finding the canal orifice may be difficult.

If careful exploration with a small file is unsuccessful, investigation of the expected position of the canal entrance with a small round bur may help. Once the canal is found, a No. 8 or 10 file should be used to try and negotiate it, using EDTA, File Eze, or RC Prep as a lubricant, and the canal prepared and filled conventionally. Success rates of 80% have been reported for canals that were hairline or undetectable on radiographs.[1] Occasionally, a total blockage of the canal is encountered, in which case the filling is placed to this level &/or an apicectomy done.

Pulp stones in the pulp chamber can usually be flicked out. If they occur in the canal use EDTA and a small file to try and dislodge them.

Fractured instruments Sometimes it is possible to get hold of the fractured portion with a pair of fine mosquitos. If not, insertion of a fine file beside the instrument may dislodge it; should this be unsuccessful a Masseran kit (p. 290) may be required. Should the fractured piece be lodged in the apical portion of the canal it may be better to fill the canal below it and keep it under observation, resorting to an apicectomy as a last-ditch solution.

1 J. O. Andreasen 1994 *Text book and Colour Atlas of Traumatic Injuries to the Teeth*, Munksgaard.

Immature teeth with incomplete roots, p. 120.

Removing old root-fillings If a single-point technique or a root-filling paste has been used removal is straightforward. If a well-condensed GP filling is present this may be softened, using a heated probe to gain purchase for a fine file to be inserted. Use of chloroform or oil of cajeput may aid softening and removal. If time is at a premium a pledget of cotton wool moistened with eucalyptus oil can be sealed in place for 1–2 weeks before removal is attempted. Apical silver points or amalgam will require an apicectomy to achieve a satisfactory apical seal if pathology is present.

Perforations can be iatrogenic or caused by resorption (p. 120). In the latter case, dressing with non-setting calcium hydroxide may help to arrest the resorption and promote formation of a calcific barrier. Increasingly MTA is being used for the repair of perforations and in surgical endodontics as a retrograde filling material with excellent results.[2] Management of traumatic perforations depends upon their size and position:

Pulp chamber floor If small, can cover with calcium hydroxide and fill with GP or GI, but if large, hemisection or extraction may be necessary.

Lateral perforation If this occurs near the gingival margin it can be incorporated in the final restoration of the crown, e.g. a diaphragm post and core crown. If in the middle 1/3, the remainder of the canal may be cleaned by passing instruments down the side of the wall opposite the perforation. Then the canal can be filled with GP, using a lateral condensation technique to try and occlude the perforation as well. Larger perforations may require a surgical approach and in multirooted teeth hemisection or extraction may be unavoidable.

Apical 1/3 It is usually worth trying a vertical condensation technique to attempt to fill both the perforation and the remainder of the canal. If this is unsuccessful an apicectomy will be required.

Ledge formation If this occurs, return to a small file curved at the apex to the working length and use this to try and file away the ledge, using EDTA or RC Prep as lubricants.

Perio-endo lesions, p. 250.

2 M. Torabinejad 1999 *J. Endod* **25** 197.

Four-handed dentistry

Working in a seated position is now the norm for all dentists. This has resulted in the dental nurse taking a more active role by working closely with the dentist. The development of four-handed dentistry is credited to Ellis Paul.[1]

Advantages and disadvantages
1 ↑ comfort for dentist and nurse
2 ↑ efficiency
3 ↑ patient comfort
4 ↑ operator visibility
5 ↓ backache
6 ↑ professional satisfaction for the dentist and dental nurse

Seating the patient Except for the old, infirm or pregnant patient, a totally supine position is preferable. Remember to warn the patient that you are about to whisk them backwards.

Seating the dentist The aim is a relaxed, undistorted, and comfortable posture, with good vision of the teeth to be treated. Adjust the dentist's stool so that the top of their thighs slope at 15° to the floor. Position the dental chair so that, with the operator's back straight, the patient's mouth is at the dentist's focal distance (mid-sternal level). Forearms should slope upwards to this point. The operator's location is between 10 o'clock and 11 o'clock relative to the patient's head. Ensure the patient's head is at the top of the headrest.

Seating the dental nurse The dental nurse must also be seated comfortably with a straight back, with their eye level 10 cm higher than the dentist's for maximum vision. The dental nurse's normal working environment is at between 2 and 3 o'clock, within easy reach of the instruments and equipment to be used.

Role of the dental nurse
• Receive, seat, and look after the patient.
• Place bib and protective glasses on patient.
• Position dental light.
• Retract patient's lips and protect their soft tissues.
• Aspirate fluids—hold aspirator in right hand.
• Hold 3-in-1 syringe in left hand whilst aspirating.
• Pass instruments to the operator.

Instrument transfer The transfer zone is just in front of, and slightly below the patient's mouth, not over their eyes. There are several techniques which enable the dental nurse to pass and receive instruments effectively from the dentist. All require practice. Each dental team needs to choose, adapt, practise, and perfect a system that safely achieves instrument transfer.[2]

1 J. E. Paul 1991 *Team Dentistry*, Dunitz.
2 J. E. Paul 1997 *Fact File: Occupational Back Pain*, BDA.

Prosthetics and gerodontology

Relevant pages in other chapters Bridges—treatment planning and design, p. 302; occlusion, p. 280; acrylic and other denture materials, p. 696; casting alloys, p. 688; impression materials, p684.

Principal sources and further reading M. R. Y. Dyer 1989 *Notes on Prosthetic Dentistry*, Wright. J. C. Davenport 1988 *A Colour Atlas of Removable Partial Dentures*, Wolfe. J. F. McCord 2002 *Missing Teeth: A Guide to Treatment Options*, Churchill Livingstone. D.W. Bartlett 2004 *Clinical Problem Solving in Prosthodontics*, Churchill Livingstone.

Treatment planning

Reasons for prosthetic replacement of missing teeth
- Restore aesthetics.
- ↑ masticatory efficiency.
- Improve speech.
- Preserve or improve health of the oral cavity by preventing unwanted tooth movements.
- Improve distribution of occlusal loads.
- Space maintenance.
- Prepare patient for complete dentures.

Disadvantages of prosthetic replacement
- ↑ plaque accumulation/changes in composition.
- Damage to soft tissues and remaining teeth, due either to poor denture design or lack of patient care.

Treatment options for the partially dentate mouth
1 No replacement of missing teeth. If the benefits of a prosthesis do not outweigh the disadvantages, then replacement is C/I. An occlusion with first premolar to first premolar present in each jaw (shortened dental arch) is usually functionally adequate. Poorly controlled epilepsy is a C/I to dentures.
2 Bridges (p. 298) are preferable for short bounded spans in well-motivated patients.
3 Removable partial dentures. Indicated for patients with satisfactory OH and whose remaining teeth have an adequate prognosis, or as a training/interim appliance prior to F/F.
4 Complete immediate dentures. These are indicated for patients who have already mastered wearing a partial denture and whose remaining teeth have a poor prognosis.
5 Extraction of the remaining teeth and provision of a denture after healing has occurred. Avoid if possible as considerable guesswork is involved in the subsequent denture and the chances of the patient coping successfully are ↓.
6 In the older, partially dentate patient it is important to assess whether the patient is likely to retain some functional teeth for the remainder of their life-span. If this is improbable, treatment could be aimed towards providing F/F dentures while the patient is still young enough to adapt, according to some authors.

Treatment planning for partial dentures
► It is important to enquire about previous denture history (just because a patient is not wearing a denture does not mean that they have not had one) and assess the reasons for failure or success. If a patient produces an extensive collection of unsuccessful dentures, unless there is an obvious and easily remedied fault, it is probably wiser to assume that you are unlikely to succeed where so many have failed and refer the patient for a specialist opinion.

- Relief of pain and any emergency treatment.
- History and exam, including a thorough clinical and radiographic assessment of remaining teeth and edentulous areas.
- Unless immediate dentures planned, extract any teeth with poor prognosis.
- OH and periodontal treatment.
- Preliminary design of partial denture.
- Carry out restorative treatment required.
- Modify design if necessary and commence prosthetic treatment (p. 346).

Treatment planning for complete dentures
- Relief of pain and any emergency treatment, including temporary modification of existing dentures, if indicated.
- History and exam.
- Investigation and treatment of any systemic problems.
- Removal of pathological abnormalities (e.g. retained roots), and pre-prosthetic surgery, if required.
- ? rebase (p. 360), copy (p. 368), or construct new dentures (p. 350).

▶ Discussing with the patient the limitations of dentures prior to their construction is more likely to be viewed as explanation, whereas leaving it until after fitting the dentures will be seen as making excuses!

Principles of removable partial dentures

Definitions

Saddle   That part of a denture which rests on and covers the edentulous areas and carries the artificial teeth and gumwork.

Connector   Joins together component parts of a denture.

Support   Resistance to vertical forces directed towards mucosa.

Retainers   Components which resist displacement of denture.

Indirect retention   Resistance to rotation about clasp axis by acting on the opposite side to the displacing force.

Fulcrum axis   Axis around which a tooth- and mucosa-borne denture tends to rock when saddles are loaded.

Bracing   Resistance to lateral movement.

Guide planes   Two or more parallel surfaces on abutment teeth used to limit path of insertion, and improve retention and stability.

Survey line   Indicates the maximum bulbosity of a tooth in the plane of the path of withdrawal.

Free-end saddle   An edentulous area posterior to the natural teeth.

Stress-breaker   A device allowing movement between saddle and the retaining unit of partial denture.

Gum-stripper   A tissue-borne partial denture which can 'sink'.

Dysjunct denture   Has complete separation between tooth- and mucosa-borne parts.

Swinglock denture[1]   Has a labial retaining bar or flange which is hinged at one side of the mouth and locks at the other.

Sectional denture   Made in two or more sections which are then fixed together with screws or other devices.

Classification

Kennedy   Describes the pattern of tooth loss:
1. Bilateral free-end saddles.
2. Unilateral free-end saddle.
3. Unilateral bounded saddle.
4. Anterior bounded saddle, only.

Any additional saddles are referred to as modifications (except Class IV), e.g. Class I modification 1 has bilateral free-end saddles and an anterior saddle.

Craddock   Describes the denture type:
1. Tooth-borne.
2. Mucosa-borne.
3. Mucosa- and tooth-borne.

1 M. Chan 1998 *Dental Update* **25**, 80.

Acrylic versus metal dentures

Approximately 75% of the dentures provided in the UK have an acrylic connector and base. Although metal bases are generally preferred, because the greater strength of metal permits a more hygienic design, an acrylic base is indicated for:

- Temporary replacement, e.g. following trauma or in children.
- Where there is inadequate support from the remaining teeth for a tooth-borne denture.
- When additions to the denture are likely in the near future.

However, where financial constraints C/I a metal base, attention to the following may avoid the production of a gum-stripper:

- Wide mucosal coverage to provide maximum support.
- Keep base clear of the gingival margins wherever possible.
- No interdental extensions of acrylic.
- Point contact and wide embrasures between natural and artificial teeth.
- Labial flanges for extra retention and bracing.
- Additional support from wrought SS rests.

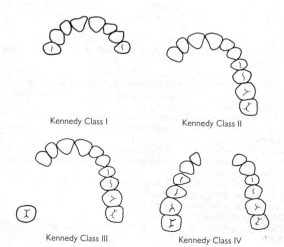

Kennedy Class I

Kennedy Class II

Kennedy Class III

Kennedy Class IV

Components of removable partial dentures

Saddles can be made entirely of acrylic or have a sub-framework of metal overlaid by acrylic.

Rests are an extension of the denture onto a tooth to provide support &/or prevent over-eruption. Occlusal rests are used on posterior teeth (over either the mesial or distal marginal ridge and fossa) and cingulum rests on anterior teeth. Rests may be wrought or cast; the latter is preferred for strength and fit.

Clasps provide direct retention by engaging the undercut portion of a tooth. The action of a clasp must be resisted either by a non-retentive clasp arm above the maximum bulbosity of the tooth or by a reciprocal connector. Clasps can be classified by their position (occlusally approaching or gingivally approaching) or by their construction and material.

Cast (cobalt chrome) clasps are stiff, easily distorted and liable to #. However, provided they are limited to undercuts of 0.25 mm, the advantage of being able to cast them as an integral part of a denture framework offsets these drawbacks.

Wrought clasps are usually attached by insertion into the acrylic of a saddle. SS is the most commonly used alloy, but gold clasps are more flexible and easily adjusted (and distorted).

The stiffer the wire the smaller the undercut that can be engaged. This can be offset by reducing the diameter of the wire to ↑ flexibility (but ↑ the likelihood of #) or by increasing the length of the clasp arm (e.g. gingivally approaching clasp). Cast cobalt chrome can be too stiff for occlusally approaching clasps on premolar teeth. The actual design used depends upon:

1. Depth of undercut: 0.25 mm—cast cobalt chrome; 0.5 mm—SS wire; <0.75 mm—wrought gold.
2. Position of undercut on tooth and relative to saddle, e.g.:
   - High survey line: gingivally approaching clasp or modify tooth shape by grinding.
   - Diagonal survey line, (a) sloping down from saddle: gingivally or occlusally approaching (ring or recurved) clasp; (b) sloping up from saddle: gingivally or occlusally (circumferential) approaching clasp.
   - Medium survey line: as above.
   - Low survey line: modify tooth shape, e.g. with resin composite.
3. Position of tooth. Gingivally approaching clasps are less conspicuous and are ∴ preferred for anterior teeth.
4. Occlusion: adequate inter-occlusal space should be present or created for a clasp arm to cross a contact point between two natural teeth, to prevent occlusal disruption.
5. Shape of sulcus: frenal attachments and alveolar undercuts may prevent use of gingivally approaching clasps.
6. Periodontal health: reduced periodontal support deserves more flexible clasps to avoid overload.
7. Material of denture base. Cast clasp arms are easily cast as part of the framework but for acrylic dentures wrought clasps are more usual.

Connectors

In addition to joining parts of the denture together, the connector can also contribute to support and retention.

P/- connectors

	Patient tolerance	Indirect retention	Support	Comments
Ant. bar	-	+	-	useful for Kennedy IV
Mid. Bar	+	-	++	C/I torus
Post. Bar	++	+	-	need mucocompression
Ring	-	++	+	
Plate	+	++	++	less hygenic
Horseshoe	+	+	++	useful for multiple saddles

-/P connectors

- Lingual bar should only be used if there is >7 mm between floor of mouth and gingival margin to give 3 mm clearance from gingivae. Does not contribute to indirect retention. Usually cast. C/I if incisors are retroclined. If insufficient space can use sublingual bar.
- Sublingual bar lies horizontally in anterior lingual sulcus, but opinions differ as to patient tolerance. More rigid than lingual bar.
- Lingual plate is well tolerated and provides good support, bracing, and indirect retention if used in conjunction with rests but covers gingival margins. Can be made of cast metal or acrylic.

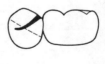

Occlusally approaching three-arm clasp
One arm is the bracing reciprocal arm
One arm is the retentive component
One arm is the occlusal rest

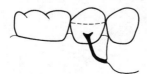

Gingivally approaching T clasp
The two most commonly used types of clasp

- Continuous clasp is really a bar which runs along the cingulae of the lower anterior teeth and is usually used in conjunction with a lingual bar. Poorly tolerated.
- Dental bar is similar to continuous clasp, but of ↑ cross-sectional area and without lingual bar. Useful for teeth with long clinical crowns. Provides support and indirect retention. May not be well tolerated.
- Buccal/labial bar is indicated when the lower incisors are retroclined.

Removable partial denture design

P/P design is carried out after assessment of the patient and with reference to any previous dentures. A set of accurately articulated study models is essential.

Surveying

Objectives:
1. Establish path of insertion.
2. Define those undercuts which may be used to retain denture.
3. Define those undercuts which require blocking out prior to finish.

If the path of insertion is at 90° to the occlusal plane insertion of the denture will be straightforward; however, where the teeth are tilted or few undercuts exist, an angulated path of insertion may be advantageous. Which provides more resistance to displacement during function is controversial.

A survey line can then be marked on the teeth to indicate their maximum bulbosity in the plane of the path of withdrawal. Where possible a proper dental surveyor should be used.

Design

1. Outline saddles   Usually straightforward. If <1/2 tooth width or if in doubt of the need to replace a missing tooth, omit.

2. Plan support   Support can be tooth only, mucosa only, or both. Tooth-borne support (occlusal and cingulum rests) should be used wherever possible, as teeth are better able to withstand occlusal loading and support will not be compromised following resorption. Tooth and mucosa support are inevitable with large or free-end saddles and where plate designs are used. Tissue-only support should be utilized when no suitable teeth are available, and is less damaging in the upper than the lower arch, because of the palatal vault.

Need to assess the role of the denture, length of the saddles, the amount of support required (? denture opposed by natural or artificial teeth), and the potential of remaining teeth to provide support (root area in bone), before a final decision is made.

3. Obtain retention   Retention can be:
Direct   E.g. clasps, guide planes, soft tissue undercuts, or precision attachments. Of these, clasps are the most commonly used. The best arrangement is to use three clasps as far away from each other as possible. Guide planes help to establish a precise path of insertion and withdrawal. Need be only 2–3 mm in length, reducing reliance on clasps.

Indirect   This is derived by placing components so as to resist 'rocking' of the denture around direct retainers, e.g. by the position of clasps and rests and the type of connector. Particularly important with free-end and large anterior saddles.

4. Assess bracing required   Bracing is provided by the connector, maximum saddle extension, and the reciprocal arms of clasps. Elimination of occlusal interferences ↓ need for bracing.

5. *Choose connector*   After consideration of above. Is there space in the occlusion to accommodate the chosen connector? Where possible the connector should be cut away from the gingival margins.

6. *Reassess*   ? as simple as possible ? aesthetic.

Instructions to technician   Should include written details and diagram. Where some confusion may arise over the precise position of a component it may be helpful to mark this directly on the cast.

Some design problems

The lower bilateral free-end saddle (Class I)   This presents a particular problem because of a lack of tooth support and retention distally, small saddle area compared to force applied, and distal leverage on abutment tooth in function (which ↑ with resorption). Possible solutions include:

1. Maximize indirect retention by placing rests and clasps on mesial aspect of the abutment tooth and using plate design.
2. Using a muco-compressive impression of saddle area to ↓ displacement in function. The altered cast technique.
3. Use fewer, smaller teeth and maximize base extension.
4. RPI system for distal abutment teeth. Mesial Rest, distal guiding Plate and mid-buccal I bar. During function the saddle moves tissue-ward and rotates around the mesial rest. The plate and I bar are constructed in such a way as to disengage from the tooth and avoid potentially harmful loading.
5. Stress-breaker design (advantages more theoretical than practical).
6. Use precision attachments (beware of overloading abutments).

Class IV   Can sometimes avoid unsightly clasps anteriorly by the use of:
- A flange engaging a labial alveolar undercut.
- A rotational path of insertion[1] utilizing rigid minor connectors that are rotated into proximal undercuts anteriorly.
- Inter-proximal undercuts, which may allow minimal display of clasps—'hidden clasps'.
- An acrylic spoon denture held in place by the tongue.

Multiple bounded saddles   A horseshoe design, which utilizes guide planes for retention, may be indicated.

---

1 Chow *et al.* 1988 *BDJ* **164** 180.

Clinical stages for removable partial dentures

1. Assessment and treatment plan, p. 336.

2. Take first impressions These are usually taken using alginate in a stock tray. For free-end saddles modify the tray first with compound or silicone putty.

3. Record occlusion If ICP is obvious the occlusion can be recorded conventionally (p. 283) at the same visit as first impressions. If ICP is not obvious, wax record blocks will be required and a separate visit. Where there are no teeth in occlusal contact, the steps involved are the same as for recording the occlusion for F/F (p. 354). If there is an occlusal stop, but insufficient standing teeth to produce a stable relationship of the casts, the procedure is as follows:

- Determine the OVD and mark the position of two index teeth with pencil.
- Define the occlusal plane using the record block on which this is easiest, e.g. tooth to tooth, tooth to retromolar pad.
- Check the record blocks in the mouth, using the mark on the index teeth as a guide, and adjust blocks if necessary.
- Record occlusion with bite-recording paste.
- Check the relationship of the index teeth on the articulated casts corresponds to that in the mouth.

4. Mounted casts are surveyed and denture designed, p. 344.

5. Tooth preparation may be required to:
- Accommodate rest seats. Rests need to be >1 mm for strength, ∴ if insufficient room in occlusion to accommodate this bulk, tooth reduction is required.
- Establish guide planes.
- Modify unfavourable survey line, e.g. ↓ bulbosity.
- Increase retention, e.g. by the addition of resin composite to create undercuts. (**NB** use microfine type to ↓ abrasion of clasp.)

6. Record second impressions using a special tray. Alginate is the most commonly used material, but elastomers are preferable for deep undercuts. It is helpful to have a wax try-in before the framework is made. This enables you to confirm tooth position so that the retentive elements for the acrylic are placed appropriately.

7. Try-in of framework
- Check extension, adaptation, and position of clasp, and rests. If casting does not fit, use of correcting fluid may reveal which areas to relieve.
- Check upper and lower separately for OVD and occlusion, and then together.
- Major faults: repeat second impressions.
- Minor faults: adjust at finish.
- Re-record occlusion, if required.
- Select tooth mould and shade.
- Altered cast technique, if required.

8. Try-in of waxed denture
- Check position of denture teeth.
- Check flange extensions/thickness.
- Check OVD and occlusion.
- Check aesthetics with patient and only proceed when patient is satisfied.
- Prescribe post-dam relief areas and management of undercuts.

9. Finish   Once any fitting surface roughness is eliminated, the dentures are tried in separately, adjusting undercuts and contacts as required. The extension, occlusion, and articulation are then adjusted if necessary. Give the patient written and verbal instructions, and a further appointment.

Rebasing P/P

Acrylic mucosa-borne dentures can be rebased at the chairside with self-cure materials, but difficulty may be experienced in removing the denture in the presence of undercuts, and the materials are generally inferior to the original denture base. Alternatively, P/P can be rebased in the laboratory by means of a technique similar to that used for F/F (p. 360). Alternatively, make a new denture. For cast metal dentures an impression can be recorded of saddle area using an elastomer or ZOE, whilst holding denture by the framework. In all cases care must be taken to avoid the introduction of occlusal errors, e.g. ↑ OVD.

Immediate complete dentures

When the remaining teeth have a poor prognosis management depends upon whether the patient is already a partial denture wearer or not.

Rx alternatives for patients with no previous denture experience
- Extract remaining teeth, wait 6 months for resorption to slow, and then construct F/F dentures. A recipe for disaster!
- Extract majority of posterior teeth leaving sufficient only to maintain OVD and occlusal relationship, and then make immediate complete dentures when resorption has slowed.
- Provide partial denture and allow patient to adapt before progressing to an immediate complete denture. The best solution.

Rx alternatives for partial denture wearer
- A 'creeping partial denture' to which teeth are added as required. This allows a gradual progression towards edentulousness and is preferable for the elderly patient.
- Immediate complete denture. This has the advantage that the form and position of the natural teeth can be copied and is said to promote better healing and reduce resorption, but frequent adjustments and early replacement are necessary.
- Overdenture (p. 370).

Types of immediate complete denture
- *Flanged* Either full or part (extended 1 mm beyond maximum bulbosity of ridge).
- *Open face* No flange, artificial teeth sit over (or just into) the socket of natural predecessor.

Flanged dentures are preferable as they afford better retention and make subsequent rebasing easier. However, where a deep labial undercut exists into which it would be impossible to extend a flange, the choice is either surgical reduction or an open-face denture. Most patients choose the latter.

Clinical procedures
1. *Assessment* Warn the patient about the effects of resorption and the need for early rebasing/replacement.
2. *Primary impressions* (as for P/P, p. 346).
3. *Secondary impressions* in alginate or silicone.
4. *Recording occlusion.* Where there are sufficient posterior teeth remaining a wax wafer should suffice, and this can be taken at the same visit as impressions are recorded. Otherwise, record blocks will be required.
5. *Try-in* This will be limited to those teeth that are already missing. Check fit, extension, and stability, etc. In addition, need to prescribe:
   – type of flange required;
   – any proposed changes in position of anterior artificial teeth compared to natural teeth.
6. *Extraction* of remaining teeth as atraumatically as possible.
7. *Finish* Repeated removal and insertion of the denture should be avoided, therefore adjustments should be limited to making the patient

comfortable. They should be instructed not to remove the denture before the review appointment in 24 h.

- *Review.* The fitting and occlusal surfaces are adjusted as required. If dentures are unretentive they will require temporary reline (see below).
- *Recall.* Regular inspection of immediate dentures is important as rapid bone resorption means that they will require rebasing early. However, this should be deferred, if feasible, for at least 3 months after the extractions. A possible regimen is 1 week, 1 month, 3 months, 9 months, and then yearly.

Laboratory procedures These are similar to F/F except that the plaster teeth are removed and the cast trimmed, before final processing.

Surgical procedures, p. 386 and 426.

Problems

- *Denture unretentive* Use a temporary reline material (replaced regularly) to tide patient over initial 3 months and then reline with heat-cure acrylic.
- *Gross occlusal error* Adjust occlusal surface of one denture until even contact attained. This denture can then be replaced after initial resorption has occurred.

Principles of complete dentures

Retention   The resistance of a denture to displacement. Dependent upon: **1** peripheral seal; **2** contact area between denture and tissues; **3** close fit; **4** viscosity/volume of saliva. Neuromuscular control has more to do with stability than retention.

Stability   The ability of denture to resist displacing forces during function. Influenced by forces acting on polished and occlusal surfaces, as well as the form of the supporting tissues.

Neutral zone   The area where the muscular displacing forces are in balance.

Ways to optimize retention and stability

- Maximum extension of denture base (as far as the surrounding musculature will allow). The upper denture should extend distally over the tuberosities and onto the compressible tissue just anterior to the vibrating line on the palate. The lower denture should extend the full depth and width of the lingual pouch, and halfway across the retromolar pad. **NB** Over-extension will result in a denture that is displaced in function.
- As close an adaptation of denture base to mucosa as possible, to maximize the surface tension effects of saliva.
- Placement of the teeth in the neutral zone. More important in -/F. The better retention of F/- often allows some latitude in this respect.
- Correct shape of the polished surfaces so that muscle action tends to re-seat the denture.
- A good border seal. This is achieved by ensuring that the flanges fill the entire sulcus width and by placing a post-dam on compressible tissue.
- Balanced occlusion free from interfering contacts.

Patient assessment   This should include:
- Previous dental history, including the age of the patient, when they became edentulous, number and degree of success of previous dentures, and their opinion of present F/F.
- EO examination of skeletal pattern and biological age.
- IO examination for signs of any pathology, and an assessment of ridge form, compressibility of mucosa, tongue size, tonicity of the lips, and the volume and viscosity of saliva.
- An evaluation of their present F/F. What to copy and what to correct.
- Personality.

Common denture faults   These are, in order of decreasing prevalence:[1]
- Lack of freeway space.
- Failure to reproduce closely enough the features of previous successful dentures.
- Occlusal errors.
- Incorrect adaptation and extension.

1 R. Yemm 1985 *BDJ* **159** 304.

Impressions for complete dentures

▶ Tissues must be healthy before final impressions are recorded. If necessary use tissue conditioner in present F/F (p. 360).

Classically, two sets of impressions are recorded of the edentulous mouth. The purpose of the first is to record sufficient information for a special tray to be made in which to record the second or master impression. In practice, many use the first impression recorded in a stock tray for construction of the denture. With a careful technique this may suffice for some patients but, especially for those with retention problems, second impressions in a special tray are advisable.

First impressions

These are recorded using an (edentulous) stock tray, and alginate, elastomer (both preferable for undercut or flabby ridges), or composition. A line should be marked on the impression to indicate to the technician the desired extension of the special tray. In the upper, the posterior limit should be the hamular notches and the vibrating line, and in the lower the retromolar pads.

Special trays can be made in self-cure or light-cure acrylic. The space left for the impression depends upon the material to be used: ZOE = 0.5 mm; elastomer = 0.5–1.5 mm (depending on viscosity); plaster = 2 mm; alginate = 3 mm. For trays with >1 mm space use greenstick stops to aid positioning.

Second impressions

These aim to record the maximum denture-bearing area and to develop an effective border seal the functional width and depth of the sulcus. The special tray should be modified by reducing any over-extension and the peripheries adapted by the addition of greenstick tracing compound. It is important that the trays are not perforated and that you can demonstrate a peripheral seal with the upper tray before you take your impression. Gently manipulate the patient's soft tissues and ask them to slightly protrude their tongue to imitate functional movements.

Muco-compressive versus muco-static A muco-compressive impression technique is sometimes advocated to give a wider distribution of loading during function and to compensate for the differing compressibility of the denture-bearing area, thus preventing # due to flexion. ZOE or composition are used. However, dentures made by this method are less well retained at rest, which is the greater proportion of time. Alginate and plaster are said to be more muco-static. Tissue adaptation following a period of use probably reduces the clinical difference between the two techniques.

Special techniques

Neutral zone impression technique This is used for recording the neutral zone in patients with limited natural retention for -/F.
• Record second impressions and occlusion.
• A fully extended acrylic baseplate is made on the lower cast, with wire loops added which do not extend above occlusal plane.

- The upper trial denture or record block is inserted.
- Tissue conditioner is placed on the baseplate and around loops, and inserted.
- The patient is asked to swallow, purse lips, and say 'Ooh' and 'Eee'.
- The impression is removed and trimmed until it can be fitted on to the articulator to replace the lower occlusal rim.
- A mould of the impression is made into which wax is poured.
- The wax is cut away so that each denture tooth can be positioned within the zone recorded to make the trial denture. The polished surfaces should replicate the impression.

Flabby ridge Classically occurs under a F/- opposed by natural lower teeth. If mild, then an impression recorded with alginate or elastomer in a tray perforated over the flabby area may suffice. For more severe cases a two-stage technique is required, using a special tray with a window cut out over the flabby tissue. First, an impression is recorded in the tray with ZOE and the paste trimmed away from the flabby area. This is then re-seated and low-viscosity elastomer or impression plaster placed into the window to complete the impression. **NB** Combination type cases should have the dentures constructed on a semi-adjustable articulator to minimize occlusal displacing forces

Functional impression Tissue conditioner is placed inside the patient's existing denture. After several days of wear a functional impression is produced.

Common impression problems and faults

- A feather edge indicates under-extension. This can be corrected by the addition of greenstick to the tray and repeating.
- Tray border shows through impression material. The tray should be reduced in the area of over-extension and the impression repeated.
- Air blows. If small, can be filled in with a little soft wax. If large, retake the impression.
- Tray not centred. This is often at least partially due to using too much material so that it is difficult to see what is where. Remember to line up the tray handle with the patient's nose (except for ex-boxers).
- Retching. A calm and confident manner is necessary for successful impressions. Gain the patient's confidence by attempting the lower first and use a fast-setting, viscous material. Distraction techniques may help, e.g. wriggling the toes on the left foot and the fingers of the right hand at the same time (the patient, not the operator!).
- Patient with dry mouth: ZOE is C/I; use elastomer instead.
- Areas where tray shows through in otherwise good impression. Can be overcome by prescribing a tin-foil relief when dentures being processed.

Recording the occlusion for complete dentures

When recording the occlusion the aim is to provide the technician with information for constructing trial dentures, including:

Vertical dimension   The FWS is the space between the occlusal surfaces of the teeth when the mandible is in the rest position. In the majority of patients it is 2–4mm. The OVD for an edentulous patient can ∴ be determined by measuring their resting face height and subtracting a FWS. Resting face height is assessed using:

- A Willis gauge, to measure the distance between the base of nose and the underside of the chin. Is only accurate to ±1mm.
- Spring dividers, to measure the distance between a dot placed on both the chin and the tip of the patient's nose. This method is less popular with patients and is C/I for bearded gentlemen (or ladies!).
- The patient's appearance and speech.

Position of the occlusal plane   This should be placed so that ~1–2mm (↓ with age) of tooth are visible below the patient's upper lip at rest. The occlusal plane should lie midway between the ridges parallel to the inter-pupillary and the alatragal lines. At rest the tongue should rise just above the lower occlusal plane posteriorly.

Horizontal jaw relationship   Record the more reproducible RCP. In the natural dentition, ICP is ~1mm forward of RCP, ∴ some prosthetists advise adjusting the finished dentures to allow the patient to slide comfortably between the two positions.

Position of the anterior and posterior teeth Ideally,   the artificial teeth should lie in the space occupied by the natural dentition. The extent to which it is possible to compensate for a Class II or III malocclusion depends upon the retention afforded by the ridges. In the natural dentition the upper incisors lie ~10mm anterior to the incisive papilla. With resorption this comes to lie on the ridge crest, ∴ the artificial teeth should be placed labial and buccal to the ridge, to give adequate lip support and a naso-labial angle of ~90°.

Mould and shade of artificial teeth   Posterior teeth should be narrow to ↑ masticatory efficiency. Low cusped teeth are preferred, but cuspless teeth are useful for patients with poor natural retention or a 'wandering' ICP. When considering the colour, mould, and arrangement of the anterior teeth the patient's age, facial appearance, and most importantly their opinion, must be taken into account. If you disagree about the suitability of their choice, document it.

Type of articulator to be used for setting-up the teeth   Most textbooks advocate adjustable or average value articulators for F/F dentures. However, most dentures are made on simple hinge articulators to the satisfaction of the majority of patients, probably because they are able to adapt to the occlusion that results. An average value type will give some degree of balanced articulation which can then be refined in the mouth and will avoid the introduction of occlusal interferences, and is the preferred method.

Practical procedures

The occlusion is recorded using wax rims mounted on rigid acrylic or shellac bases. A heated wax trimmer, or a plaster knife and a bunsen burner, are required to adjust the rims. As head posture can affect FWS, position the patient so that the Frankfort plane is horizontal.

1. Check fit of bases. If poor, can either repeat second impressions, or take a ZOE or low viscosity elastomer impression with the base and proceed.
2. Adjust upper record block to give adequate lip support.
3. Trim occlusal plane of upper rim.
4. Trim lower record block to obtain correct lip support and bucco-lingual position of posterior teeth.
5. Adjust lower rim so that it meets upper evenly in RCP, with 2–4 mm of FWS.
6. Mark centre lines.
7. Locate rims in RCP, e.g. with bite-recording paste.
8. Prescribe mould and shade of artificial teeth for try-in.
9. Consider using a facebow to mount the maxillary cast on the articulator

Common pitfalls

- Inaccuracies caused by poorly fitting bases.
- Rims contacting prematurely posteriorly and flipping-up anteriorly, or vice versa.
- Failure to provide adequate FWS. This is less likely to occur if the rest position is recorded with only one denture or rim in position.
- Attempting to correct too much when replacing old worn dentures and exceeding the adaptive capacity of the patient.

Trial insertion of complete dentures

Trial dentures are constructed by setting-up the prescribed teeth in wax on acrylic or shellac bases. Both the dentist and patient must be satisfied before the dentures are processed in acrylic.

Clinical procedures

Check the trial dentures
On and off the articulator. Comparison with the patient's existing dentures is helpful to see if the features to be copied or modified have been successfully incorporated.
- Singly in the mouth. To check extension, stability, and the position of the teeth relative to the soft tissues.
- Together in mouth. Examine vertical dimension, occlusion, aesthetics, and phonetics ('S' sound will be affected by an ↑ or ↓ FWS).

Seek the patient's opinion   Some advocate getting patients to sign an acceptance slip before going to finish.

Prepare post-dam   This should be placed just anterior to the vibrating line on the palate, which can be assessed by asking patient to say 'Aah'. The degree of compressibility of the tissues is assessed and the depth of the post-dam cut accordingly (usually ~1 mm). The post-dam is prepared on the upper cast with a wax knife in the shape of a cupid's bow.

Complete prescription to the technician This should include:
- Any changes in posterior tooth position or anterior tooth arrangement.
- For fibrous undercuts >4 mm and bony undercuts >2 mm, decide whether they are to be plastered out or the flange thickened for adjustment at finish.
- Tin-foiling for relief of hard or nodular areas, if required.
- Gingival colour and contour.
- Denture base material. This is usually heat-cure acrylic; however, metal bases are indicated for patients with a history of fractured dentures.
- Identification marker, which is preferably legible.

Common problems and possible solutions

- Over-extension of flanges. Reduce.
- Under-extension of flanges. Try a temporary wax addition to flange first, to check effect of extending it. If this is satisfactory a new impression is required.
- Teeth outwith neutral zone. Remove offending teeth and replace with wax which can be trimmed until correct.
- Incorrect OVD. If too small, can increase by adding wax to the occlusal surfaces of teeth, but if too large, will need to replace lower teeth with wax and re-record OVD.
- Occlusal discrepancy or anterior open bite or posterior open bite. Replace lower posterior teeth with wax and re-record OVD.
- Too little of upper anterior teeth visible. Reset anterior teeth to correct position and ask lab to adjust occlusal plane accordingly.
- Too much of upper anterior teeth showing. The effect of reducing the length of the incisors can be judged by colouring incisal region with a black wax pencil and then indicating desired change in position to lab.

- Inadequate lip support. An increase in support can be assessed by adding wax to the labial aspect of the upper try-in.

A new try-in will be required if large errors are being corrected or if any doubt still exists about the occlusion.

Fitting complete dentures

Some adjustment of completed dentures is inevitable following processing. On average, a 0.5 mm increase in height occurs and a slight shift in tooth contact posteriorly. The main steps are:

Adjustment of fitting surface   First, smooth any roughness and if necessary gradually reduce the bulk of the flanges in areas of undercut until the denture can be easily inserted without compromising retention.

Check occlusion   The vertical dimension of the dentures is maintained by contact between the upper palatal and lower buccal cusps, ∴ adjustment of these should be avoided if possible.
1. Get patient to occlude and check contact with articulating paper. If contact uneven, or heavy contacts seen, adjust the fossae.
2. For cusped teeth only, place articulating paper between occlusal surfaces and ask patient to make small lateral movements and adjust Buccal Upper and Lower Lingual (BULL rule) cusps only to remove any interferences.
3. Remove any interferences to protrusive movements.
4. Balancing contacts are desirable, but not essential unless they can be established easily by minor adjustments to working side contacts. Some authorities suggest providing even occlusal contact only at the time of fitting, allowing the patient to adapt to their new dentures before trying to achieve balanced articulation.

Advice to the patient   Verbal and written instructions should be given.
- Most patients take some time to adapt to their new dentures. During this time a softer diet is advisable.
- If pain is experienced the patient should try to continue wearing their dentures and return for adjustment as soon as possible so that affected areas can easily be seen.
- Although patients should be encouraged not to wear their dentures at night, adaptation may be speeded up if they are worn full-time for the first 1–2 weeks.
- When the dentures are not being worn they should be stored in water to prevent them drying out and warping. Plastic denture boxes are cheap, and safer than a glass of water at the bedside.
- Cleaning, p. 362.

Review   The patient should be seen 1–2 weeks after fitting to ease the dentures and adjust the occlusion. Localization of the cause of any irritation due to a flaw on the fitting surface can be helped by:
- Pressure relief cream which is painted onto the fitting surface of the denture.
- Indelible pencil, or denture fixative powder mixed with zinc oxide, which is applied carefully to area thought to be responsible and the denture inserted. On removal the mark will have been transferred to the adjacent mucosa and should correspond with the damaged area.

If there is no obvious cause relating to the fitting surface remember that occlusal faults can cause displacement and mucosal trauma, and an excessive OVD is a common cause of generalized soreness under -/F (p. 364).
Stress the importance of regular review of all patients with dentures.

Denture maintenance

▶ Review patients with F/F annually. Regular maintenance will help prevent damage due to ill-fitting dentures and will ↑ the likelihood of early detection of oral pathology.

Problems caused by lack of aftercare of F/F As a result of resorption all dentures become progressively ill-fitting, leading to loss of retention and stability. Movement of dentures in function may result in:

- Resorption.
- Predisposition to candidal infection.
- Denture irritation hyperplasia, p. 426.
- Inflammatory papillary hyperplasia of the palate.

All of these are exacerbated by wear of the occlusal surfaces.

Rebasing

The terms rebasing and relining are commonly used interchangeably. Strictly speaking relining is replacement of the fitting surface (e.g. with a temporary material) and rebasing is replacement of most or all of the denture base.

Rebasing is indicated where the only feature of F/F that requires improvement is the fitting surface; otherwise consider replacement F/F using copy method. For rebasing the material of choice is heat-cure acrylic (p. 696), but this necessitates the patient being without their dentures while the addition is being made. Self-cure acrylic applied at the chairside appears attractive, but its properties are inferior. For a heat-cure rebase, a wash impression (ZOE or low viscosity elastomer) must be recorded inside the denture.

Technique To avoid an ↑ in OVD, record the impression for one denture at a time.

- Check occlusion and adjust if required. Note OVD.
- Remove undercuts from fitting surface.
- Correct extension and place post-dam in greenstick.
- Apply impression material and insert in mouth. Get patient to close into contact with opposing denture. Check OVD and occlusion.
- Remove and examine impression; if unsatisfactory (or if in doubt) repeat.

An alternative method for inflamed tissues is to record a functional impression (p. 353) over several days with a tissue conditioner, in which case the resulting impression needs to be cast immediately.

Tissue conditioners

These are resilient materials which give a more even distribution of loading and thus promote tissue recovery. They are particularly useful where ill-fitting dentures have caused trauma, as it is important to allow the tissues to recover before impressions for replacement dentures or a rebase are taken.

Technique Relieve any areas of pressure on the fitting surface and reduce any over-extension. A minimum thickness of 2 mm is required and the material should not be left for > 1 week. Repeated applications may be necessary. Crushed Nystatin tablets can be incorporated in the powder of Viscogel prior to mixing, if candidal infection is present.

Soft linings are indicated for
- Older patients with a thin atrophic mucosa. Usually for -/F.
- Following prosthetic surgery.
- To utilize soft tissue undercuts for ↑ retention, e.g. following hemimaxillectomy, clefts.

It is wise to make a new denture first in acrylic and adjust the occlusion, before placing soft lining. A minimum thickness of 2 mm is required, which may significantly weaken a lower denture necessitating placement of a metal strengthener on the lingual aspect. No material is ideal and soft linings are best avoided (p. 698).

Cleaning dentures

When new dentures are fitted the importance of regular, thorough cleaning with soap, water, and a brush to prevent the build-up of plaque, stain, and calculus should be emphasized. Unfortunately, few patients are sufficiently diligent, due in part to being conditioned by advertising, to expect to use a denture cleaner.

Advise patients to clean their dentures over a basin of water to act as a safety net.

Formulation	Active ingredients	Problems
Powder	Abrasives, e.g. calcium carbonate	Abrasion
Paste	Abrasives + eugenol	Abrasion + crazing
(Dentu-creme)	Abrasive + phenol oil	Abrasion + sensitivity
Hypochlorite (Dentural)	Sodium hypochlorite	Can corrode metal
Effervescent (Steradent)	Dissolves to give alkaline peroxide solution	Doubts about effectiveness
Dilute acids (Denclen)	3–5% hydrochloric acid or 5–10% phosphoric acid	Can corrode metal
Enzymatic	Proteolytic enzymes	Not widely available

Practical tips

Hypochlorite solutions are effective for acrylic dentures when used overnight, but if used with *hot* water are liable to cause bleaching, ∴ warn patient.[1] The peroxide cleaners are popular but are ineffective if used for only 15–30 min as the manufacturers advise.

	Avoid	Use
Viscogel	Acids, alkaline peroxide	Hypochlorite
Molloplast	Acids, alkaline peroxide	Hypochlorite
Coe-comfort	Hypochlorite, alkaline peroxide	Soap + water
Metal denture	Hypochlorite	Alkaline peroxide
Any denture	Household bleach	

1 C. A. Crawford 1986 *J Dent* **14** 258.

Denture problems and complaints

The most common complaints are of pain &/or looseness, which can be due to denture errors or patient factors. The latter should be foreseen and the patient warned in advance of the limitations of dentures. The wise prosthetist will tend to overestimate the difficulty of providing successful dentures. Unless the cause is immediately obvious, e.g. a flaw on the fitting surface, a systematic examination of the fitting, and polished and occlusal surfaces (including the jaw relationship) should be carried out.

Pain This can be due to a variety of causes, including roughness of the fitting surface, errors in the occlusion, lack of FWS, a bruxing habit, a retained root, or other pathology. Forward or lateral displacement of a denture due to a premature contact can lead to inflammation of the ridge on the lingual or lateral aspect, respectively. With continued resorption bony ridges become prominent and the mental foramina exposed, which can lead to localized areas of specific pain.

Pain from an individual tooth on P/P
- Excessive load &/or traumatic occlusion.
- Leverage due to unstable denture.
- Clasp arm too tight.
- Inadequate lining under amalgam restoration failing to insulate against a galvanic couple with metal denture.

Looseness This more commonly affects the lower than the upper denture.

Denture faults	**Patient factors**
Incorrect peripheral extension	Inadequate volume or amount of saliva
Teeth not in neutral zone	Poor ridge form
Unbalanced articulation	↓ adaptive skills, e.g. elderly patient
Polished surfaces unsatisfactory	

Burning mouth This can be due to: **1** local causes: e.g. ↑ OVD or sensitivity to acrylic monomer, or be unrelated to the denture (e.g. irritant mouth washes); **2** systemic causes: e.g. the menopause, deficiency states, cancerophobia, xerostomia.

Speech

Patient's complaint	Possible cause
Difficulty with f, v.	Incisors too far palatally
Difficulty with d, s, t	Alteration of palatal contour
	Incorrect overjet and overbite
s becomes th	Incisors too far palatally
	Palate too thick
Whistling	Palate vault too high behind incisors
Clicking teeth	↑ OVD
	Lack of retention

Cheek biting Check first that teeth are in neutral zone. If satisfactory, ↓ buccal 'overjet', i.e. reduce buccal surface of lower molars (provided normal bucco-lingual relationship).

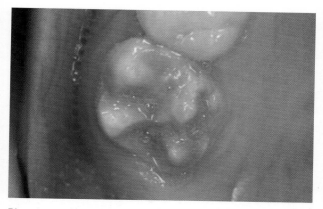

Plate 1(a) Upper first permanent molar in a patient with molar incisor hypomineralization, prior to restoration.

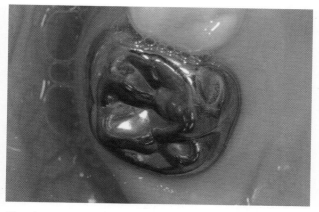

Plate 1(b) The same tooth following placement of a stainless steel crown.

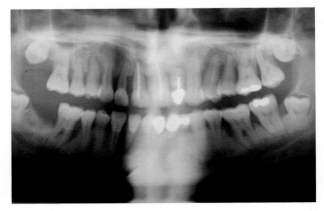

Plate 2 DPT of a diabetic smoker aged 35 with chronic periodontitis.

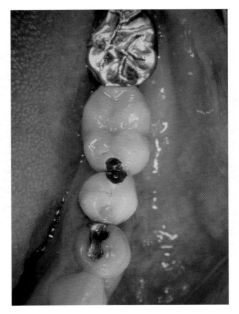

Plate 3 Fixed movable bridge replacing the lower left first permanent molar.

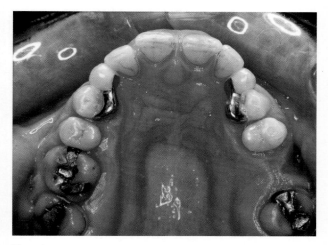

Plate 4 Adhesive cantilever bridgework replacing missing upper canines.

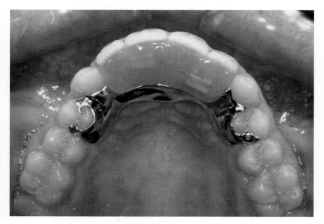

Plate 5 Sectional partial denture.

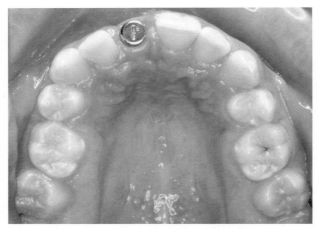

Plate 6 Implant placed to replace the upper right central incisor.

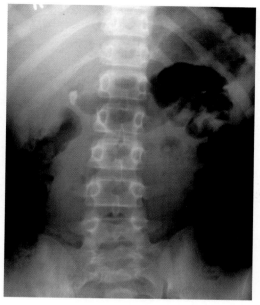

Plate 7 Chest X-ray showing inhaled tooth. This is a mandatory investigation for an inhaled tooth. Refer immediately for removal.

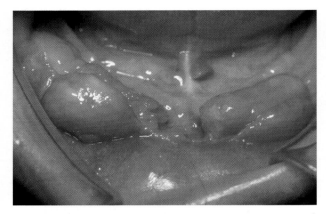

Plate 8 'Denture' hyperplasia. These soft irritation induced masses are benign.

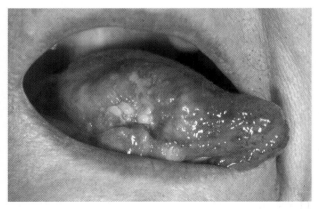

Plate 9 Squamous cell carcinoma of tongue. This has a typical appearance *and* a typical 'feel'. Always palpate the lesion.

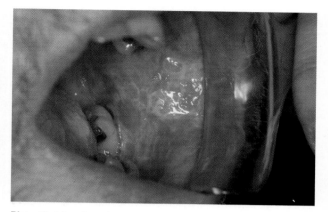

Plate 10 Lichen planus showing a typical reticular (lacy, white lines) pattern.

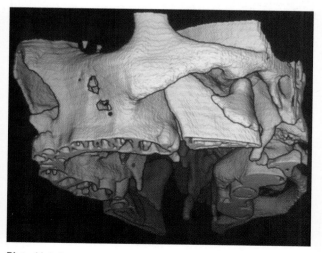

Plate 11 3-dimensional scan of fractured condyle showing overlap and displacement.

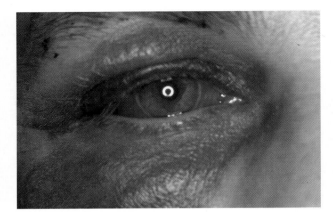

Plate 12 Black eye. The combination of circumorbital ecchymosis with medial *and* lateral subconjunctival haemorrhage means this is a much more substantial injury than it first appears.

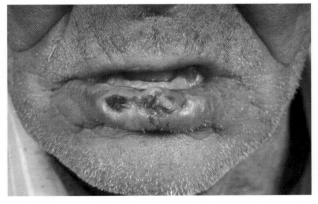

Plate 13 Squamous cell carcinoma of lip showing a typical position and appearance.

Retching
- Map out extent of sensitive area on palate using a ball-ended instrument and firm pressure, and check extension of denture.
- Palateless dentures may be a solution, but their retention is poor.
- Training dentures. These can take the form of a simple palate to which teeth are added incrementally, starting with the incisors.
- Implants (p. 428) and a fixed prosthesis.

The grossly resorbed lower ridge   Resorption is progressive with time, which is a good argument for avoiding rendering young patients edentulous. The mandible resorbs more quickly than the maxilla, which exacerbates the problem of retention for -/F. Management is dependent upon the severity of the problem and the patient's biological age.
- Minimizing destabilizing forces upon the lower denture, e.g. (1) maximum extension of denture base; (2) ↓ number and width of teeth; (3) ↑ FWS; (4) lowering occlusal plane.
- Neutral zone impression technique (p. 352).
- Surgery (p. 426).
- Implants (p. 428).

Recurrent fracture   Apart from carelessness, this is usually caused by occlusal faults or fatigue of the acrylic due to continual stressing by small forces. Flexing of the denture can occur with flabby ridges, palatal tori, and following resorption. Notching of a denture, e.g. relief for a prominent frenum, can also predispose to #. Treatment depends upon the aetiology, but in some cases provision of a metal plate or a cast-metal strengthener may be necessary.

Candida and dentures

Candida is a common oral commensal. It becomes pathogenic if the environment favours its proliferation (e.g. dentures, antibiotic alteration of the bacterial flora) or the host's defences are compromised.

Denture stomatitis

Also known as denture sore mouth, a misnomer because the condition is usually symptomless. Classically, seen as redness of the palate under a F/- denture, with petechial and whitish areas. 90% of cases due to *Candida albicans*, 9% to other candida, and < 1% to other organisms, e.g. *Klebsiella* spp.

Incidence   A common condition, having been reported in 30–60% of patients wearing F/F. It affects F more commonly than M, in a ratio of 4:1, and usually affects the upper denture-bearing area only.

Aetiology is still not completely understood.
- Infection with *Candida* spp.
- Poor denture hygiene.
- Night-time wear of dentures.
- Trauma is often cited as a contributing factor to denture stomatitis, BUT
  – it occurs more commonly under F/- than -/F;
  – it can affect patients wearing F/- only;
  – it is also found under well-fitting orthodontic appliances.
- Systemic factors can predispose to candida infection, e.g. iron and vitamin deficiency, steroids, drugs which cause xerostomia, and endocrine abnormalities.
- A high sugar intake provides substrate for candida to multiply. It has been postulated that the upper denture-bearing area is more commonly affected because it is related to the more serous nature of saliva from the submandibular glands and the poorer fit of -/F, which allows saliva to reach the underlying mucosa more easily.

Management
- Leave dentures out. Though not a realistic solution to most patients, they should be encouraged to remove their dentures at night.
- Improved denture hygiene, e.g. brushing fitting surface and soaking in hypochlorite cleanser.
- Reduce sugar intake.
- Antifungals (p. 628). Nystatin suspension 100 000 units/ml, 1 ml qds (**NB** pastilles contain sugar) or Amphotericin suspension 100 mg/ml, 1 ml qds are the first choice. 2% Miconazole gel is more expensive and should ∴ be reserved for patients with candida which is unresponsive to other agents, or associated with angular cheilitis.
- If suspect systemic factors exacerbating condition, refer to GMP.
- Coexisting papillary hyperplasia of palate may need surgical reduction.

Angular cheilitis,   p. 438.

Denture copying

Successful function with complete dentures depends to a marked degree upon the patient's ability to control them. This ability is learnt during a period of denture use. When replacement dentures become necessary, it is helpful if the new appliances require as little adaptation as possible to the existing skills. This is generally considered to be particularly important for the older patient. Not only may skills have been developed over a long period, but also the ability to relearn may be diminished. So-called denture copying techniques provide a more reliable method for provision of replacements.

Treatment planning

Before undertaking treatment it is essential to decide which features of the previous dentures are satisfactory, and which require modification, and by how much. Consider:

- Fitting surface—if this is the only feature that requires improvement, then rebasing is a possibility.
- Polished surface shapes.
- Occlusal surface, jaw relationship, OVD. The effect of an increase in OVD can be assessed by self-cure addition to the existing dentures, but remember that this irreversibly alters them.
- Anterior tooth size, arrangement, relation to lips.
- Posterior tooth mould and arch width (relation to tongue and cheeks).

Copying complete dentures

A number of techniques have been described. They vary in the materials used, and these in turn affect the acceptability of laboratory work, and the clinical freedom to incorporate 'corrections'. In general, copies of the old appliances are used as substitutes for record blocks, and as special trays. A typical method involves the following stages:[1]

1. Clinic

- Correct under-extension with greenstick tracing compound.
- Record impressions with silicone putty of polished surface and teeth, using large disposable tray. Complete mould with second mix of putty to record fit surface (use a separating medium—Vaseline or, better, emulsion hand cream).
- Open mould, clean dentures, and return to patient.
- Send putty moulds to laboratory.

2. Laboratory

- Fabricate self-cure acrylic baseplates on the silicone model of the fit surface.
- Pour wax into remaining space.
- After cooling remove completed copy, cut off sprues, and polish.

3. Clinic

- Employ the copies ('replica record blocks') to record required changes in denture shapes (see treatment planning), by adding or removing wax.

1 R. Yemm 1991 *Int Dent J* **41** 233.

- Record working impressions in low viscosity silicone *with adhesive* to aid retention on base.
- Record jaw relationship with 'bite recording paste'.
- Select shade/moulds for new teeth.

4. Laboratory
- Cast impressions and articulate.
- Set-up, cutting away modified replica rims to substitute new teeth (rather like setting up an immediate denture!).
- Wax-up, including borders defined by working impressions.

5. Clinic
- Try-in stage.

6. Laboratory
- Finishing stages as normal.

7. Clinic
- Normal insertion stage (and subsequent review).

Other methods use alternative materials (e.g. alginate for impressions of existing dentures, wax, and shellac to form the copy dentures). Choice will depend on acceptability to both clinic and laboratory. In no instance, however, is an all-wax copy regarded as being acceptable, since rigidity is inadequate for use as an impression tray.

Copying partial dentures for immediate dentures[1]

In patients with successful P/P, for whom extraction of the remaining teeth is planned, the transition to complete dentures can be facilitated by using a copy technique.

Clinic 1 Correct under-extended flanges with greenstick and then take impressions of the dentures with putty in stock trays (see F/F technique). Record an alginate impression of the opposing arch, if no denture is planned for that arch.

Lab 1 Wax/shellac or acrylic replica of partial denture is constructed.

Clinic 2 Use the replica denture to develop the prescription and then record a wash impression inside the base with a light-bodied silicone. Record the occlusion using bite registration paste. Finally, take an overall impression in a stock tray with the modified replica denture *in situ*.

Lab 2 The impression is cast and used as a base for articulating the wax replica with the cast of the opposing arch. The teeth prescribed are then set up, and the wash impression retained in the replica, for the try-in.

Try-in and Finish as for complete immediate dentures, p. 348.

1 J. R. Drummond 1983 *BDJ* **155** 297.

Overdentures

An overdenture (OD) derives support from one or more abutment teeth by completely enclosing them beneath its fitting surface. It can be a partial or complete denture.

Advantages

- Alveolar bone preservation around the retained tooth.
- Improved retention, stability, and support.
- Preservation of proprioception via PDL.
- Improved crown to root ratio, which ↓ damaging lateral forces.
- ↑ masticatory force.
- Additional retention possible using attachments.
- Aids transition from P/P to F/F.

Disadvantages

- RCT probably required.
- To avoid excessive bulk in region of retained tooth, denture base may need to be thinned, which ↑ likelihood of #.
- ↑ maintenance for both patient and dentist.

Indications

- Motivated patient with good oral hygiene.
- Because of ↓ retention and stability of -/F and ↑ rate of mandibular resorption, ODs are particularly useful for -/F or free-end saddle.
- Cleft lip and palate.
- Hypodontia.
- Severe toothwear.

Choosing abutment teeth

- Ideally: bilateral, symmetrical with a minimum of one tooth space between them.
- Order of preference: canines, molars, premolars, incisors.
- Healthy attached gingiva, adequate periodontal support (> 1/2 root in bone), and no or limited mobility.
- Is RCT required and if so is it feasible?

Preparation of abutment teeth

Alternatives include:
1. Removal of undercuts only.
2. Preparation of crown for thimble/telescopic gold coping.
3. RCT, tooth cut to dome shape, and access cavity restored with amalgam or an adhesive restoration.
4. RCT and gold coping over root face.
5. RCT and precision attachment.

Precision attachments[1] are useful for ↑ retention of dentures or bridges, especially in cases with tissue loss (e.g. trauma or CLP), but they ↑ loading on abutment teeth, and are expensive and difficult to rebase and repair. Usually of two parts, which are matched to fit together. One part is

1 H. W. Preiskel 1984 *Precision Attachments in Prosthodontics*, Quintessence.

attached to the abutment tooth and the other to the denture. A variety of attachments are available, including stud/anchor (e.g. Rotherman eccentric clip), bar (e.g. Dolder), and magnets.

Since precision attachments require the highest technical skill and are highly dependent on patient and professional maintenance, it is wise to first use a basic OD and then reassess the need for additional retention. Hybrid dentures are partial dentures that utilize precision attachments (either intra- or extracoronal) on the abutment teeth for retention. Implants which are inserted in edentulous areas can be used with a precision attachment to increase retention.

Clinical procedures

1. Assessment (clinical examination, study models, radiographs, etc.).
2. RCT if required.

If abutment preparation is limited to crown reduction:

3. The steps involved are as for immediate dentures, with the abutment teeth reduced less on cast than is planned clinically. At the visit during which the final dentures are to be fitted, the abutment teeth are prepared and the dentures relined with self-cure acrylic to improve their adaptation.

If precision attachments or copings to be used:

4. The teeth are prepared and an impression of the abutments, including post holes, taken. In the lab, dies are prepared and transfer copings (usually metal) made. The transfer copings are tried on the abutments, and if satisfactory an overall impression is recorded to accurately locate the copings to the remainder of the denture-bearing area. Alternatively, a two-stage technique using a special tray with windows cut out over abutments can be used.
5. Regular review (6-monthly) and maintenance is necessary for success.

Problems

The most important are:

- Caries of abutment teeth, ∴ need good oral and denture hygiene and topical fluoride, e.g. toothpaste, applied to the fitting surface of the denture. Patients should be encouraged to remove their denture at night.
- Periodontal breakdown.

Gerodontology

(or Gerodontics or Gerontology)

Definition Dentistry for the elderly. For those who have not reached pensionable age, the elderly is anyone over 65. Others suggest that it is >75 yrs of age. Rather than arbitary cut-offs, biological age should be considered.

Epidemiology Two factors are mainly responsible for the increasing relevance of dentistry for the elderly: an increase in the proportion of the elderly in the population and the improvements in dental health that have resulted in more people keeping their natural teeth for longer. By 2001 the proportion aged >75 yrs will have ↑ by 22%. It is estimated that by 2001, 10% of adults will be edentulous, compared with 25% in 1983.

Problems The major overall problems are:
• Age changes, both physiological and pathological.
• Disease and drug therapy (Chapter 11).
• Delivery of care.

Restorative problems include:
• Root caries, which can occur following exposure of root surfaces by gingival recession, in association with changes in diet, ↓ self-care, and ↓ salivary flow. Details of management are given p. 29. Prevention of root caries in susceptible patients is possible using either a topical fluoride mouthrinse or fluoride-containing artificial saliva, e.g. Luborant or Saliva Orthana.
• Toothwear (p. 310) is especially prevalent when partial tooth loss has occurred.
• Pulpal changes, including sclerosis (p. 332) and ↓ repair capacity.

Periodontal problems include:
• Reduced manual dexterity, making OH procedures difficult. Epidemiological studies of the periodontal needs of the elderly population are still sparse and some trends may be masked by a high rate of edentulousness. The available evidence suggests that, although older patients develop plaque more quickly, the need for periodontal treatment ↑ up to middle age, and thereafter the majority can be maintained by regular non-surgical management.

Prosthetic problems include:
• Reduced adaptive capacity; ∴ if teeth are unlikely to last a lifetime, the transition to at least partial dentures should be made whilst the patient is able to learn the new skills necessary.
• Age changes in the denture-bearing areas, including bone resorption and mucosal atrophy.

Age changes

Age changes are defined as an alteration in the form or function of a tissue or organ as a result of biological activity associated with a minor disturbance of normal cellular turnover.

In general

↓ microcirculation↓ cellular reproduction, ↓ tissue repair, ↓ metabolic rate, ↑ fibrosis. Degeneration of elastic and nervous tissue. These result in reduced function of most body systems.

Dental

Oral soft tissues   A ↓ in the thickness of the epithelium, mucosa, and sub-mucosa is seen. Taste bud function ↓. With age, an ↑ occurs in the number and size of Fordyce's spots (sebaceous glands), lingual varices, and foliate papillae. Recent evidence suggests that stimulated salivary flow rate does not fall purely as a result of age. However, medications or systemic disease can affect salivary output.

Dental hard tissues   Enamel becomes less permeable with age. Clinically, older teeth appear more brittle, but there is no significant difference between the elastic modulus of dentine in old or young teeth. The rate of secondary dentine formation reduces with age, but still continues. Occlusion of the dentine tubules with calcified material spreads crownwards with age.

Toothwear is an age-related phenomenon and can be regarded as physiological in many cases. However, excessive and pathological wear can be caused by parafunction, abrasion, erosion (dietary, gastric, or environmental), or a combination of these factors.

Dental pulp   ↑ fibrosis and ↓ vascularity mean that the defensive capacities of the pulp ↓ with ↑ age, ∴ pulp capping is less likely to succeed. Also ↑ secondary dentine and ↑ pulp calcification.

Periodontium   ↑ fibrosis, ↓ cellularity, ↓ vascularity, and ↓ cell turnover are found with ↑ age. Whether gingival recession is pathological or physiological (developmental) is still hotly debated.

Systemic

Immune system   A ↓ in cell-mediated response and ↓ in number of circulating lymphocytes leads to an ↑ incidence of autoimmune disease as well as a ↓ in the older patient's defence against infection. Also an ↑ in neoplasia is seen. Steroid treatment for autoimmune disease may complicate dental treatment.

Nervous system   Ageing involves both a physiological decline in function and dysfunction associated with age-related disease (e.g. strokes, parkinsonism, trigeminal neuralgia). A ↓ in acuity compounds the problem.

Cardiovascular   Hypertension and ischaemic heart disease worsen with age. Anaemia is more common in the elderly. In general, the greatest problems arise when a GA is required, or the practice is on the second floor.

Pulmonary system   Lung capacity ↓ with age and chronic obstructive airways disease ↑ in prevalence.

Endocrine system Diabetes is more common.

Muscles ↓ bulk, slower contractions, and less precision of control occur.

Nutrition Poverty, impaired mobility, ↓ taste acuity, and ↓ masticatory function can result in nutritional deficiencies in the elderly. These can manifest as changes in the oral mucosa.

Mucosal disease, which is more common with increasing age
- Oral cancer, p. 452.
- Lichen planus, p. 466.
- Herpes zoster is more common with ↑ age due to a ↓ in T-cell function. Neuralgia occurs more frequently after an attack in the elderly.
- Benign mucous membrane pemphigoid, p. 444.
- Pemphigus, p. 442.
- Candida is seen more frequently in the older age groups due to an ↑ proportion of denture wearers and ↑ immune deficiencies.

This list is obviously not exhaustive.

Dental care for the elderly

The basis for delivery of care to the older patient has been, and is likely to continue to be, via the GDP.

General management problems

Medical and drug history (Chapter 11)   It is wise to check any complicated medical problems with the patient's GMP or physician. Unfortunately, many doctors are only familiar with the dental treatment they have personally received, ∴ give details of what is proposed.

Communication   with the elderly requires patience and understanding. Often older patients will try to cover up deafness, poor eyesight, and lack of comprehension, so it is better to err on the side of over-stressing an important point or instruction, but avoid sounding patronizing. It is often helpful to enlist the assistance of a relative or friend of the older patient.

Oral hygiene   may be compromised by arthritis &/or a stroke. Advise an electric toothbrush or modifying the handle of an ordinary toothbrush to make it easier to grip, e.g. with elastoplast or bicycle handlebar grips. Alternatively, self-cure acrylic can be used to make a custom grip for a toothbrush.

Delivery of care

Dental practice   Consideration should be given to:
• Access for a wheelchair or Zimmer frame. This is easy to arrange when a purpose-designed practice is being built, but can pose considerable problems for the established practice. In the surgery it is important to allow sufficient space around the dental chair.
• Timing of appointments; e.g. for a diabetic patient these need to be arranged around meals and drug regimens, and early morning visits are probably C/I for arthritic patients as it may take them a couple of hours to 'get going'.
• Positioning of the patient. Many elderly patients are unhappy to be recumbent in the dental chair. In addition, this position is C/I for those with cardiovascular or pulmonary disease. Adjust dental chair gradually as rapid movement from a flat to upright position can result in postural hypotension.

Domiciliary care   An estimated 12–14% of the elderly population are bedridden or housebound to such a degree that they cannot visit their GMP or GDP. Unfortunately, although the dental needs of this group are high the uptake of dental care is low, due to the low priority placed on such care and the difficulty experienced in obtaining it. Hygienists can now make domiciliary visits.
• *Site*   The kitchen is probably the most suitable room, with access to water and heat. However, it is wise to defer to the patient should they prefer another location for the improvised surgery. Care must be taken to protect the floor and work surfaces from any spillages.
• *Seating*   Where possible the patient should be seated in their wheelchair, or a straight-backed chair placed against a wall with a cushion for additional head support. When a patient is bedridden

there is no choice, but the dentist(s) should take frequent rests from bending over, to prevent back strain.
- *Equipment* The expenditure on this will be determined by the volume of such work undertaken. Portable dental units are available, but costly. However, the outlay could be shared by several practices or PCT. A mothercare or fishing-tackle box is useful for holding small items.
- *After-care* This is particularly important. It is the dentist's responsibility to ensure that the relatives or carers appreciate the need for good oral and denture care and how to carry it out. In the bedridden, chlorhexidine can be applied to the teeth by cotton swabs.

▶ Take a chaperone.

Key points
- Can treatment be carried out successfully?
- Consider maintenance required by any proposed treatment. Elaborate procedures which fail may leave the patient worse off.
- The objective is to maintain optimum oral function. Sometimes retention of a few teeth can be disadvantageous.
- Medical crises (e.g. a period in hospital) can result in a very rapid change in a previously stable oral state, e.g. rapid caries attack, loss of denture-wearing skill through lack of use.
- Avoid sudden changes in occlusion. The shape/form of dentures should not be changed anteriorly. During restorative work refrain from introducing significant occlusal change. If necessary to extract teeth, do so a few at a time, with additions to existing dentures.

Some clinical techniques of particular value in elderly
- Adhesive restorations, e.g. GI for root caries.
- Acid-etch bridgework is less destructive to abutments and is ∴ more fail-safe.
- Gradual tooth loss, with additions to existing P/P, is less demanding of a ↓ adaptive capacity.
- Replacement dentures should be made with careful regard to existing appliances. Use of copying techniques again ↓ amount of adaptation required.
- If recording the occlusion proves difficult, use cuspless teeth.
- Mark dentures with the patient's name.

Oral surgery

Principal sources: G. Dimitroulis 1997 *A Synopsis of Minor Oral Surgery*, Wright. K. Riden 1998 *Key Topics in Oral and Maxillofacial Surgery*, Bios. D. Mitchell 2004 *An Introduction to Oral and Maxillofacial Surgery*, OUP. J. Pedlar and J. Frame 2001 *Oral and Maxillofacial Surgery: An Objective Based Textbook*, Churchill Livingstone.

Additional background Pathology: J. V. Soames and J. C. Southam 1999 *Oral Pathology*, 3rd edn, OUP.

Third molars: NICE 2000 *Guidance on Removal of Wisdom Teeth*. MacGregor 1985 *The Impacted Lower Wisdom Tooth*, OUP. Kwon and Laskin 1997 *Clinicians' Manual of Oral and Maxillofacial Surgery*, 2nd edn, Quintessence.

Principles of surgery of the mouth

The mouth is a remarkably forgiving environment in which to operate, because of its excellent blood supply and the properties of saliva. It is compromised less than could be expected by its teeming hordes of commensal organisms. This does not, however, constitute *carte blanche* for ignoring the basic principles of surgery, although these can and should be modified to suit the nature and the site of the surgery.

Asepsis and antisepsis, p. 382.

Analgesia Thankfully, nowadays all patients should expect and receive painless surgery, both perioperatively and post-operatively. Analgesia and anaesthesia, Chapter 13.

Anatomy and pathology are the interdependent building blocks of surgery. Know the anatomy and you can understand or even devise the operation. Know the pathology and you know why you are doing it, what can be sacrificed, and what must be preserved.

Access For all minor and certain major oral surgical procedures, access is through the mouth via intra-oral incisions. Extra-oral surgery, Chapter 10.

Incisions for dento-alveolar surgery are full thickness, i.e. mucoperiosteal flaps; for mucosal and periodontal surgery split thickness flaps are raised (pp. 238 and 244). For mucoperiosteal flaps, although the base does *not have* to be longer than its length, this design improves the blood supply to the flap and should be used where this is a concern. Improved access via a large flap, allowing minimally traumatic surgery, virtually always outweighs the trauma of additional periosteal stripping.
  Always plan the incision mindful of local structures. *One cut*, at right angles, through mucoperiosteum to bone, is the aim. Do not split interdental papillae. Try to cut in the depth of the gingival sulcus. Raise the flap cleanly, working subperiosteally with a blunt instrument, moving from easily elevated areas to the more difficult (p. 384).

Retraction of the raised flap should be gentle and precise. It is the assistant's duty to prevent trauma to the tissues by sharp edges, overheated drills, or bullish surgeons.

Bone removal by drills must be accompanied by sterile irrigation to prevent heat necrosis of bone, damage to soft tissues, and clogging of the bur. When using chisels to remove bone remember the natural lines of cleavage of the jaws and make stop cuts (chisel technique, p. 400).

Removal of the tooth/root is carried out using *controlled force*.

Debridement is removal from the wound of debris generated by both the pathology and the operation. It is as important as any other part of the operation. Subperiosteal bone dust is a common cause of pain and delayed wound healing.

Haemostasis and *wound closure* are covered on p. 392.

Post-operative oedema is, to some degree, inevitable; it is minimized by gentle efficient surgery, which is more important than such measures as ice packs and peri- or post-operative steroids, although these can help.

Asepsis and antisepsis

Asepsis is the avoidance of pathogenic microorganisms. In practical terms, 'aseptic technique' is one which aims to exclude all microorganisms. Surgical technique is aseptic in the use of sterile instruments, clothing, and the 'no touch' technique.

Antisepsis is an agent or the application of an agent which inhibits the growth of microorganisms while in contact with them. Scrubbing up and preparation of operative sites are examples of antisepsis.

Disinfection is the inhibition or destruction of pathogens, whereas **sterilization** is the destruction or removal of **all** forms of life. Pre-packaged sterile supplies and the use of an autoclave (121 °C for 15 min or 134 °C for 3 min) for resterilizable equipment are the only really acceptable techniques in dentistry. Disinfection using gluteraldehyde or hypochlorite are second choices, for use where true sterilization is not feasible. There are strict restrictions on the use of gluteraldehyde which limit its usefulness outside hospitals. It is not possible to render the mouth aseptic and it is fruitless to try; there are, however, three basic techniques which are of value:

Avoid introducing infection This is achieved by *always* using *sterilized* instruments, and wearing gloves.

Avoid being infected yourself by the operative site Wear gloves, face, and eye protection.

Reduce the contaminating load to the site By pre-extraction cleaning of teeth, use of chlorhexidine mouthrinse, and prophylactic antimicrobials, when appropriate.

Cross-infection and its control

Much attention has been focused on this problem in recent years, first with hepatitis B and its related agents, then with HIV, and now with prions. Although screening is possible in some instances, this is of little real value since the majority of individuals with communicable viral particles *are asymptomatic* and hence not identifiable. Therefore safe practice mandates the use of sound cross-infection control as part of everyday practice on *all* patients.

Aerosols are easily created and are a potential source of cross-infection. Minimize wherever possible by high vacuum suction. Wear glasses and a mask if exposure to an aerosol cannot be avoided. Masks are routine in theatre, although of unproven value in preventing wound infection.

Cleaning and sterilizing Use disposable equipment when possible and **never** reuse. Clean instruments prior to sterilization. Use disposable or easily disinfected work surfaces. This book cover can be wiped down!

Gloves should be worn routinely. Sterile gloves for surgery.

Immunization against Hep B is available. Get it and get all staff with clinical contact to do likewise.

Waste disposal It is everyone's responsibility to ensure sharps are carefully placed in rigid, well-marked containers and disposed of by an appropriate service. Dealing with potentially contaminated impressions and appliances, p. 687. Treatment of the known high-risk patient, p. 748.

Needlestick injuries   If this happens to you, rinse wound under running water and record date and patient details. In hospital, follow local policy; in practice, contact local public health laboratory. DH guidance in the UK recommends universal source testing for Hep B, C, and HIV after an appropriate risk assessment.

Forceps, elevators, and other instruments

Extraction forceps come in numerous shapes and sizes. The choice of forcep is largely down to individual preference or, more frequently, availability. 'Universal' forceps are straight-bladed upper or lower forceps used to grip the roots of teeth to allow a controlled extracting force. 'Eagle beak' forceps are upper and lower molar forceps which engage the bifurcation of molar teeth allowing a buccally directed extraction force. 'Cowhorns' are designed to penetrate the molar bifurcation either to be used in a figure of eight loosening pattern or to split the roots. Most forceps come with a deciduous tooth equivalent.

Elevators used to dilate sockets to facilitate extraction or to remove dental hard tissue by themselves. These are the instruments which should **always** be used to remove impacted teeth. They should be used with gentle (finger pressure) forces. The commonly used patterns are Couplands No. 1, 2, and 3, Cryers right and left, and Warwick–James right, left, and straight.

Scalpel A Bard–Parker handle with a No. 15 blade is the usual.

Periosteal elevators A number are available; the Howarths, originally designed as a nasal rasparatory, is a favourite. McDonalds and 'No 9' are others.

Retractors Tongue, cheek, and flap retractors are needed and are legion in number; Dyson's tongue retractor, Kilner's cheek retractor, Bowdler–Henry's rake retractor, and the Minnesota flap retractor are favourites. Lack's is an all-purpose retractor (really a bent bit of metal)!

Chisels versus burs Depends upon your training. Generally, burs (No. 8 round T-C for bone removal, medium taper fissure T-C for tooth division) are kinder on the conscious patient and the best bet for the inexperienced. Chisels are more appropriate in theatre and are particularly useful (3 mm and 5 mm T-C tipped) for disto-angular third molars and upper third molars.

Curettes The Mitchells (no relation) trimmer is probably the most valuable instrument in this category.

Needle holders and sutures vary more than any of the above, depending on your location. The usual suture size for IO work is 4/0; the material may be non-absorbable (silk) or absorbable (Dexon®, Vicryl®). It is difficult to justify the continued use of any non-absorbable IO suture for routine use.

Scissors Remember to keep dissecting scissors, e.g. McIndoe's, separate from suture-cutting scissors, and keep both sets sharp.

Dissecting forceps are designed to hold soft tissue without damaging it; Gillies dissectors are popular. College tweezers are *not* dissecting forceps and are used to lift up sutures prior to removing them.

Aspirator Sterile/disposable suction tip small enough to get into the defect.

The extraction of teeth

The extraction of teeth must be viewed as a minor surgical procedure, ∴ the medical history will be pertinent, e.g. bleeding diathesis, at risk from bacteraemia, etc. More common and specific considerations are the sex, age, and build of the patient. Extractions in children are technically simple; it is the child who is most likely to be a problem, whereas stoical old men who may not bat an eye at the procedure often have teeth aptly described as 'glass in concrete'. Malpositioned teeth present problems of access and isolated teeth, especially upper second molars, tend to be ankylosed. Heavily restored and root-filled teeth tend to be very brittle. In all these cases a pre-extraction X-ray can help.

Extraction of teeth begins with *positioning* After LA has taken, the patient is positioned supine at the height of the operator's elbow for upper teeth, and sitting with the operator behind for (right-handed dentists) lower extractions on the right and in front for lower extractions on the left. The position is reversed for left-handers, but unfortunately the world seems biased against this group, and many dental chair systems seem to preclude comfortable positioning for them.

Common technique The socket is dilated either using an elevator between the bone of the socket wall and the tooth or by driving the forceps blades into the socket. The blades of the forceps are applied to the buccal and palatal/lingual aspects of the tooth and pushed either along the root of the tooth or, in certain molar extractions, into the bifurcation. The tooth is then gripped in the forceps and, maintaining a consistent and quite substantial *vertical* force, the tooth is moved depending on its anatomy:

1, 2, 3 have conical roots—rotate then pull.

4, 5 have either two fine roots or a flattened root—move bucco-palatally until you feel them 'give', then pull down and buccally.

6, 7 have three large divergent roots—these are moved buccally while maintaining upward pressure, but frequently need a variety of rocking movements before they are sufficiently disengaged to complete extraction.

$\overline{\textbf{1, 2, 3}}$ can usually be removed with a simple buccal movement, but sometimes need to be rocked or even rotated.

$\overline{\textbf{4, 5}}$ are rotated and lifted out.

$\overline{\textbf{6, 7}}$ are two-rooted and can usually be removed by a controlled buccal movement. Remember to support the patient's jaw.

Deciduous teeth are extracted using the same principles, but while permanent molars can be removed using forceps which engage the bifurcation, these should *not* be used on deciduous teeth.

Third molars (p. 398)

As with all operative techniques in dentistry, the doing is worth a thousand words. To become competent there are three golden rules: practice, practice, and practice.

Complications of extracting teeth

Access   Small mouths present an obvious, but usually manageable problem. Crowded or malpositioned teeth may need trans-alveolar approach. Trismus, if due to infection, e.g. submasseteric abscess, should be managed in hospital where facilities for external drainage and airway protection are available.

Pain   Has the LA worked? Try further LA as regional block, infiltration, or intraligamentary injection. Is it pain or pressure? If pressure, reassure and proceed. If pain, and other signs of adequate LA are present, then acute infection is the most likely culprit. Can the extraction wait by using delaying tactics such as draining an abscess? The vast majority can and very few adult extractions really justify a GA.

Inability to move the tooth   Don't worry; it happens to us all. Have you got an X-ray? If not, get one and look for: bulbous or diverging roots, very long roots, ankylosis, or sclerotic bone. Do not press on regardless; it will work sometimes but shows lack of consideration and will cost you in time and goodwill in the long run. Most 'solid' teeth have an easily identifiable cause, e.g. diverging roots, and raising a flap and using a trans-alveolar procedure (p. 394) will quickly and easily remedy this.

Breaking the tooth   is a common occurrence and may even assist extraction if, e.g., the roots of a molar are separated. More often, unfortunately, the crown #, leaving a portion of root(s) *in situ*. It is quite acceptable to leave small (<3 mm) pieces of deeply buried apex, but provide antibiotics, tell the patient, and review. Larger pieces of root must be removed as they have a high incidence of infective sequelae (p. 408).

# of alveolar &/or basal bone   Breaking the alveolar bone is relatively common. If # only involves the alveolus containing the extracted tooth, remove any pieces of bone not attached to periosteum and close the wound. Rarely, the alveolus carrying other teeth will be involved, in which case remove tooth by a trans-alveolar procedure and splint remaining teeth (p. 116). Basal bone # is rare; ensure analgesia (LA &/or systemic analgesics) and arrange reduction and fixation (p. 498).

Loss of the tooth   Stop and look; in the mouth, is it under the mucoperiosteum or in a tissue space: these can usually be milked out. Look in the suction apparatus. Is it in the antrum (p. 422) or even the ID canal? Has it been swallowed or inhaled? Chest X-ray is mandatory if not found plate 7.

Damage to other teeth/tissues and extraction of the wrong tooth   Prevent by confirming with the patient the tooth to be removed and making careful notes. Plan the operation; do not use inappropriate instruments or ones which you don't know how to use. If the wrong tooth is extracted, replant if feasible and proceed to remove the correct tooth. Tell the patient and make careful notes.

Dislocated jaw   Reduce (p. 502); **Bleeding** (p. 390); **pain, swelling**, and **trismus** are common sequelae, and discussed on p. 400.

Post-operative bleeding

Bleeding disorders are covered on p. 528.

Principles of management of post-operative bleeding.

1 Support the patient. If hypotensive and tachycardic, establish IV access and replace lost blood volume.
2 Diagnose each cause, nature, and site of blood loss.
3 Control the bleeding point.

Classically, post-op bleeding is described as: immediate (primary), reactionary, and secondary.

Immediate   When true haemostasis has not been achieved at completion of surgery.

Reactionary   Occurs within 48 h of surgery and is due to both general and local rise in BP opening up small divided vessels which were not bleeding at completion of surgery.

Secondary   Occurs ~7 days post-op and is usually due to infection destroying clot or ulcerating local vessels. In practice, bleeding following removal of teeth is common and usually simple to diagnose. The patients are seldom shocked or hypotensive but are often very anxious and nauseated by the taste, smell, and sight of blood, and by blood in the stomach, which is irritant. Bleeding usually comes from one or all of three sources: **1** gingival capillaries; **2** vessels in the bone of the socket; and **3** a large vessel under a flap or in bone, such as the inferior alveolar artery. The first two are by far the more common.

Management

Reassure the patient they won't bleed to death. Remove accompanying entourage and get the patient to an area with reasonable facilities. Take a drug history (anticoagulants?). *Wear gloves and apron*: patients often vomit. (If patient has to wait to be seen they should bite firmly on a clean handkerchief or gauze, rolled to fit the area the bleeding seems to be coming from.) In good light, with suction, clean the patient's face and mouth, remove any lumps of clot, and identify the source of bleeding. Is it from under a flap? If from a socket, squeeze the gingivae to the outer walls of the socket between finger and thumb; if bleeding stops it is from a gingival vessel. In these cases, LA and suturing are needed. If bleeding continues it is from vessels in bone, which need some form of pack.

Technique

Give LA if needed, and have assistance with suction. If flap involved remove old sutures, evacuate clot, identify bleeding point, and place a tight suture around it. Bleeding should be much ↓; if not, repeat until it is, then close wound and have the patient bite on a swab for at least 15 min. If it is a gingival bleed a tight interrupted or mattress suture will compress the capillaries, again followed by a swab to bite on. If bleeding is from the depths of the socket, the clot may need to be removed and replaced by a pack or supported by a resorbable mesh (oxidized cellulose) &/or agents such as tranexamic acid, adrenaline, or epsilon aminocaproic acid soaked into the mesh. If removing clot and packing the socket, remember this will delay healing and predispose to infection, so use BIPP or Whitehead's varnish packs. If all else fails, all the above measures plus a pressure pack, analgesia, a sedative antiemetic, and a night in a hospital bed will do the trick. Patients requiring this degree of treatment should be investigated haematologically and for liver disease.

Suturing

Every dentist should master the basic skills of suturing.

Materials Most sutures are suture material fused to a needle, although threaded reusable needles are used in some countries. Needles may be round-bodied, cutting or reverse cutting. Straight, curved, or J-shaped. Almost all IO work is done with a 16–22 mm curved cutting or reverse cutting needle held in a needle holder. Suture material may be resorbable (Dexon®, Vicryl®, or Monocryl®) or non-resorbable (silk, nylon, prolene, or Novafil®). Monofilament suture (e.g. nylon) causes less tissue response than braided (e.g. silk).

Skin is best closed with nylon, prolene, or Novafil®. *Mucosa* and *deep tissues* best closed with an absorbable. *Vessels* are tied off using resorbables, except major veins and arteries, which are transfixed and tied with silk. BSS can be used for skin but must be removed *early*. Suture strength is described as 0 (thickest) to 4/0 (commonest in IO use) to 11/0 (thinnest for microvascular work).

Types of stitch are shown in the diagram.

Suture technique Closure of a wound or incision should, whenever possible, be without tension, by closing deep layers and over supporting tissue. Hold the needle in the needle holder ~2/3 of the way from its tip. Suture from free to fixed tissue taking a bite of 2–3 mm on both sides. Leave the sutured wound edges slightly everted in apposition. Except when swaging tissue to bone, e.g. when arresting haemorrhage or when tying vessels, do not overtighten the suture as wound margins become swollen, and you need not allow for this.

Knot tying The two most useful are the square (reef) knot and the surgeon's knot (see diagram).

Instrument tying is easy to learn from a book but needs considerable practice to perfect. The knot is started by passing the suture once (square knot) or twice (surgeon's knot) around the tip of the needle holders; the knot is tightened and then locked by passing the suture around the needle holder in the opposite direction once. It is possible to control the suture tension by completing the knot in three loops instead of two.

Hand tying is invaluable for those wishing to develop surgical expertise or involved in major maxillofacial surgery. It takes a substantial amount of time and practice and is impossible to learn from a book. Get a sympathetic senior to demonstrate.

Suture removal is not someone else's job to be casually forgotten about. Do the stitches need to be removed? In inaccessible sites, difficult patients, or areas in which scar quality is less important, a resorbable suture should be used. An alternative is a tissue glue, e.g. Dermabond®, Indermil®. Facial skin sutures should be removed at 3–5 days. When removing sutures use *sharp* scissors (avoid 'stitch cutters' if you can), lifting up and cutting a bit of suture that has been in the tissue, thus avoiding dragging bacteria through the incision on removal.

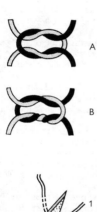

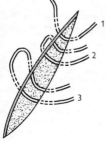

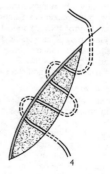

A Reef knot.
B Surgeon's knot.

1 Simple interrupted suture.
2 Horizontal mattress suture.
3 Vertical mattress suture.
4 Continuous subcuticular suture.

Dento-alveolar surgery: removal of roots

Does the root need to be removed? If large, being extracted for pulpal or apical pathology, is symptomatic, is an impediment to denture construction, or is in a patient in whom risk of minor local infection is not tolerable (e.g. immunocompromised or at risk from IE) then the answer is yes.

Non-surgical methods The use of root forceps or elevators may allow simple removal of roots close to the alveolar margin. When using root forceps ensure the root can be seen to be engaged by the blades. Elevators can be used to direct a root along its path of withdrawal providing (a) one exists, and (b) an elevator can be introduced between bone and root. Do not waste time persisting with non-surgical methods if your initial attempt is unsuccessful.

Surgical methods Plan your operation. Do you know why the root cannot be delivered, exactly where it is, and about any adjacent structures? If not, get an X-ray.
(a) The flap: if endentulous incise along the crest of the ridge, if dentate in the gingival margin. Flaps may be envelope, two-sided, or three-sided. Relieving incisions make reflection of the flap easier but must be avoided in the region of the mental nerve ($\overline{45}$) and are better avoided around the buccal branch of the facial artery (mesial root $\overline{7}$). Include an interdental papilla at either side of the flap and start vertical cuts 2/3 of the way distal to the included papilla. Big flaps heal as well as small ones; the important consideration is access.
(b) Identify obstructions to the path of withdrawal of the root; these are either removed or the root is sectioned to create another path of withdrawal, depending on which approach is the least traumatic.
(c) Remove the minimum amount of buccal bone compatible with exposing the maximum diameter of the root and a point of application for an elevator (No. 8 round T-C surgical bur).
(d) Elevate by placing an elevator between bone and tooth (remember to apply to the convex surface of curved roots) and direct the root along its natural path of withdrawal.
(e) Finally, debride and close the wound.

Special cases
1 Small apical fragments: use an apicectomy approach.
2 Multirooted teeth: always divide the roots, as this makes life much easier.
3 Cannot find the root: re-X-ray and look in the soft tissues. The root may have been displaced into another cavity or even be in the aspirator; look carefully but remember discretion is the better part of valour. Tell the patient.
4 Patient refuses operation: it's their body; record your advice and their decision.

Under GA Mallet and chisel can replace bur and the 'broken instrument' technique can be used. This involves using a straight instrument or elevator guided through the bone using the mallet, and either then being used as an elevator or being placed in contact with the tooth or fragment, which is delivered by a sharp blow. Use with care.

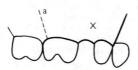

Outline of two-sided flap in heavy shade.
X Retained root or similar.
a Line of additional incision to convert to three-sided flap.

Dento-alveolar surgery: removal of unerupted teeth

The teeth most commonly requiring removal, other than third molars, are maxillary canines and premolars, supernumaries, and mandibular canines and premolars. Rarely, permanent or deciduous molars may be impacted or submerged.

Maxillary canines (p. 160, 162) The canine may lie within or across the arch, buccally or, most frequently, palatally. Assessment requires a careful examination, palpation, and X-rays (either two films at 90° or the parallax technique, p. 162).

Techniques Buccal impactions are approached via a buccal flap, palatal via a palatal flap, and cross- or within-arch impactions need a combination of the two. Buccal flaps are as previously described (p. 394). Palatal flaps involve the reflection of the full thickness of the mucoperiosteum of the anterior hard palate, the incision running in the gingival crevice from 6̲ to 6̲ for bilateral canines or to the contralateral canine region for single impactions. The neurovascular bundle emerging from the incisive foramen is often sacrificed, with no noticeable morbidity. **Never** incise the palate at 90° to the gingival crevice and **always** use an envelope flap, otherwise you will section the palatine artery. Remove bone over the bulge of the crown of the tooth until the maximum bulbosity of the crown and the incisal tip are exposed. If the root curvature and path of withdrawal are favourable, the entire tooth can be elevated out. If not, section at the cervical margin with a tapered fissure bur and winkle the pieces out separately. Debride the socket and close with vertical mattress sutures to minimize haematoma formation.

Mandibular canines Most lie buccally, and can be elevated or removed with root forceps. Unerupted, deeply impacted buccal or lingual canines rarely need to be removed. If necessary a degloving incision provides good access.

Maxillary premolars Most lie palatally. If partially erupted and conically rooted, they are simply elevated. Otherwise, a similar approach to that used for palatal canines is used. Premolars within the arch are approached buccally, sectioned, and removed piecemeal.

Mandibular premolars are often angled lingually. The 'broken instrument' technique can be invaluable. Otherwise, an extended buccal flap is raised to visualize and protect the mental nerve, buccal bone is removed, and the tooth sectioned at its cervical margin. The crown is then displaced downwards into the space created and the root elevated upwards.

Submerged deciduous molars If must be removed, they are approached buccally and sectioned vertically, then elevated along the individual roots path of withdrawal.

Supernumeraries (p. 70) These are removed using the approach used for the tooth they impede or replace. This can be a surprisingly difficult operation, usually because of difficulty in finding and identifying the supernumary.

Dento-alveolar surgery: removal of third molars

Not all wisdom teeth need to be removed.[1] Those which have space to erupt into functional occlusion should be left to do so, and those which are deeply impacted and asymptomatic are best left alone. Decisions about surgery vary widely.[2]

Aetiology As the last tooth to erupt, the third molar is most liable to be prevented from doing so in a crowded mouth. *Causes*: soft Western diet doesn't create space by contact point abrasion, inherited tooth–jaw size incompatibility, and possibly an evolutionary tendency towards decreased jaw size.

Symptoms Pain, swelling, pericoronitis (p. 408), and sometimes a foul taste. Mostly due to localized infection, less commonly due to caries or resorption of second molar or cyst associated with third molar. Third molars covered by bone are very unlikely to become infected, whereas those where the crown has breached mucosa will almost inevitably do so. Infections in older, less vascular bone are more difficult to treat.

Indications for removal Recurrent pericoronitis, unrestorable caries in 7 or 8, external or internal resorption, cystic change, periodontal disease distally in 7. The prevention of LLS crowding on its own is **not** an indication, nor is vague TMJ pain.

Timing Symptoms are most common in the late teens and twenties; bone is soft, spongy and elastic in this age group, so this is the usual and most favourable time to operate. Prophylactic removal of symptomless third molars is currently hard to justify.[3]

Choice of anaesthetic Bilateral impacted third molars are more kindly treated under GA, as are those where surgery may be technically more difficult, e.g. disto-angular 8s. LA &/or sedation is appropriate for most unilateral impactions not presenting particular difficulty. Consider medical history.

Assessment Look first: unerupted or partially erupted? Take pre-op X-ray (DPT is ideal).

Assess angulation (vertical, mesio-angular, disto-angular, horizontal, or transverse); depth of impaction from the alveolar crest to the maximum diameter of the crown; degree of impaction (and against what); root shape; bone density; the relationship to the ID canal; and the presence of any other pathology or complicating factors.

Plan the path of withdrawal. What impedes it? How much bone needs to be removed to provide a point of application for an elevator? How much to clear the path of withdrawal? Can this be done less traumatically by sectioning the tooth? In what direction?

Warn the patient about pain, trismus, swelling, and the possibility of damage to the ID and lingual nerves.

1 NICE 2000 www.nice.org.uk.
2 M. Brickley 1993 *BDJ* **175** 102.
3 University of York 1998 *Effectiveness Matters* **3** (2).

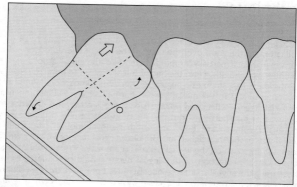

Diagram showing a schematic of planning for third molar removal.

Dento-alveolar surgery: third-molar technique

Technique

Mandible A buccal flap is incised along the external oblique ridge (lies well lateral to the arch) over the crest of the ridge if unerupted, or in the gingival margin if partially erupted. Extend to the distal aspect of the second molar and down into the buccal sulcus. Cut on to bone to create a full thickness flap. If a mesio-angular or horizontal impaction, extend the incision around $\overline{7}$ to the mesial border, but beware the buccal branch of the facial artery. Reflect and retract flap. There is now good evidence to suggest that manipulation from the lingual aspect results in unnecessary lingual nerve morbidity. Bone and tooth removal should ∴ be from a buccal approach. An attached mucosa disto-lingual flap for visibility which does not encroach on the lingual nerve is reasonable. Wide exposure and subperiosteal protection of the lingual nerve should be undertaken by those using the lingual split technique. Remove bone to provide a point of application for an elevator and clear obstruction to the path of withdrawal. This can be done with chisels or a bur. With a bur this is done by creating a disto-buccal gutter, exposing the maximum bulbosity of the tooth. If needed the bur can then be used to section the $\overline{8}$ to provide an unimpeded path of withdrawal.

With chisels, place mesial and distal stop cuts around the tooth and split off a collar of buccal and distal bone to expose the bulbosity of the crown. This can then be extended into a lingual split, taking off a piece of lingual plate and allowing the tooth to be elevated lingually. Whichever technique is used, it is important to remember that if it has been done properly a minimum of directed force via an elevator will deliver the tooth or fragment out along its path of withdrawal. If this cannot be done, look carefully for another obstruction. Once the tooth is removed debride the socket, remove the follicle, and close the wound with loose sutures to allow for swelling. Achieve haemostasis with pressure.

Maxilla A flap similar to that in the mandible can be used for inaccessible wisdom teeth but many can be approached using a 'slash' incision (from disto-palatally on the tuberosity to disto-buccally at the second molar and into the buccal sulcus). Reflect and retract the flap. Bone removal can usually be effected by a hand-held chisel. The much softer bone rarely causes any problem with elevation, but care has to be taken to prevent displacement into the pterygoid space. The 'slash' incision often needs no closure, whereas a conventional incision will need repositioning with sutures.

Post-operatively

Pain can be quite severe and responds best to NSAIDs. Peri-operative LA works well and leaves patients pain-free but numb for the duration. Trismus is due to pain and muscle spasm and can be ↓ by adequate analgesia (p. 596). It has obvious but often forgotten connotations for meals post-op. Swelling can also be ↓ by high-dose peri-operative steroids. There is no evidence that ice-packs help, although they are often used.

Haemorrhage can usually be controlled by biting on pressure packs. Rarely, it may be necessary to re-explore the wound. Antibiotic prophylaxis is probably beneficial.[1]

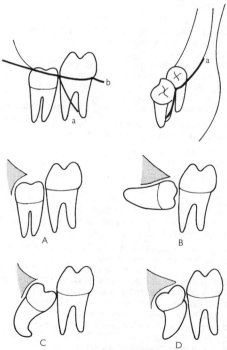

a Outline of incision for raising a third-molar buccal flap.
b Modification to create an envelope flap.
A Vertically impacted third molar.
B Horizontally impacted third molar.
C Mesio-angular impaction of a third molar.
D Disto-angular impaction of a third molar.
(Source: after Moore 1976.)

1 1995 *Journal Oral and Maxillofacial Surgery* **53**.

Dento-alveolar surgery: apicectomy

There are four surgical aids to endodontics: apicectomy, root hemisection, endodontic (diodontic) implants, and removal of extruded endodontic paste.

Apicectomy

This is by far the commonest. It is a *second line* treatment after failure of, or as a supplement to, orthograde endodontics (which has an 86–96% success rate in expert hands).[1]

Indications

- Impossible to prepare and fill apicial 1/3 of tooth, e.g. pulpal calcification, curved apex, open apex.
- Irretrievable broken instrument in canal.
- Post crown on tooth with apical pathology (only if post crown has sealed the coronal root and crown margin).
- Root perforation.
- Fractured and infected apical 1/3.
- Persistent infection due to apical cyst or other lesion requiring biopsy.

Assessment IO X-ray, best possible root filling *in situ*, free from acute infection, crown sealed with good quality restoration.

Remember Non-surgical retreatment: 72% success; apicectomy and RRF: 60%, apicectomy no RRF: 51%.[1]

Technique This operation is best performed under LA. Ensure an area of two tooth widths either side of the tooth being treated is anaesthetized, and give palatal infiltration. In the mandible, give a block plus infiltration to aid haemostasis. If associated with infection, prophylactic antibiotics, e.g. amoxicillin 1 g 1 h pre-op and 6 h post-op, or metronidazole 400 mg 1 h pre- and 6 h post-op can help.

Flaps may be two- or three-sided, semilunar, or sublabial; the latter two avoid post-op recession but give inferior access. Reflect and retract well above the apex (there is often a bulge or perforation of the cortical plate to aid location of the apex). A bony window is created to visualize the apex, which is often found sitting in a mass of granulation tissue. Excise the apical 1–2 mm and currette out the cystic and granulation tissue. Pack the cavity with bone wax or adrenaline-soaked ribbon gauze, identify the canal and prepare it with a 1/2-round bur or ultrasonics (depending on availability). Seal with "super EBA," "IRM" or "MTA" and debride. Close, using interrupted or vertical mattress sutures.

Special points in apicectomy

Warn patients about post-op swelling. Lower incisors present an access problem eased but not erased by a degloving incision and experience. Think twice about the mental nerve in lower premolar apicectomies. Think hard about alternatives to apicectomy of 6. Don't think at all about 7, 8. Remember the buccal and palatal roots in <u>4</u>; section the buccal root low to see the palatal. Apicectomy of 6̲ is fine provided the palatal root can be treated by an orthograde approach, is hemisected, or you are happy to deal with breaching the antrum.

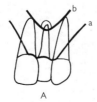

A An approach to apicectomy.
a Outline of incision for three-sided flap, good access, best flap for the novice.
b Outline of semilunar flap incision.
B An approach to apicectomy, a window is created in the buccal cortex to expose the apex, which is resected, leaving a smooth raw bony cavity.

Dento-alveolar surgery: other aids to endodontics

Root perforations are approached as for apicectomy; however, multirooted tooth perforations, unroot-fillable roots, or untreatable periodontal pockets may be dealt with by

Root hemisection This simply involves raising a flap around the tooth, identifying and horizontally sectioning the root, and atraumatically elevating it out. The wound is closed and a cleanable undersurface sealed with Super EBA, IRM, or MTA left.

Endodontic (diodontic) implants have not received widespread acceptance. A sterile alloy implant passes through the prepared root canal into periapical bone, transfixing the tooth. Such implants have been superseded by single-tooth osseintegrated implants (p. 428).

Removal of extruded paste Usually, all that is required is an apicectomy approach. However, careless use of 'paste only' techniques can result in paste in the floor of the nose, the antrum, or the ID canal. The nasal floor can be approached sublabially or intranasally, the antrum by standard methods (p. 422), and the ID canal by sagittally splitting the buccal cortex of the mandible.

Prognosis Single-rooted tooth apicectomies should succeed 58–96% of the time. The range is due to an ill-defined definition of 'success' and operator technique. Multirooted teeth, revision apicectomy, and perforation repair have a much lower success rate.

Dento-alveolar surgery: helping the orthodontist

Many minor oral surgical procedures, e.g. extraction of 4s or removal of 8s, are carried out at the instigation of an orthodontist. This page concerns itself with the specific procedures of frenectomy, pericision, tooth exposure, and tooth repositioning.

Frenectomy This is of value in closing a median diastema only if gentle traction on the upper lip and fraenum produces blanching in a palatal insertion around the incisive papilla. It follows that the excision of the frenum must include those fibrous insertions, which leaves a raw area of alveolus after excision—this can be dressed with Surgicel, BIPP, or a periodontal pack. It is a different operation from preprosthetic fraenectomy and is performed for a different reason.

Pericision is simply incising supra-alveolar periodontal fibres to prevent relapse when derotating teeth.

Tooth exposure Orthodontic traction is the treatment of choice for malpositioned, unerupted canines and incisors if the apices are in good position for eruption. The essential aspect of the operation is to remove any sacrificable impediments to tooth movement. Bonding an eyelet and gold chain or other bracket technique has a lower incidence of reoperation, but needs the orthodontist in theatre.

Technique Palatal teeth are exposed by a palatal flap. Remove bone carefully with chisels, expose the greatest diameter of the crown and the tip. (Moving the tooth is counter-productive, ∴ don't do it.) Excise palatal mucoperiosteum generously, it grows back; bond a bracket if you're going to. Firmly pack the wound with, e.g., Whitehead's varnish and ribbon gauze and secure, or use an acrylic dressing plate with periodontal paste dressing. Close the remainder of the flap with vertical mattress sutures. Buccally located teeth are approached by a buccal flap, in order to preserve attached gingiva, and bonding should be done at operation. The flap can be repositioned coronally with the elastics or chain tunnelling subgingivally. Teeth within the arch are approached buccally removing crestal bone as needed.

Tooth repositioning (transplantation) Although there are claims of success rates as high as 93%, few people match this and most would transplant only when exposure and orthodontic movement were rejected. The most commonly transplanted tooth is the maxillary canine. It is essential to measure the available space and compare this with the erupted contralateral tooth or a good X-ray estimation, as it is not acceptable to grind down healthy teeth at operation to accommodate the retrieved tooth. If the tooth appears to be too big for the available space then orthodontic Rx is required to create space. As this is often the reason the patient rejected exposure, an impasse is sometimes reached.

Technique The tooth is exposed by buccal or palatal flap, and once it is certain that it can be removed atraumatically, the deciduous tooth, if present, is extracted and a new socket surgically prepared with a bur. The tooth is reimplanted without force, the flaps sutured, and a close-fitting but **not** cemented splint placed. Functional splinting is continued for 7–10 days and the tooth root-filled as soon as possible after surgery. Regular follow-up is essential to allow early detection of root resorption.

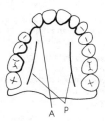

A Outline (heavy black line) of the incision for a palatal flap raised to expose a buried right maxillary canine.
p Position of the palatine arteries. Do not attempt a palatal 'relieving' incision; exposure is achieved by the length of the envelope flap.
(Source: after Moore 1976.)

Dento-facial infections

▶ Infection associated with teeth is rarely, if ever, treated *definitively* by antibiotics and analgesics.

The vast majority of infections in this area requiring surgical treatment are bacterial, usually arising from necrotic pulps, periodontal pockets, or pericoronitis. Can be life-threatening if allowed to progress, e.g. to the fascial spaces of the neck or the cavernous sinus, or as a focus for infective endocarditis (p. 530).

Microbiology Culture of dento-facial infections usually produces several commensal organisms, of which anaerobes are the most important. The predominant species *Bacteroides* (anaerobe) and streptococci (aerobe and anaerobe) are usually sensitive to the penicillins. Resistance is reported rarely. *Bacteroides* is nearly always sensitive to metronidazole. Remember the aerobic pathogens in established infection (don't just rely on metronidazole, and haemophilus and staphylococci near the antrum (p. 422).

Diagnosis Usually simple and clinical based on pain, swelling, temperature, and discharge.

Apical abscess Teeth with an apical abscess are TTP and non-vital. They may be discoloured or crowned and have a history of trauma or RCT. Pain and TTP are often diminished when the intrabony pus tracks through the soft tissues and discharges, usually in the buccal sulcus (exceptions are 2̲, and palatal roots of maxillary molars which discharge palatally, and 1̅2̅ which often discharge on the chin). May be associated periostitis with severe thickening.

Rx Drainage of pus either via the root canal, by incision of any fluctuant abscess, or by extraction under LA or GA. Palatal or buccal abscesses can be drained quite simply under LA by infiltrating a small amount of LA *between* the abscess cavity and the overlying mucosa, then incising the abscess. Explore using blunt closed forceps and keep patent either by excising an elipse of tissue or inserting and suturing a small rubber drain; this is particularly important in the palate. Cover the procedure with 'best guess' antibiotics such as amoxicillin 500 mg tds PO for 5–7 days, or metronidazole 400 mg tds PO for 5–7 days, or both.

Periodontal abscesses arise in a pre-existing periodontal pocket (p. 222). Initial treatment involves incision and drainage, followed by elimination of the pocket, unless extraction is considered the only option.

Pericoronitis is inflammation and infection of a gum flap (operculum) overlying a partially erupted tooth, usually a 8̅ often traumatized by an overerupted 8. Rx: involves removal of the opposing 8̲, irrigation under the operculum with saline or chlorhexidine, and antibiotics (see above) if necessary. Nearly all third molars associated with pericoronitis need removal.

Dry socket is osteitis of a socket following tooth removal. Commonest in the mandible after removal of molars, especially 8̅. Predisposing factors are smoking, surgical trauma, LA, history, bone disease, the pill, or immunodeficiency.

Diagnosis Pain onset after (usually 2–4 days) extraction, similar in nature but *worse* than the preceding toothache. The socket looks inflamed and exposed bone is usually visible. Rx is to gently clean the socket by irrigation and dress the exposed bone with Alvogyl, BIPP, or ZOE packs (provide remarkable analgesia but are a horror to remove). Topical metronidazole is an alternative.[1] Chlorhexidine &/or hot salt mouthwashes may help. NSAIDs are the systemic analgesic of choice (p. 612). Prophylactic anaerobicidals such as metronidazole reduce the incidence of this condition.[2]

Actinomycosis (p. 200) Persistent low-grade infection, multiple sinuses. Rx: drainage and up to 6 weeks amoxicillin 500 mg tds. Doxycycline 100 mg od is an alternative.

Staphylococcal lymphadenitis Especially seen in children; small occult skin or mucosal breach allows ingress. May mimic a 'slapped face' due to exotoxin. Drain and give flucloxacillin 125–500 mg qds (depending on age, p. 610).

Atypical mycobacteria Lymphadenitis with no obvious cause. Cold nodes, non-febrile patient. Drain or excise. Culture for up to 12 weeks. Do **not** start antituberculous therapy as many atypical mycobacteria are resistant and side-effects are common and significant. Clarithromycin most useful 'conventional' antibiotic. Excision of nodes is definitive Rx.

1 L. Mitchell 1984 *BDJ* **156** 132.
2 J. Rood 1979 *Br J Oral Surg* **17** 62.

Biopsy

A biopsy is a sample of tissue taken from a patient for histopathological examination.

Types of biopsy Biopsies may be incisional or excisional. Examples of incisional biopsies are fine-needle aspirate (really cytology), punch biopsy, trephines, and 'true-cut' needle biopsy. The commonest technique by far, however, is to excise an ellipse of tissue that includes a portion of the lesion and surrounding normal tissue. Excisional biopsy provides after the fact information on the excised sample (reserve for lesions < 0.5 mm).

What should be biopsied? Nearly everything that is worth excising is worth histological review, and so all excised specimens should be examined histopathologically. Any soft tissue lesion not amenable to accurate clinical Δ (by a reasonably trained eye) should be biopsied. All red lesions of oral mucosa and most white patches should be biopsied. If you think 'should I biopsy this?' then do it; you will always get some unpleasant surprises.

Special considerations Frozen sections are biopsy specimens taken during major surgery, either when the extent of the procedure will depend on the histological Δ of the lesion or to verify clearance of excision. It is essential to contact the pathology lab before the patient goes to theatre to warn them. Advance warning is also necessary for certain special tests, e.g. immunohistochemistry.

How it is done Tell the patient you need a piece of tissue to help make the Δ. LA or GA. For simple incisional biopsy, stabilize the tissue to be sampled. Transfixing with a 3/0 BSS helps avoid crush artefact, and orientates the specimen. Cut an ellipse of tissue, including lesion and normal surrounding tissue, lift up and dissect out, then close primarily with sutures.

Biopsy and oral cancer Incisional biopsy carries a (theoretical) risk of shedding malignant cells into the circulation. The alternative is to subject a patient to mutilating surgery before definitive Δ. If you suspect an oral malignancy, refer before biopsy because most consultants have a preferred approach. This also allows integrated Δ and counselling.

Specimens are best laid out on paper if small or pinned out on a cork board if large. This allows orientation and decreases shrinkage artefact, which can be considerable. Usual preservative is 10% formalin; ask if you are not sure, as some specimens are needed fresh. Consider a specimen for culture as well (e.g. lymph node biopsy). Make a diagram of the specimen on the pathology form to accompany the clinical details. A photograph of the operative site can help.

▶ Tell the pathologist what you are thinking!

Cryosurgery

Cryosurgery is the therapeutic use of extreme cold.

Equipment   The coolants (usually nitrous oxide or liquid nitrogen) act via a cryoprobe, a tubing system in which the coolant is not in direct contact with the tissues. The probe tip is applied to the lesion with an intervening layer of lubricant jelly; this gives rise to an 'iceball', which is essential for success. Liquid nitrogen can also be directly sprayed onto lesions and, rarely, bone can be immersed into liquid nitrogen prior to reuse as a framework for grafting.

Mechanism   Cell death and subsequent tissue necrosis by cellular disruption, dehydration, enzyme inhibition, and protein denaturation follow application of extreme cold. Indirect effects include vascular stasis and an immune response.[1] There is a curious lack of infection and scarring following cryosurgery.

Indications   Some vascular malformations and haemangioma (not the same thing) respond very well. Areas of leukoplakia unsuitable for excision, and provided they have not already undergone malignant change, may respond. Occasionally, malignant change following cryosurgery of leukoplakia is reported, so some controversy surrounds the technique. Extensive hyperplastic lesions, e.g. palatal hyperplasia under F/-, may respond. Viral warts respond in most instances and some advocate its use for mucoceles. Superficial basal cell carcinoma is frequently treated with cryosurgery, usually liquid nitrogen spray, although its use in more aggressive malignancy is controversial, as is its use following enucleation of keratocysts. Intractable facial pain is one of the more accepted uses, the freezing of peripheral nerves being followed by a period of analgesia which extends beyond the original post-op numbness.

Technique
- Warn the patient about the procedure, post-op oedema (which can be severe), and a slough which forms over frozen sites. There is sometimes depigmentation of skin lesions.
- LA for larger lesions or if biopsy needed. (LA may ↑ effectiveness of iceball.)
- Select a probe tip suitable for the lesion; overlap ice zones if the lesion is large.
- Use KY jelly to improve contact between probe and tissues.
- Usual freeze–thaw cycles are ~1 min, repeated at least twice.
- Do not remove probe until defrosting has occurred.
- Careful follow-up and check the histology of the lesion, except when using cryoanalgesia.

Simple analgesics and chlorhexidine mouthwash post-op often help.
   The treatment of frank malignancy by cryosurgery remains controversial, but freeze–thaw cycles used must be in excess of the usual (up to 3 min) and tissue temperatures monitored.

1 V. Popescu 1980 *J Max-fac Surg* **8** 8.

Non-tumour soft-tissue lumps in the mouth

Abscess (p. 408). Generalized gingival swelling and gingivitis (p. 212).

Brown 'tumour' Not a tumour but a giant cell lesion sometimes found in soft tissue but more commonly within bone (p. 416). It occurs 2° to hyperparathyroidism, although this Δ is usually suggested after enucleation on finding giant cells in a fibrous stroma histologically. Check bone biochemistry (Ca^{2+}, PO^{4+} ↓, alkaline, phosphatase ↑, PTH ↑). If hyperparathyroidism is confirmed and treated, these lesions regress.

Dermoid cyst Developmental cyst commonest at the lateral canthus of the eye, but next most often found in the midline of the neck above mylohyoid, where it causes elevation of the tongue. Rx: complete but conservative excision.

Congenital epulis By definition present at birth; usually presents as a pedunculated nodule. Histology reveals large granular cells. Rx: complete but conservative excision.

Peripheral giant cell granuloma (giant cell epulis) Deep red gingival swelling, probably caused by chronic irritation. Histology reveals a vascular lesion with multinuclear giant cells. Rx: excision with stripping of periosteum and curettage of underlying bone.

Pregnancy epulis An ↑ inflammatory response to plaque during pregnancy causes a lesion indistinguishable from a pyogenic granuloma. Onset usually in 3rd month. Rx: none (other than OHI) if possible, as it regresses after delivery. If very troublesome, simple excision; but it may recur.

Pyogenic granuloma Red fleshy swelling, often nodular, occurring as a response to recurrent trauma and non-specific infection. Histology shows proliferation of vascular connective tissue, ∴ bleeds easily. Rx: excision, debride area, good OH.

Fibroepithelial polyp An over-vigorous response to low grade recurrent trauma. May be cessile or pedunculated and range from small lumps to lesions covering the entire palate. Excise with base. Histology shows dense collagenous fibrous tissue lined by keratinized stratified squamous epithelium.

Irritation (denture) hyperplasia A very common hyperplastic response to repeated trauma, e.g. following denture-induced ulceration. Classically, seen as rolls of tissue in the sulcus related to a denture flange. Histology is similar to fibroepithelial polyp. Rx: complete excision with temporary removal of dentures allows healing. Consider simple preprosthetic measures and replace F/F.

Mucoceles Usually mucous extravasation cysts, where saliva leaks from a traumatized duct and pools, creating a compressed connective tissue capsule. Rarely, they are mucous retention cysts. Mostly affect lower lip—similar swellings in the upper lip are often minor salivary gland tumours (p. 510). Rx: excision with associated damaged glands and duct.

Ranula   Mucoceles of the floor of the mouth, arising from the sublingual gland. Tend to recur if marsupialized. A plunging ranula crosses deep to mylohyoid and appears as a neck and floor of mouth swelling. Rx: excision of cyst and associated sublingual gland, submandibular gland may have to be excised if the duct is damaged.

Granulomata   Lumps characterized by the histological finding of granulomata may be caused by Crohn's disease (p. 468) or its localized variant orofacial granulomatosis, sarcoidosis (p. 455), or implanted foreign bodies such as amalgam.

Haemangioma   Developmental lesion of blood vessels. Present at birth, they can grow with the child, remain static, or regress. Blanch on pressure. Do **not** biopsy. 80% spontaneously regress; Rx for those that don't: laser or cryotherapy.

Lymphangioma   Rarer developmental lesion, this time of lymphatics. May present as an enlarged tongue or lip. Rx dificult; some can be beneficially excised. Sclerosant DK432 sometimes benefits.

Vascular malformations   Developmental lesions of blood vessels which *do not* regress but grow with patient. Characterized by rate of blood flow in lesion. Rx: interventional radiology and surgery.

Warts/squamous papillomata   Main aetiological factor is HPV. True warts are rare in the mouth and usually transmitted from skin warts. Found in those with STD or AIDS, but most have no such link.
Papillomas are common in the mouth; appear as multiply papillated pink or white asymptomatic lumps. Rx: excision biopsy (if on a stalk—ligate or diathermy base as they contain a prominent vessel).

Non-tumour hard-tissue lumps

Cysts (p. 418); benign tumours (p. 420); malignant tumours (p. 452).

Tori are bony exostoses found in both jaws. *Torus palatinus* is found in the centre of the hard palate; *torus mandibularis* on the lingual premolar/molar region of the mandible. Rx: reassurance that these developmental anomalies cause no harm (they are *not* part of the Gardener syndrome, p. 758). Rarely, excision for denture construction is indicated.

Giant cell granuloma (p. 415) This can present as an intrabony swelling or symptomless radiolucency. Carefully enucleate.

Brown 'tumour' (p. 414) Again, imitates the giant cell granuloma; difference is in bone biochemistry.

Paget's disease of bone Relatively common over the age of 55 and affects the skull, pelvis, and long bones, as well as the jaws. Although aetiology is uncertain both the measles and respiratory syncytial virus have been implicated. The maxilla is more frequently affected than the mandible. Hypercementosis of roots makes extractions difficult in this group. There is a replacement of normal bone remodelling by a chaotic alternation of resorption and deposition, with resorption dominating in the early stages. Bone pain and cranial neuropathies can occur. X-rays show a 'cotton wool' appearance. Biochemistry shows an ↑ alkaline phosphatase and urinary hydroxyproline. Avoid GA; use prophylactic antibiotics and plan extractions surgically. Diphosphonates and calcitonin are used in treatment.

Fibrous dysplasia Areas of bone are replaced by fibrous tissue. Onset in childhood; ossifies and stabilizes with age. Jaw involvement usually presents as a painless hard swelling. Characteristic X-ray appearance is of 'ground glass' bone. Histology shows fibrous replacement of bone with osseous trabeculae which look like irregular 'Chinese characters' Rx: skeletal resculpting after stabilization of growth &/or orthognathic surgery/orthodontics.

Cherubism Hereditary, and presents at 2–4 yrs. It is a bilateral variant of fibrous dysplasia. In addition to the histological pattern for fibrous dysplasia there are also multinucleated giant cells. Natural history is not well understood, may burn out or regress. Skeletal resculpting after cessation may be necessary.

Cysts of the jaws

Cysts are abnormal epithelium-lined cavities which often contain fluid but only contain pus if they become too infected. Jaw cysts predominantly arise from odontogenic epithelium and grow by a means not fully understood but involving epithelial proliferation, bone resorption by prostaglandins, and variations in intracystic osmotic pressure.

Diagnosis

Many are detected as asymptomatic radiolucencies on X-ray; others present as painless swellings, almost always of the buccal cortex. Infected cysts present with pain, swelling, and discharge. Vitality test associated teeth. Take a DPT and a periapical film when possible to screen for size and coexisting pathology. Transillumination rarely helps, but aspiration is sometimes useful and can help distinguish some lesions. Rarely, cysts may present with a pathological #, especially of the mandible.

Treatment

(a) Enucleation with 1° closure is commonest and generally the Rx of choice. It consists of removing the cyst lining from the bony walls of the cavity and repositioning the access flap. Any relevant dental pathology is treated at the same time, e.g. by apicectomy.

(b) Enucleation with packing and delayed closure is used when badly infected cysts, particularly very large ones, are unsuitable for 1° closure. Pack with Whitehead's varnish or BIPP.

(c) Enucleation with 1° bone grafting. Rarely useful.

(d) Marsupialization. This is the opening of the cyst to allow continuity with the oral mucosa; healing is slower than with enucleation and a cavity persists for some time. It is useful to allow tooth eruption through the cyst or where enucleation is C/I.

▶ Always submit cyst lining for histopathology.

Types of cysts

Many classifications exist, few are helpful.

Inflammatory dental cysts are very common. Described as apical or lateral depending on position in relation to tooth root, or residual if left behind after tooth extraction. Necrotic pulp is the stimulus, and the epithelium comes from cell rests of Malassey. Rx: enucleation plus endodontics or extraction.

Eruption cysts, p. 68.

Dentigerous cysts form around the crown of an unerupted permanent tooth and arise from reduced enamel epithelium. May delay eruption. Rx: marsupialization or enucleation, depending on position.

Keratocysts are lined by parakeratinized epithelium derived from the remnants of the dental lamina and are thought to replace a missing tooth. They have a fluid filling with a protein content <4 g/dl. Aspiration of samples for biochemistry and cytology for parakeratinized squames can be helpful. It is important to identify these cysts, as outpouching walls and 'daughter' or 'satellite' cysts make them more liable to recur. Their multiloculated appearance on X-ray may confuse them with an ameloblastoma (p. 420). Rx: careful enucleation, &/or cryotherapy &/or Carnoy's solution, or aggressive curettage of the cavity. Rarely, excision is needed if recurrent.

Calcifying epithelial odontogenic cysts are rare and distinguished by areas of calcification and 'ghost cells' on histology. Rx: enucleate.

Solitary bone cysts are usually an incidental finding on X-ray and devoid of a lining, but may contain straw-coloured fluid. They probably arise following breakdown of an intraosseous haematoma, and are distinguished by a scalloped upper border on X-ray where the cyst pushes into cancellous bone between teeth but spares the lamina dura. Opening the cyst, gentle curettage, and closure heals these 'cysts'; associated teeth need no Rx.

Aneurysmal bone cysts are expansile lesions full of vascular spongy bone. Present as a symptomless swelling, unless traumatized, when bleeding causes pain and rapid expansion. Small ones can be carefully enucleated, but larger aneurysmal bone cysts need excision and possible reconstruction since they will recur if incompletely excised.

Fissural cysts are not associated with dental epithelium but arise from embryonic junctional epithelium. They are rare and include incisive canal cysts, incisive papilla cysts, and nasolabial cysts. Rx: enucleation.

Benign tumours of the mouth

Non-odontogenic tumours

Epithelial

Squamous cell papilloma (p. 415) Resembles a white or pink cauliflower and is caused by papilloma virus. Usually presents on the palate. Does not undergo malignant change. Excise.

Connective Tissue

Fibroma Very rare. Benign fibrous tumour, usually pink and pedunculated. Excise with a narrow margin.

Lipoma Soft, smooth, slow growing yellowish lump composed of fat cells. Enucleate or excise with narrow margin.

Osteoma Smooth, hard, benign neoplasm of bone. Usually unilateral and covered by normal oral mucosa. Not situated in the classical position of tori (p. 416). Gardener syndrome (p. 758).

Neurofibroma Rare tumour of the fibroblasts of a peripheral nerve. Usually affects the tongue; may be part of von Recklinghausen disease (p. 761). Can undergo sarcomatous change. Excise with a small margin.

Neurolemmoma (schwanomma) Tumour composed of Schwann cells (cells of the axonal sheath). Rx: excision; nerve fibres can sometimes be preserved due to eccentric tumour growth.

Granular cell myoblastoma Rare tumour of histiocyte origin, usually arising as a nodule on the tongue. Excise with a margin.

Ossifying fibroma May be neoplasm or developmental anomaly. It is a well-demarcated fibro-osseous lesion of the jaws. Presents as a painless slow-growing swelling, expanding both buccal and lingual cortices. X-ray shows a radiolucent area, circumscribed by a radiopaque margin. Histology is similar to fibrous dysplasia. Enucleation or conservative excision is curative. A faster-growing but equally benign version occurs in children.

Odontogenic tumours

Many of these are fascinating (to some) rarities. Only the more important are discussed.

Ameloblastoma One of the commoner odontogenic tumours. Commonest in men and Africans, and in the posterior mandible. There are three basic types: unicystic, polycystic, and peripheral. The unicystic type is the least aggressive; the polycystic and peripheral types show a tendency to invade surrounding tissue, whereas the unicystic expands it. Metastases are very rare. Histologically, two types are seen: plexiform and follicular. Rx: unicystic can be enucleated provided a rim of enclosing bone is removed as well; the other types require excision with a margin.

Adenoameloblastoma Tends to occur in the anterior maxilla in females. Rx: conservative excision, as recurrence is not a problem.

Calcifying epithelial odontogenic tumour (Pindborg tumour) Characteristically, a radiolucency on X-ray with scattered radiopacities. Needs excision with a margin.

Myxoma Occurs in both hard and soft tissues. Those arising in the jaws are tumours of young adults arising within bone and can invade the surrounding tissue extensively. Characteristically, has a 'soap bubble' appearance on X-ray. Histology reveals spindle cells in a mucoid stroma. These tumours need excision with a margin of surrounding normal bone.

Ameloblastic fibroma Rare; affects young adults and appears as a unilocular radiolucency on X-ray, causing painless expansion of the jaws. Enucleation is usually curative.

Odontomes Not true neoplasms, but malformations of dental hard tissues. Classically, they are classified as *compound* when they are multiple small 'teeth' in a fibrous sac, and *complex* when they are a congealed irregular mass of dental hard tissue. These are best regarded and treated as unerupted, malpositioned, or impacted teeth, and removed using standard dento-alveolar techniques when required (p. 396).

Disturbances in tooth formation can lead to isolated abnormalities of enamel, dentine, and cementum. Cementomas are worthy of mention because they create extreme difficulty in tooth removal. Dens in dente, p. 74.

The maxillary antrum

These are the largest of the four paired paranasal air sinuses, lying in each half of the maxilla between the alveolus inferiorly, nasal cavity medially, and orbits superiorly.

Antral pathology often mimics symptoms attributable to maxillary teeth. Δ is by exclusion of dental pathology, nasal discharge or stuffiness, tenderness over the cheeks, and pain worse on moving the head. Occipito-mental X-rays (15° and 30°) may reveal antral opacity, fluid level, or # (p. 496). To define fluid level, repeat film with head tilted. Other X-rays: DPT for cysts and roots and CT scans for tumours, pansinusitis, and blow out #.

Extractions and the antrum The proximity of maxillary cheek teeth to the antral floor makes it easy for roots and even teeth to be displaced into the antrum. It also predisposes to # of the alveolar process during 6 7 8 extraction. Displaced roots can be retrieved either by an extended transalveolar approach similar to that for removing roots (useful when the roots are lying under the antral lining) or via a *Caldwell–Luc* approach.

Maxillary sinusitis

Acute sinusitis usually follows a viral URTI which has ↓ cilia activity, and is due to bacterial superinfection (usually mixed; anaerobes, haemophilus, staphylococci, and streptococci). Less commonly, due to foreign body, e.g. roots, water. Poor drainage via the osteum exacerbates the situation. Δ as above and confirmed by proof puncture if necessary. Rx: erythromycin 500 mg PO qds or doxycycline 100 mg PO od. Decongestants, e.g. oxymetazoline or xylometazoline. **Chronic sinusitis** may then develop, particularly if a foreign body or poor drainage is present. Mucosal lining hypertrophies and may form polyps. A post-nasal discharge (drip) is often present. Rx: aimed at reventilation of the sinus. Foreign bodies, if present, should be removed via an incision in the canine fossa (above the premolars) and creation of a bony window into the antrum (Caldwell–Luc). Ventilation is provided either by intra-nasal antrostomy or (ideally) by endoscopic enlargement of the osteum &/or drainage of anterior ethmoids, depending on cause (functional endoscopic sinus surgery—FESS, p. 432).

Oro-antral fistula

Is the creation of a pathological epithelium-lined tract between the mouth and maxillary sinus. This most often occurs following the extraction of isolated molar teeth when the fistula tends to persist. Post-extraction reflux of fluids into the nose or minor nosebleeds are a diagnostic pointer. Confirm by getting patient to attempt to blow out against a closed nose; air bubbles through the fistula. Occasionally antral mucosa prolapses through the socket. Rx: many small fistulae are asymptomatic and close spontaneously. Closure if Δ is made at time of extraction: close the socket by suture or buccal advancement flap, give antibiotics and decongestants as above, and advise not to blow nose. Closure if Δ is made >2 days after extraction: place on antibiotics, etc., for 2 weeks and review after 6. Many will have closed. If not, repair by:

1 **Buccal advancement flap** Excise fistula to prepare a line of closure over bone and raise a broad-based buccal flap. Incise periosteum to

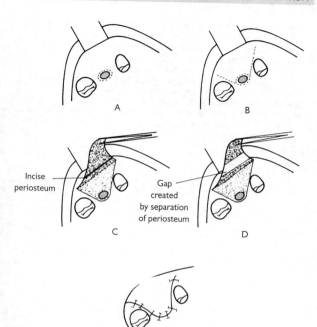

The buccal advancement flap (after Rehrmann).

Steps:

A Excise the fistulous tract; easiest with a No. 11 blade.

B Outline (dashed) of incision for a full thickness mucoperiosteal buccal flap.

C Reflect full thickness mucoperiosteal flap and incise the periosteal layer ONLY. This makes it possible to mobilize the flap.

D 'Stretch' the flap to assess the degree of elasticity once the restraining effect of the periosteum is lost.

E The flap is advanced across the fistula and sutured to palatal mucosa *over bone*.

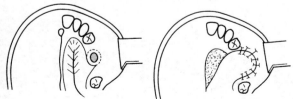

The palatal rotation flap (after Ashley).

A Excise fistula; outline palatal flap based on greater palatine artery.

B Mobilize and rotate palatal flap, suturing its leading edge to buccal mucosa over bone. Leave donor site to granulate under surgical dressing or pack.

allow mucosa to stretch over the socket and close, **over bone**, with vertical mattress sutures. Use antibiotics, etc., remove sutures at 10 days. *Disadvantages*: thin tissue may break down; reduces sulcus depth.

2 **Palatal rotation flap** Excise fistula as above. Dissect a palatal mucoperiosteal flap based on palatine artery, rotate over socket, and suture in similar fashion. *Disadvantages*: bare bone left to granulate; difficult flap to rotate without distortion.

3 **Buccal fat pad flap** If after raising the buccal advancement flap the periosteal incision is opened with artery forceps, the buccal fat pad is exposed. This can be easily mobilized as a pedicled flap to suture into and obtund the defect.

Sinus lift operation (p. 504)

Minor preprosthetic surgery

When teeth are extracted alveolar bone resorbs, ∴ should aim to preserve alveolar bone whenever possible, either by not extracting teeth (over-dentures, p. 370) or by using a minimally traumatic technique.

At time of extraction of remaining teeth   Extract carefully, compress the sockets, remove only small unattached pieces of bone, cover any exposed areas of bone with gingival flaps, and surgically remove roots *only* when necessary (infected, loose, >1/3 root length). Consider interseptal alveolotomy if ridge is prominent and heavily undercut (e.g. Class II). This consists of creating a labial osteomucosal flap by dividing the septae and extending bone cut at the <u>3</u> region through the buccal plate and collapsing-in the bone flap. Prominent fraena should simply be excised. Attempts at decreasing the rate of ridge resorption have been made by leaving roots under mucosal flaps and by implanting hydroxyapatite or biocoral cones into extraction sockets.

Problems in denture wearers

▶ Only use surgery when denture faults and psychogenic disorders have been excluded. Screen jaws with DPT.

Retained roots and bone sequestrae   are removed using standard transalveolar technique, except in the maxilla where buried canines may be removed using an osteoplastic flap (where bone is raised on a mucoperiosteal hinge).

Small bony irregularities   can be smoothed with a bur but consider ridge augmentation if extensive.

Fibrous (flabby) ridges   ↓ by raising a flap of attached gingiva to repair the defect, excise remaining soft tissue ridge, and repair with flap raised first. Fibrous tuberosities can be dealt with similarly.

Fibrous bands and irritation hyperplasia   should be excised. Results are improved if palatal mucosal grafts are used to repair the defects and minimize scarring.

Tori   can be reduced with a bur under a local flap. Or resected with a combination of bur and chisel.

Muscle attachments   to the mylohyoid ridge or genial tubercles can be displaced by resecting the bone from the mandible with a chisel and dissecting away the muscles. Genioglossus and geniohyoid should be reattached to the labial sulcus.

Ridge augmentation   (p. 504) The use of subperiosteally injected porous hydroxyapatite as an outpatient procedure under LA is useful in a very limited number of cases, mainly due to ridge type. In this technique, a subperiosteal tunnel is raised along the crest of the ridge and filled with a hydroxyapatite/saline sludge. It is very dependent on the shape of the ridge, and works best with concave ridges as opposed to the more often seen feather-edge ridge. *Problems*: migration of particles after periosteal elevation. Biocoral is replacing particulate hydroxyapatite for this purpose.

Sulcus deepening   (p. 504) When adequate vertical and horizontal basal bone exists but there is a shortage of ridge &/or attached gingiva, these procedures can help. Depends on: (a) dissecting away non-attached mucosa to leave a raw 'new' sulcus; (b) lining this new sulcus with skin or mucosa; (c) *securing the new depth with a 'stent'*—a denture or baseplate lined with tissue conditioner or impression compound, which is held in place by nylon sutures for 10–14 days, then replaced immediately by a new denture with a soft lining extended to the new sulcus and worn continually for the first 3 months.

Implantology

The 'screw-in tooth' has arrived!

History Numerous procedures for oral implants have been described, including subperiosteal, endosseous, and submucosal. All have been strongly advocated by bands of enthusiasts and have one thing in common: failure. Genuine advances in the discipline have come about, thanks to a major contribution by Bränemark: 'osseointegration'. All current implants are based on this now well-accepted concept.

Osseointegration is the direct abutment of bone to implant surface such that osteoblasts can be seen on electron micrographs to be growing on the implant surface. In addition, a tight fibrous/epithelial attachment above the crestal bone between gingiva and implant is essential. Finally, the implant must be designed to resist displacement and evenly dissipate occlusal loads.

Types of implant Large range. Materials are titanium or hydroxyapatite-coated titanium. Bioceramic or gold are less common. May be inserted transmucosally or in two stages (see below). Attached mucoperiosteum is 'best' perimplant tissue.

Indications Edentulous mouths unable to retain dentures, partially dentate for bridge abutments, single anterior tooth replacement, and maxillofacial prostheses post cancer surgery or trauma. If implants survive first 2 yrs there is a 98% success rate with dramatic improvement in all functional parameters.[1] Success mandible > maxilla (bone quality). Irradiated bone should receive hyperbaric O_2 preoperatively.

Techniques Joint planning between oral surgeon and restorative dentist is essential for success.[2] Conventional denture modification should have been tried, a balanced occlusion should be creatable, and a high standard of OH is mandatory. The surgical procedure is highly equipment-dependent, and the surgeon needs to be trained in the particular technique used. Most commonly, this involves:

1 Fixture installation. A gingival–mucosal flap is raised, based lingually, and a receiving channel is prepared in bone, using matched spiral drills. The entrance to the fixture site is counter-sunk and, depending on the type of implant, it is either pressed into place or, if the channel is threaded, a fixture is screwed in. In two-stage procedures the implant is covered by the flap at the end of the procedure. When placing multiple implants a direction indicator is helpful for achieving parallelism. Bone over-heating must be avoided by constant irrigation. In two-stage procedures, a healing period of 4 months in the mandible and 6 months in the maxilla is recommended. In one-stage procedures a connecting bar can be fitted within 2 weeks but load-bearing or retentive studs should be avoided for 4–6 months.

2 In two-stage procedures, abutment connection is then carried out by punch excision of mucosa overlying the implants, removal of cover screws, and insertion of the abutment. A post-op surgical pack is

1 R. Adell 1983 *J Prosthetic Dent* **49** 251.
2 BAOMS/BSSPD 1995 Guidelines on Standards for the Treatment of Patients Using Endosseous Dental Implants, BDJ.

usually used, prosthetic procedures starting about 2 weeks after abutment connection.

Implant salvage/bone augmentation   The principles of GTR (p. 240) can be used to allow bone formation around osseointegrated implants either to ↑ bone height or bulk, or to cover an exposed side of the implant.

Craniofacial implants   (p. 521)

Transmandibular implants   (p. 504)

Lasers

Definition Light amplification by the stimulated emission of radiation. Light consists of packets of photons transmitted in electromagnetic waves (visible light 400–700 nm). Laser energy is produced by light stimulation of active media to generate collimated light energy at a specific frequency. The active media determines the characteristics of the laser.

Clinical lasers

These consist of two main groups, *hard* and *soft* lasers.

Hard lasers work principally by thermal effect, although certain benefits such as decreased scarring and pain are thought to be due to the photo-chemical effects of the laser beam.

Carbon dioxide laser A hard laser in common use in the hospital service. Main role is as a cutting beam which seals small vessels as it cuts. Also used to evaporate benign white patches of oral mucosa. Used as continuous wave or pulsed beam at 10–20 watts of energy.

KTP laser Similar to carbon dioxide laser, giving initially painless wounds. Becomes painful after 48–72 h, however.

Argon laser Produces a light beam which is selectively absorbed by haemoglobin and melanin, ∴ particularly useful for pigmented and vascular lesions.

Neodymium–Yttrium aluminium garnet (Nd–Yag) laser Originally marketed as a hard laser with a relatively low power output; now available as a soft dental laser.

Tuneable dye laser Expensive variable frequency laser.

Soft lasers Thought to work by stabilizing cell membranes by a non-thermal photochemical process, increasing cellular metabolism by a minor thermal change, and possibly by inducing endorphin release.

Helium–Neon The red aiming beam on hard lasers, classroom pointers, and the 'Terminator's' weaponry. Part of the soft laser group, it has no cutting effect but seems to act photochemically on cells.

Neodymium–Yag A system using this active media is now marketed for use in dentistry and is purported to ↑ cell turnover, ↓ inflammatory response, inhibit oedema, ↑ rate of cell regeneration, e.g. peripheral neurones, and ↓ wound scarring. All this without any recognized side-effects. Many of these claims have yet to be widely validated.

Summary

Lasers are available for a range of uses in dentistry; they are expensive and require special safety precautions. Some benefits can be achieved in other ways and some have yet to be proven. They are a tool, not a magic wand.

Minimally invasive surgery

While some specialties such as orthopaedics and gynaecology have been using endoscopic technology for many years, a recent surge in fibre-optic technology coupled with the 'discovery' of the laparoscope by general surgeons made minimally invasive (minimal access) surgery one of the hot topics of the late 1990s.

One of the spin-offs of the sudden uncontrolled ↑ in the number of laparoscopic operations was bad publicity about some of the adverse outcomes following this type of surgery, and questions about surgeons' training. One very positive result of this has been the development of surgical skills laboratories (remember phantom heads?), structured courses, and a real interest in training and education.

In the field of oral and maxillofacial surgery minimally invasive surgery has yet to make a significant impact. Current examples include:

Temporomandibular joint arthroscopy Uses specialized small rigid endoscopes with a fibre-optic light source which can be placed in the TMJ space (usually upper joint space) through a tiny incision in the preauricular skin. The joint is distended by a throughflow of sterile irrigant which exits via a needle placed about 1 cm anterior to the arthroscope. Reasonable visualization is possible but significant surgery is fairly limited.

Functional endoscopic sinus surgery (FESS) Rigid endoscopes with angled viewing ports allow visualization and a certain amount of surgery of the paranasal sinuses. Biopsy and sampling of a wide range of paranasal tissues is possible and specific surgical expansion of the osteum may prove to be the ideal treatment for chronic sinusitis. This technique has been rapidly developed by many ENT enthusiasts but indications for its use will take a few more years to become stabilized.

Endoscopically assisted internal fixation Internal fixation of facial # is now widely accepted and standard practice; however, some areas, particularly of the mandible, are very difficult to access safely. Condylar neck # and some angle # may be more easily treated using a modified trocar system and light source.

Endoscopically assisted face and brow lifting Aesthetic facial surgery by its very nature requires distant and minimalist scars. Endoscopic brow lifting from the anterior scalp is reasonably straightforward and popular in France and the USA. Long-term stability is awaited. Endoscopic facelifting makes a tedious operation more so.

NB While flexible fibre-optic scopes play quite an extensive role in examination of the upper aerodigestive tract, the extent to which significant head and neck surgery can be performed is currently limited.

Oral medicine

Principal sources   Much of the skill of oral medicine lies in the clinical recognition of lesions, ∴ a colour atlas of oral mucosal disease is invaluable, e.g. C. Scully 1999 *Slide Interpretation in Oral Diseases*, OUP. Related subjects are **oral pathology**: J. Soames 1999 *Oral Pathology*, 3ed OUP; **temporomandibular joint**: R. Gray 1995 *Temporomandibular Disorders: A Clinical Approach, BDJ*. Although the authors of the latter have a slightly different approach, this is a thoughtful, informative, and useful book.

Bacterial infections of the mouth

Caries (p. 28); periodontal disease (p. 206); dento-facial infections (p. 408). This page refers primarily to mucosal infections.

Scarlet fever May be due to a delayed type hypersensitivity to streptococcal erythrogenic toxin. Usually causes an URTI. The sore throat is accompanied by a skin rash, general malaise, and fever. The oral mucosa is reddened and the tongue undergoes pathognomonic changes; the dorsum develops a white coating through which white oedematous fungiform papillae project—the 'strawberry tongue' of scarlet fever. Later the white coating is shed and the dorsum becomes smooth and red with enlarged fungiform papillae—'raspberry tongue'. Rx is directed towards the systemic condition with high-dose penicillin. The oral manifestations resolve within 14 days.

Tuberculosis A re-emerging infectious disease caused by *Mycobacterium* tuberculosis. It is commonly seen in immunocompromised patients, including elderly persons; although 1/3 of global population is affected by TB, oral involvement with it is rare. When it does occur it is usually 2° to open pulmonary infection or coexisting HIV. The oral lesion presents as a deep painful ulcer, gradually increasing in size. Any part of the oral mucosa may be involved, although the posterior aspect of the dorsum of the tongue is the commonest site. PCR may facilitate definitive Δ, especially in cases with unusual presentation. Histopathology shows necrotizing granuloma with giant and epithelioid cells and a Ziehl–Neelsen stain reveals mycobacteria. Refer to a chest physician for management as combination chemotherapy is required.

Syphilis All phases (1°, 2°, and 3°) affect the mouth.

1° lesion A chancre (a firm ulcerated nodule) develops at the site of inoculation, usually the lips or tongue. This lesion is highly infectious and *Treponema pallidum* can easily be isolated. There is usually marked cervical lymphadenopathy which resolves spontaneously in 1–2 months.

2° lesion Develops 2–4 months after the 1° with a cutaneous rash, condylomata and ulceration of the oral mucosa. This oral involvement occurs regardless of the site of 1° infection, with superficial grey, sloughy ulcers known as mucous patches or snail-track ulcers. These are also highly contagious and *T. pallidum* can be easily isolated. Syphilis serology is positive at this stage. The ulcers generally clear up within a few weeks, although there may be recurrences.

3° lesion Develops several years later and is marked by gumma formation. This is a necrotic granulomatous reaction usually affecting the palate or tongue, which enlarges and ulcerates and may lead to perforation of the palate. In the past, syphilis of the tongue was associated with malignant change, often presenting as a leukoplakia. It is not entirely clear whether it was the condition or its Rx which caused this. Lesions are non-infectious.

Congenital syphilis Classical appearance of saddle nose, frontal bossing, Hutchinson incisors (peg-shaped with notch), and mulberry (Moon) molars.

Gonorrhoea 15 times more common than syphilis. This is a result of orogenital contact with an infected partner and presents as a non-specific stomatitis or pharyngitis with frequent persisting superficial ulcers caused by *Neisseria gonorrhoeae*. Swabs may reveal Gram −ve intracellular diplococci. Rx is with high-dose penicillin; STD should be referred to a genitourinary medicine specialist.

Viral infections of the mouth

Herpes simplex   Although oral infection with herpes simplex types 1 and 2 have been described, type 1 remains the dominant pathogen. Antibodies indicating past infection are virtually ubiquitous in adults. There are two oral manifestations.

Primary herpetic gingivostomatitis   varies widely in severity (↑ with age). In infancy is often mistakenly attributed to 'teething'. Presents with a single episode of widespread stomatitis with vesicles which break down to form shallow painful ulcers, enlarged, tender cervical lymph nodes, halitosis, coated tongue, fever, and a general malaise for 10–14 days. Although generally self-limiting, rare complications include herpetic encephalitis. Δ: based on the clinical features and history, although the virus can be grown in cell culture. Microscopically ballooning degeneration of epithelial cells with intranuclear viral inclusions 'Lipshutz bodies' are seen. A fourfold ↑ in convalescent phase antibodies is also diagnostic, *but* give the Δ only retrospectively. Rx: topical and systemic analgesia (Benzydamine, paracetamol), a soft or liquid diet with extra fluid intake, and prevention of 2° infection (chlorhexidine mouthwash) is usually adequate in healthy patients. Severely ill or immunocompromised patients should receive systemic aciclovir.

Secondary herpes (herpes labialis, cold sore)   is a reactivation of the 1° infection which is believed to lie dormant in the trigeminal ganglion. Precipitating factors include trauma, e.g. during removal of 8 and immuno-suppression and, less commonly, exposure to sunlight, stress, or other illness. Usually recurs on the skin of lip or nose supplied by one branch of trigeminal nerve, classically at the mucocutaneous junction, or rarely as an IO blister. Prodromal phase over 24h where there is a prickling sensation on the lips followed by vesiculation and pain. Lesions may respond to topical aciclovir 5% cream. Should consider systemic aciclovir (p. 628) in the immunosuppressed.

Herpes (varicella) zoster   is neurogenic DNA virus which causes chickenpox as a 1° infection and shingles as a reactivation.

Chickenpox   Classically an itchy, vesicular, cutaneous rash which may rarely affect the oral mucosa.

Shingles   is confined to the distribution of a nerve, the virus staying either in the dorsal root ganglion of a peripheral nerve or the trigeminal ganglion. Always presents as a unilateral lesion never crossing the midline. Facial or oral lesions may arise in the area supplied by the branches of the trigeminal nerve. Δ: pre-eruption pain, followed by development of painful vesicles on skin or oral mucosa which rupture to give ulcers or crusting skin wounds, in the distribution outlined above. These usually clear in 2–4 weeks, but apparent resolution is often followed by severe post-herpetic neuralgia which may continue for years. Rx: symptomatic relief for chickenpox. There is some evidence to suggest that aggressive early Rx of shingles with aciclovir ↓ the incidence and severity of post-herpetic neuralgia in immunocompromised patients. Refer to an ophthalmologist if the eye is involved.

Coxsackievirus is an RNA virus causing 2° oral mucosal conditions.

Herpangina Caused by Coxsackie A virus (A1 + A6, A8, A10, A12, A16, or A22) is confined to children and presents with widespread small ulcers on the oral mucosa with fever and general upset. Clinically it resembles herpetic stomatitis, but with no *gingivitis* and only moderate cervical lymphadenitis. May be preceded by sore throat and conjunctivitis. Can also be mistaken as 'teething'. Self-limiting in 10–14 days. Fairly rare.

Hand, foot, and mouth disease Caused by Coxsackie virus (usually A16) and is also confined to children. A papular, vesicular rash appears on the hands and feet in conjunction with nasal congestion and oral mucosal vesicles. These break down, leaving painful superficial ulcers, particularly on the palate. The gingivae are rarely involved. It is self-limiting in 10–14 days. Rx as herpetic stomatitis. Quite common.

Human papilloma virus has been associated with squamous cell papilloma (p. 415), condyloma acuminatum (multiple white/pink nodules), focal epithelial hyperplasia (multiple painless papules), and verruca vulgaris (white exophytic lumps). The last three are very rare. Rx: local surgery and interferon.

Measles The prodromal phase of measles may be marked by small white spots with an erythematous margin on the buccal mucosa, known as Koplik spots. A few days later the maculo-papular rash of measles appears, usually behind the ears, then spreading to the face and trunk.

Glandular fever (infectious mononucleosis) is seen mostly in children and young adults and spread by infected saliva. It varies widely in severity and presents with sore throat, generalized lymphadenopathy, fever, headaches, general malaise, and often a maculo-papular rash. There may be hepatosplenomegaly. Oral manifestations may mimic 1 herpetic gingivostomatitis, with widespread oral ulceration, and in addition petechial haemorrhages, especially at the junction of hard and soft palate (pathognomonic), and bruising may be present. The cause is usually Epstein–Barr virus (EBV) and, less commonly, cytomegalovirus (CMV). Toxoplasmosis can give a similar picture. Δ: initially monospot test, Paul–Bunnell test to exclude EBV, and acute and convalescent titres for CMV and toxoplasmosis. Be aware that early HIV infection can mimic this condition. Rx: symptomatic as for 1° herpes, except toxoplasmosis, which may respond to sulfa drugs; seek expert advice. **NB** Ampicillin should not be given to patients with a sore throat who may have glandular fever as it inevitably produces an unwanted response, ranging from a rash to anaphylaxis. Opportunistic infection on the tongue mucosa by EBV is thought to be the pathological mechanism behind 'hairy leukoplakia'.

Reiter's disease Causative agent unknown but appears to be post-infective response. Consists of urethritis, arthritis, conjunctivitis &/or oral ulcers or erosions. Predominantly affects young males and is associated with HLA B27 in 80% of patients—leukocytosis and ↑ ESR are common.

Oral candidosis (candidiasis)

Although over 100 *Candida* species can be isolated only a handful are clinically important. *C. albicans* and *C. dubliniensis* are by far the most important. It is found in the mouths of more than 40% of the symptom-free population. Overt infection occurs when there are local or systemic predisposing factors, ∴ the prime tenet of management is to look for and treat these factors. Candidosis is conveniently divided into:

Acute candidosis

Acute pseudomembraneous candidosis (thrush) Commonest in infancy, old age, and the immunosuppressed or debilitated (e.g. radiotherapy, cytotoxics, steroids, diabetes, cancer, HIV, and haematological malignancy), or those on broad spectrum antibiotics. Δ: appears as creamy lightly adherent plaques on an erythematous oral mucosa, usually on the cheek, palate, or oropharynx. Occasionally symptomless, but more commonly cause discomfort on eating. These plaques can be gently stripped off, leaving a raw under-surface and, with Gram staining, show candidal hyphae. In infancy, widespread oral candidosis can be associated with a livid facial rash and an associated nappy rash. Colonization of a breast-feeding mother's nipples can lead to mutual recolonization. Rx: nystatin SF suspension 100 000 units rinsed then swallowed qds 10 days, or nystatin pastille 1 qds, are cheap and usually effective preparations. Chlorhexidine mouthwash is an effective adjunct to Rx. Amphotericin and miconazole are more expensive (and mutually antagonistic) alternatives. Fluconazole 50 mg od is the systemic drug of choice. *C. glabrata*, *C. tropicalis*, and *C. knusel* are fluconazole resistant, ∴, candida subtyping should be performed for resistant cases.

Acute atrophic (erythematous) candidosis is an opportunistic infection following the use of broad-spectrum antibiotics, sometimes inhaled steroids, and in patients with HIV as well as those with xerostomia. It is painful and exacerbated by hot or spicy foods. The oral mucosa has a red, shiny, atrophic appearance and there may be coexisting areas of thrush. Rx: eliminate cause (if due to inhaled steroids rinse mouth with water after inhaling), otherwise as above. Gargling with 1:50 dilution of Amphotericin B is effective in Rx of oral candidosis of asthmatic patients Rx with inhaled steroids.

Chronic candidosis

Chronic atrophic candidosis (denture stomatitis) (pp. 124, 366) Reported prevalence of denture stomatosis: 10–75%.

Angular cheilitis is a combined staphylococcal, streptococcal, and candidal infection, involving the tissues at the angle of the mouth, often with an underlying precipitating factor, e.g. iron deficiency and B_{12} deficiency anaemia. Therefore, haematological deficiency should be investigated with a FBC red cell folate, B_{12}, and glucose. Anecdote suggests an inadequate OVD can also predispose, but correction of this alone will not resolve the condition. Often associated with chronic atrophic candidosis. Clinically, see red, cracked, macerated skin at angles of the mouth, often with a gold crust. Infecting organisms can be identified on culture of swabs of the area, although it is usual to make a clinical Δ. Rx: miconazole cream, which is active against all three infecting organisms. Rx needs to be prolonged, up to 10 days after resolution of clinical lesion, and carried out in conjunction with elimination of any underlying factors.

Median rhomboid glossitis   is no longer considered to be an anatomical abnormality but a form of chronic atrophic candidosis affecting the dorsum of the tongue. Seen in patients using inhaled steroids and smokers. Some patients have lesions in the centre of the dorsum of tongue and palate (kissing lesions). Rx only if symptomatic as discomfort can be improved with topical antifungals, but the appearance cannot.

Chronic hyperplastic candidosis (candidal leukoplakia)   More commonly seen in smokers. Typically presents as white patch on the oral commissural buccal mucosa bilaterally. Although there is an ↑ risk of malignant change (see p. 450), the initial approach *after ensuring the diagnosis microbiologically and histopathologically* is to eradicate the candidal infection. Candidal hyphae can be seen in the superficial layers of the epidermis, one reason why eradication is so difficult. Rx: systemic antifungals such as fluconazole and itraconazole, while expensive, are indicated in an attempt to remove the infecting organism. Often associated with iron, folate, and B_{12} deficiency, and smoking, which should be corrected. Most lesions will resolve after such Rx; if not, reassess degree of dysplasia.

Chronic mucocutaneous candidosis   A rare syndrome complex with several subgroups, including: **candidal endocrinopathy,** where skin and mouth lesions occur in conjunction with endocrine abnormalities, **granulomatous skin candidosis,** a **late-onset predominantly male-affecting group,** and an **AIDS-associated group.** Rx: fluconazole, and itraconazole (p. 628).

Histoplasmosis   This and other rare fungal infections have occasional oral manifestations.

Recurrent aphthous stomatitis (ulcers)

This is the term given to a fairly well-defined group of conditions characterized by recurrent oral ulceration. There are three subgroups:

Minor aphthous ulcers A very common condition (~25% of population) affecting ~80% of RAS patients. Usually appears as a group of 1–6 ulcers at a time, of variable size (usually 2–5 mm diameter). Mainly occur on non-keratinized mucosa and heal within 1–2 weeks without scarring. Prodromal discomfort may precede painful ulcers. Exacerbated by stress, local trauma, menstruation, and may be an oral 'marker' of iron, B_{12}, or folate deficiencies. In some cases are a manifestation of Crohn's disease, ulcerative colitis, or gluten enteropathy. Aetiology, although not fully understood, is almost certainly autoimmune. There is a familial history in 45% of cases. Rx: prevent superinfection with chlorhexidine mouthwash and relieve pain (simple analgesics, benzydamine mouthrinse). Topical tetracycline and steroid preparations are sometimes useful (p. 616). It is important to look for and treat any underlying deficiency or coexisting pathology.

Major aphthous ulcers Seen in 10% of RAS patients. A more severe variant with fewer, but larger ulcers > 10 mm which may last 5–10 weeks and most commonly affect keratinized mucosa. Associated with tissue destruction and scarring, and any site in the mouth and oropharynx may be affected. There is an even higher association between major aphthae and gastrointestinal and haematological disorders. They are also seen in AIDS. Seldom a cyclical pattern. Rx: as for minor aphthae, plus topical or systemic steroids (p. 616).

Herpetiform ulcers Least common. A descriptive term, as these ulcers have nothing whatsoever to do with infection with the herpesvirus. Manifest as a crop of small but painful ulcers which usually last 1–2 weeks, the commonest site being the floor of mouth, lateral margins, and tip of tongue. They heal without scarring and may occur on both keratinized and non-keratinized surfaces. Rarely, merge to form a large ulcer which heals with scarring. Rx: as for minor aphthous ulceration.

Behçet disease A severe refractory systemic vasculitis of unknown aetiology, characteristically affecting venules. All organs of the body can be concurrently or consecutively affected. It has a world wide distribution but is most prevalent in the Far East, along the *Silk Route*, and in the Middle East. In the UK a prevalence of 0.064 in 10 000 has been reported from Yorkshire. It is a disease of young adults, and rare before age of 10 yrs and after 50 yrs. More common and more severe in males. It is associated with HLA subtype Δ clinical due to absence of laboratory tests and based on presence of recurrent oral ulcers and two of the following: recurrent genital ulceration, eye lesions (uveitis), or skin lesions (erythema nodosum, folliculitis). Good evidence that prophylactic Rx with Azathioprine can prevent blindness. Steroids are mainstay. Rx: ophthalmic referral if eye involved. Monoclonal anti-TNF and similar agents may be of benefit and controlled studies are still in progress. Thalidomide is effective but neuropathy is a major side-effect.

Oral ulcers See p. 480.

Vesiculo-bullous lesions— intraepithelial

Vesicle is a small blister a few millimetres in diameter.

Bulla is a larger blister.

Intraepithelial bullae are caused by loss of attachment between individual cells (acantholysis).

Subepithelial bullae separate the epithelium from the underlying corium.

Ulcer is a breach in the mucous membrane.
Immunopathology: immunofluorescence is a prime diagnostic test. Direct immunofluorescence is performed on fresh biopsy specimen. Indirect is performed on a serum sample.

Erosions are shallower than ulcers.
Because the vesiculo-bullous lesions constitute a defined group with examples from several different pathological processes, they are a favourite examinations topic. One method of classifying this group is into intraepithelial and subepithelial, according to where the blisters form.

Pemphigus is a chronic skin disease which is lethal if not Rx. Oral mucosa is affected in 95% of patients with pemphigus vulgaris and may be the initial presentation of pemphigus in 50%. Autoimmune in aetiology, there are circulating autoantibodies to epithelial intercellular substance. Acantholysis and intercellular IgG &/or C3 are typical (autoantibodies against desmoglein adhesion molecules of squamous epithelium) and cause separation of epithelium above the basal cell layer, and oedema into this potential space produces a superficial, easily burst, fluid-filled bulla. Rupture leaves a large superficial, easily infected ulcer. The first identifiable lesions are quite often found in the mouth, especially on the palate, although these are usually seen as ulcers because the bullae break down rapidly. It is mainly a disease of middle age (F > M), with ↑ incidence in Jews and Arabs. Rarely, it may be drug-induced. Δ: stroking the mucosa produces a bulla (Nikolsky's sign), but this is inducing pathology for the sake of Δ. Other methods are by direct or indirect immunofluorescent techniques (biopsy samples need to be fresh. Rx: systemic steroids &/or azathioprine, dapsone, mycophenolate mofetil, or gold; also cyclophosphamide, especially in refractory and severe cases.

Benign familial chronic pemphigus differs from the above by having a strong family history, with onset of the disease in young adults.

Viral infections, p. 436.

Epidermolysis bullosa (simplex is most common form) Other variants are subepithelial. Due to genetic defect in basement membrane proteins. Skin blisters due to mild trauma, leading to scarring and disfigurement. Caries and periodontal disease are common due to inability to maintain good OH. Simplex type is due to mutations in *K5* or *K14* gene, leading to disruption of basal cells and formation of bullae.

Vesiculo-bullous lesions—subepithelial

Angina bullosa haemorrhagica A fancy name for localized oral blood blister of unknown aetiology, although steroid inhalers may predispose. Δ: exclude other bullous conditions. Rx: puncture &/or reassure (must differentiate from pemphigus/pemphigoid).

Benign mucous membrane pemphigoid Commonest in females > 60. Presents as mucous membrane bullae which rupture and heal with scar formation. Rare to see skin bullae. Conjunctiva may be affected and if scarring occurs can lead to loss of vision, ∴ regard oral signs as a warning to prevent ocular damage. The natural history is of a long-lasting disease which persists with periods of activity and inactivity alternating and may be quiescent for several years. More common than pemphigus and pemphigoid. Δ: again direct and indirect immunofluorescence is used, the antibodies being found at the level of the basement membrane. The bullae are blood-filled and tense and may be found in conjunction with atrophic gingivitis (p. 212). Rx: topical steroids, systemic steroids, or dapsone. Refer to ophthalmology.

Pemphigoid affects > 60-yr age group. Subepithelial bullae form which are firm and less likely to break down than those in pemphigus due to autoantibodies to epithelial basement membrane. The oral mucosa is only affected in ~20% of patients. May be an external 'marker' of internal malignancy or a drug-related immune response.

Dermatitis herpetiformis is a rare chronic condition of unknown aetiology, but often associated with gluten sensitivity with autoantibodies against reticullin, gliadin, endomysium, and transglutaminase. Oral lesions seen in 70% of patients with skin lesion. Commoner in middle-aged men; it affects both skin and mucous membranes; bullae in the mouth break down to leave large erosions. Rx: dapsone may be used both diagnostically and therapeutically. Gluten-free diet helps. Sulfapyridine is an alternative to dapsone.

Lichen planus affects both skin and mucous membranes. Bullous lichen planus is a rare variant in which subepithelial bullae form and break down, leaving large erosions. See also p. 466.

Epidermolysis bullosa This is a rare skin disease which exists in numerous different forms. The dystrophic autosomal recessive form is most likely to present with oral manifestations and appears shortly after birth. Associated with bullae formation after minor trauma to skin or mucosa; these break down leaving painful erosions. Healing is with scarring, resulting in difficulty in eating, speaking, and swallowing as scar tissue limits movement. Skin involvement can lead to destruction of extremities and may be overtaken by carcinomatous change. Prognosis varies widely depending on type. Phenytoin and steroids may help some varieties.

Erythema multiforme This is a group of signs and symptoms of multifactorial aetiology; the most severe form is known as Stevens–Johnson syndrome (p. 761). Affects skin and mucous membranes with an acute onset, usually in young adult males, and is probably due to deposition of immune complexes. It is associated with exposure to certain drugs (sulfas, barbiturates) or infecting organisms (herpes, mycoplasma) in a susceptible individual (hormonal changes). Δ: from clinical features which include 'target lesions', concentric rings of erythema on the palms, legs, face, or neck. The oral mucosa is covered in bullae which break down, the lips and gingivae becoming crusted with painful erosions. There is usually a fever. It is a self-limiting condition in 3–4 weeks but can recur once or twice a year.

Management   Hospitalization may be required in severe forms. Biopsy; virological studies to exclude herpes; identify and avoid precipitating factors; aciclovir or calciclovir may be needed if it is related to herpes. Improve OH with 0.2% chlorhexidine MW. Severe form: Rx with steroids. Minor form: Rx with topical steroids.

Linear IgA disease   is rare, identified pathologically. May be variant of dermatitis herpetiformis.

White patches

Numerous conditions manifest as white patches of the oral mucosa; some of these are transient, such as thrush (p. 438) or chemical burns (e.g. aspirin). More are persistent, and there exists some confusion over the terminology applied to these white patches.

White spongy naevus This is a rare condition affecting keratin. A benign, familial disorder inherited as autosomal dominant. It appears as asymptomatic diffuse soft, uneven thickening of the superficial layer of the epithelium, which characteristically has no definite boundary and may affect any part of the mouth. Histology shows hyperplastic epithelium with gross intraepithelial oedema. Rx: neither exists nor is required.

Frictional keratosis This is a white patch due to hyperplastic hyperkeratotic epithelium induced by local trauma, e.g. sharp tooth and cheek biting. It is managed by removal of the source of the friction, which will generally allow complete resolution of the lesion. If this doesn't happen, biopsy is indicated. Can be seen as self-mutilation in psychiatric disorders or learning disability.

Smokers' keratosis Characteristically a white patch affecting buccal mucosa, tongue, or palate. Appears as discrete white patch. Due to a combination of low-grade burn and the chemical irritants of smoke, and seen particularly in pipe smokers. There is little evidence that these patches are premalignant and they resolve on stopping smoking.

Stomatitis nicotina Affects palate; numerous red papules on a white/grey base. The papules have a dark 'head' which is the opening of a distended minor salivary gland.

'Syphilitic leukoplakia' A white patch on the dorsum of the tongue is one of the classical appearances of tertiary syphilis (p. 434). Active disease must be treated; however, this will not resolve the area of leukoplakia, which has a propensity to undergo malignant change. Δ is usually suggested by histology, serology, or dark ground microscopy of smears.

Chronic hyperplastic candidosis/candidal leukoplakia, p. 439.

Lichen planus, p. 466.

Lupus erythematosis, p. 466.

Leukoplakia, p. 450.

Hairy leukoplakia, p. 476.

Panoral leukoplakia is where the entire oral mucosa appears to be undergoing hyperplastic field change. Risk of malignant change.

Oral carcinoma Occasionally, oral cancer may appear as a white patch, as distinct from a leukoplakia becoming malignant.

Skin grafts may appear as a white patch in the mouth—and are a trap for the unwary in exams.

Renal failure can produce soft, oval white patches which resolve on Rx of renal failure.

Darier's disease   A rare skin condition whose oral lesions (present in ~50%) are coalescing white papules on gingivae and palate.

Pachyonychia congenita   A rare genetic condition affecting nails, skin, and sweat glands. Oval, benign white patches on tongue are common.

Pigmented lesions of the mouth

In many respects the pulling together of pigmented lesions of the oral mucosa is artificial, as they are not related by pathology or Rx. Pigmented lesions are, however, a popular exam question and with this in mind we offer the following well-recognized conditions.

Δ is aided by whether the pigmentation is localized, or generalized throughout the mouth.

Localized

Foreign body amalgam tattoo is the commonest, a localized dense blue/black area of mucosal pigmentation. May result from implantation at time of restoration or from broken filling. Radio opaque. May be palpable but often not. Amalgam tends to become granular and fragmented and if removal is planned, cut out as full thickness wedge. If asymptomatic, diagnose and reassure. 'Road rash' from grit after road traffic accident or graphite from pencils can cause similar.

Local response to chronic trauma usually presents as an area of keratosis but sometimes can appear pigmented.

Ephelis a freckle of the oral mucosa. Harmless.

Pigmented naevi Rare and benign. Analogous to a mole. Mostly harmless. Most commonly seen on vermilion border of lips and palate. If < 1 cm, they do not change in size or colour.

Peutz–Jegher syndrome (p. 760) Multiple small perioral naevi.

Kaposi's sarcoma (p. 476) A radiosensitive tumour associated with AIDS.

Malignant melanoma Potentially lethal, relatively rare IO malignancy. Very dark, irregular outline, enlarges rapidly; poor prognosis. Rare variant is non-pigmented.

Generalized

Racial pigmentation of the oral mucosa varies with skin type and is obviously not pathological.

Foodstuffs A variety can cause superficial mucosal discoloration. Tobacco is the major offender, and paan in some Asian cultures.

Drugs Antimalarials, phenothiazines, cisplatin, zidorodine, busulfan, and oral contraceptives can all cause mucosal pigmentation. Commonest offender is chlorhexidine mouthwash, especially if 'blended' with tea and tobacco.

Heavy metal salts Now rare; classically deposited along the gingival margin in lead or mercury poisoning.

Endocrine associated Addison's disease, ACTH-secreting tumours, adenomatous pituitary dysfunction (Nelson syndrome), ACTH Rx. *Diagnose*: BP, electrolytes, cortisol levels, and response to ACTH stimulation (synacthen test).

Haemochromatosis Haemosiderin deposits cause hyperpigmentation. Rare.

Black hairy tongue   Caused by overgrowth of pigment-producing micro-organisms combined with benign overgrowth of the filiform papillae of the dorsum of the tongue and a lack of normal desquamation. Rx: reassurance, improve OH, tongue scrape or tongue shave depending on patient need/severity.

Premalignant lesions

There exists a group of conditions which have an ↑ risk of malignant transformation of the oropharyngeal mucosa. Although a great deal of attention has been paid to these premalignant conditions, it should be remembered that only a small number of oral cancers are preceded by them, and also that the designation 'premalignant' does not necessarily imply certain malignant transformation. Indeed, the majority of patients with so-called premalignant lesions will not go on to develop oral cancer. The ↑ risk of progression to carcinoma necessitates accurate Δ, Rx if indicated, and long-term follow-up in an attempt to pre-empt life-threatening disease.

Leukoplakia 'White patch or plaque which cannot be characterized clinically or pathologically as any other disease and is not associated with any physical or chemical agent except the use of tobacco' (WHO).

The histopathology of these lesions varies widely from the essentially benign to carcinoma-*in-situ*. They are usually characterized by a thick surface layer of keratin with thickening of the prickle cell layer of the epithelium, acanthosis, and infiltration of the corium by plasma cells; however, the most important variable is cellular atypia amongst the epithelial cells. Pointers to look for are: nuclear hyperchromatism, an ↑ nuclear/cytoplasmic ratio, cellular and nuclear pleomorphism, ↑ &/or atypical mitoses, individual cell keratinization, and focal disturbance in cell arrangement and adhesion. The degree of cellular atypia is one of the most important factors to be considered in the management of a leukoplakia. However, histology of epithelial dysplasia is not reliable, and in one study pathologists in 20% of cases could not confirm or refute their own earlier Δ of dysplasia. Furthermore there is no guarantee that the biopsy specimen is representative of the whole lesion. The second major consideration is the site, e.g. floor of mouth and ventral surface of tongue are more likely to undergo malignant change than most. Thirdly, relation to cause, e.g. buccal leukoplakia, in the preferred site for a paan quid is at high risk if the habit is not discontinued.

On average 5% of leukoplakias progress to carcinomas; however, in certain sites, e.g. floor of mouth, > 25% may progress and certain variants, e.g. 'candidal leukoplakia', have a claimed 10–40% incidence of malignant change. Δ and Rx: specialist referral is indicated—biopsy guided by toluidine blue to select most appropriate area and Rx as appropriate. Malignant transformation is more common among non-smokers (idiopathic leukoplakia): 2.4% are malignant in 10 yrs, 5% are malignant in 20 yrs, a 50–100 times greater risk than normal mouth.

Erythroleukoplakia (speckled leukoplakia) This is basically leukoplakia with areas of erythroplakia. Exhibits an ↑ risk of malignant transformation.

Erythroplakia is generally a well-demarcated, red velvety patch of the oral mucosa which histologically shows marked cellular atypia, no surface keratinization, and a degree of atrophy of the surface layer. Most of these lesions are carcinoma-*in-situ* or frank carcinoma and are found at high risk sites (> 80%).

Erosive lichen planus is a comparatively rare variant of lichen planus, which some authorities believe to be premalignant. The common forms of lichen planus have no premalignant potential.

Submucous fibrosis is a condition found particularly in those of South Asian extraction, and is thought to be a tanning of the oral mucous membrane induced by betel-quid chewing *without* the addition of tobacco (some cultures use a quid of betel leaf, areca nut, and slake lime; others add tobacco to this; the first seems to produce submucous fibrosis, the second carcinoma). The mucosa is pale, with constraining fibrous bands, and fibrosis of the submucosa occurs, making the lips and cheeks immobile and resulting in trismus. Histology shows hyalinization and acellular dense fibrous tissue with narrowed blood vessels and a lymphocytic infiltrate. There is epithelial atrophy and cellular atypia. Pathogenesis unclear; ↑ levels of copper due to areca nut chewing leading to cross-linking of collagen by upregulation of lysyl oxidase and thus ↑ fibrosis and DNA damage.

Malignant transformation is seen in 10% in 10–15 yrs. Rx: stop habit, intralesional steroids/exercise, surgery with flap reconstruction.

Dyskeratosis congenita A rare autosomal dominant condition of pigmented skin, nail dystrophy, and leukoplakia evident in childhood. White plaques have premalignant potential (p. 466).

Patterson–Brown–Kelly syndrome (Plummer–Vinson syndrome), p. 760.

Management of premalignant lesions Record site, preferably photographically. Consider site, histology, age, and health of the patient, in conjunction with aetiological factors, before deciding on long-term observation or active intervention. Completely stop patient from smoking and 60% will disappear.[1] Observation may consist of clinical examination with repeated cytology (although cytology has generally been disappointing), or biopsy if change is seen. Guided biopsy with toluidine blue may ↑ diagnostic accuracy. Rx options: laser excision, cryotherapy, surgical excision, topical bleomycin, after removal of any identifiable aetiological factors. Follow-up at 3-monthly intervals.

▶ It is impossible to predict the behaviour of a patch of leukoplakia with precision.

1 J Pindburg 1980 *Oral cancer and precancer*. Wright, Bristol.

Oral cancer

Cancer of the mouth accounts for ~2% of all malignant tumours in northern Europe and the USA, but ~30–40% in the Indian subcontinent. > 90% of these are SCCs. Globally it is the 6th commonest cause of cancer-related death. > 2000 new cases of oral cancer are registered per year in the UK and each year half that number die from or with the disease. Oral cancer is largely preventable. Overall mortality rate is 50%. Recent survival data suggests that the UK has the best survival figures for diagnosed oral cancer at all stages.

Site The floor of the mouth is the commonest single site, and when combined with lingual sulcus and ventral surface of tongue, creates a horseshoe area, accounting for over 75% of carcinomas seen in European or American practice. M > F, although this difference is less marked than it has been in the past, possibly due to changes in smoking habits between the sexes. It is an age-related disease, with 98% of patients > 40 yrs.

Aetiology Main aetiological factor in cancer of the lip is exposure to sunlight, as with skin cancer. It is estimated that the risk of developing lip cancer doubles every 250 miles nearer the equator. Excessive alcohol and tobacco use are the important factors in the aetiology of cancer of the mouth showing a 'synergistic effect'. Perhaps the most clear-cut aetiological factor is the chewing of tobacco and paan. Late-stage syphilis is now an exceedingly rare risk factor. Immunosuppression, e.g. renal transplant, HIV patients have ↑ risk of this and other tumours.

Clinical appearance Most often seen as a painless ulcer, although may present as a swelling, an area of leukoplakia, erythroleukoplakia or erythroplakia, or as malignant change of long-standing benign tumours or rarely in cyst linings. Pain is usually a *late* feature when the lesion becomes superinfected or during eating of spicy foods. Referred otalgia is a common manifestation of pain from oral cancer. The ulcer is described as firm with raised edges, with an indurated, inflamed, granular base and is fixed to surrounding tissues.

Staging The **TNM** classification is most commonly used;

T	primary tumour	**N**	cervical nodes
T1	<2 cm diameter	**N0**	no nodes
T2	2–4 cm diameter	**N1**	single node < 3 cm
T3	>4 cm diameter	**N2**	single 3–6 cm node (N2a), multiple
T4	massive, invading		nodes (N2b) or contralateral
	beyond mouth		node(s) (N2c)
		N3	node > 6 cm
		M	distant metastases
		M0	absent
		M1	present

Survival Dependent on site, stage, and comorbidity. The presence or absence of extracapsular spread of tumour in metastatic cervical nodes is the most important single prognostic factor.

Histopathology Almost always SCC. Characteristically shows invasion of deep tissues with cellular pleomorphism and ↑ nuclear staining. The presence of a lymphocytic response may have prognostic value, as does the manner of invasion (pushing or spreading). Can spread via local infilt-ration or lymphatic system (cervical nodes), and late spread via blood stream. However, histologically similar tumours can show quite different biological behaviour and this is a focus of currrent research.

Verrucous carcinoma A distinctive exophytic, wart-like lesion which grows slowly, is locally invasive, and is regarded as a lower-grade SCC, characterized by folded hyperplastic epithelium and a lower degree of cel-lular atypia. Surgical excision &/or radiotherapy is the Rx. Inadequate radio-therapy has been reported to induce more aggressive behaviour.

Other tumours Malignant connective tissue tumours (sarcomas) are rare in the mouth, but fibrosarcoma and rhabdomyosarcoma are seen in chil-dren. Osteosarcoma of the jaws has a slightly better prognosis than when found in long bones.

Salivary gland tumours, p. 510. Malignant melanoma, p. 514.

Management of oral malignancy, p. 516.

Abnormalities of the lips and tongue

Although many diseases of the oral mucosa will involve the lips and tongue, there are a number of conditions specific to these structures, due in part to their highly specialized nature. The tongue is a peculiar muscular organ covered with specialized sensory epithelium and the lips form the interface between skin and mucosa.

The tongue

Ankyloglossia (tongue tie)   The commonest of the developmental variations of the tongue and may be associated with microglossia. Rx: frenectomy.

Macroglossia   Congenital; Down syndrome, Hurler syndrome, Beckwith–Weidemann syndrome. Benign tumours (e.g. lymphangioma), or acquired; acromegaly, amyloidosis, p. 526. Surgical reduction of the tongue is bloody, but sometimes worthwhile.

Fissured tongue   Deep fissuring of the tongue is not pathological in itself (affects 3% of tongues) but may harbour pathogenic microorganisms. Commoner in Down syndrome patients than average population. Different fissure patterns are identified by various delightful names such as scrotal tongue. The Melkerson–Rosenthal syndrome is a deeply fissured tongue in association with recurrent facial nerve palsy and swelling. Rx: reassurance for most, referral for Melkerson–Rosenthal.

Hairy tongue   A peculiar condition of unknown aetiology probably due to elongation of the filiform papillae, which may or may not be accompanied by abnormal pigmentation. Sometimes responds to podophylin paint, a thorough scrape, or surgical shave.

Median rhomboid glossitis,   p. 439.

Geographic tongue (benign migratory glossitis, erythema migrans)   This peculiar inflammatory condition of unknown aetiology involves the rapid appearance and disappearance of atrophic areas with a white demarcated border on the dorsum and lateral surface of the tongue, giving it the appearance of moving around the tongue surface. It is due to temporary loss of the filiform papillae. Several clinical variants exist. Familial pattern is common. 4% have psoriasis. Rx: reassurance about benign self-limiting nature.

Depapillation   of the tongue also appears in a number of haematological and deficiency states and in severe cases may also appear lobulated.

Sore tongue (glossodynia)   May occur in the presence or absence of clinical changes; however, it should be remembered that even the presence of glossitis may not explain the symptoms of sore or burning tongue. Main causes of glossitis are iron deficiency anaemia, pernicious anaemia, candidosis, vitamin B group deficiencies, and lichen planus. Sore, but clinically normal tongue is a common problem and often psychogenic in origin; however, the first line of Rx is to exclude any possible organic cause, e.g. haematological deficiency states and unwanted reactions to self-administered or professionally administered medicines or mouthwashes.

The lips

Granulomatous cheilitis (orofacial granulomatosis) This is characterized by swelling of the lips and is histologically similar to Crohn's disease (non-caseating granuloma being found on biopsy but no systemic features). Intralesional steroids, e.g. triamincinolone, 40 mg into affected lip, may help.

Persistent median fissure This may be found as a developmental abnormality but is usually secondarily infected, which is extremely difficult to eradicate. May be associated with granulomatous cheilitis.

Sarcoidosis A chronic granulomatous condition which can affect any body system. Lip swelling, and gingival and palatal nodules occur. Heerfordt syndrome p. 758. Biopsy reveals non-caseating granuloma with inclusion bodies. CXR : hilar lymphadenopathy. Serum adenosine deaminase, angiotension converting enzyme level is ↑. Ask an ophthalmologist to exclude uveal tract involvement. Rx: steroids, intralesional or systemic.

Actinic cheilitis Sun damage to the lower lip causes excessive keratin production and ↑ mitotic activity in the basal layer. Premalignant. Advise sun blocks.

Exfoliative cheilitis Similar to above but of unknown aetiology.

Dry sore lips Except when accompanied by frank cheilitis, this is usually entirely innocent and can be treated symptomatically. Common causes are lip licking, exposure to wind or sunlight. It is also a manifestation of viral illness. Rx: lip salves.

Peutz–Jegher syndrome, p. 760.

Herpes labialis, p. 436.

Mucocele, p. 414.

Allergic angio-oedema Severe type I allergic response affecting lips, neck, and floor of mouth. Usually an identifiable cause. Rx: mild—antihistamine PO; severe—as anaphylaxis, p. 570.

Hereditary angio-oedema Defect of C_1-esterase inhibitor. Lip, neck, floor of mouth swelling, and swelling of feet and buttocks. Precipitated by trauma. Rx: acute attacks—fresh frozen plasma (contains C_1-esterase inhibitor. Prophylaxis, stanozalol.

Kawasaki disease This systemic vasculitis affecting children < 5 yrs causes death in the UK in < 4% (USA and Japan ~0.1%).[1] It can be treated if diagnosed. The criteria include red, dry cracked lips, strawberry tongue, and erythematous oropharyngeal mucosa, bilateral conjunctivitis, cervical lymphadenopathy, generalized rash, and fever. If suspected refer to a paediatrician.

---

1 N. Curtis 1997 *BMJ* **315** 322.

Salivary gland disease—1

The salivary glands consist of the major glands, the paired sublingual, submandibular, and parotid glands, and the minor salivary glands present throughout the oral mucosa, but particularly dense in the posterior palate and lips.

Xerostomia Dry mouth can be both a sign and a symptom. Note that some patients complain of a dry mouth when, in fact, they have an abundance of saliva. True xerostomia predisposes the mouth, pharynx, and salivary glands to infection and caries. Common causes include irradiation of the head and neck, drugs (e.g. tricyclic antidepressants), anxiety states, and Sjögren syndrome. Rx is aimed at the underlying cause. Symptomatic relief with carboxymethylcellulose saliva, e.g. Glandosane spray or Saliva—Orthana, helps. Optimal OH is essential. SF (containing sorbital) chewing gum may help. Pilocarpine systemically ↑ salivary flow at expense of unwanted effects.

Sialorrhoea/ptyalism Rare, although apparent sialorrhoea can occur with drooling due to inflammatory conditions of the mouth, or neurological disorders which inhibit swallowing. Rare causes include mercury poisoning and rabies. Problems with swallowing may be overcome by surgical repositioning of the major salivary ducts. Propantheline 15mg tds will reduce salivary flow.

Sialadenitis Inflammation of, usually, the major salivary glands. **Acute bacterial sialadenitis** presents as a painful swelling, usually with a purulent discharge from the duct of the gland involved. It may also develop as an exacerbation of **chronic bacterial sialadenitis,** which often exists as a complication of duct obstruction. Both conditions are almost always unilateral and common infecting organisms are oral streptococci, oral anaerobes, and *Staph. aureus*. Rx: exclusion or removal of an obstructing calculus. Plain radiographs with reduced exposure may reveal calculus, but 50% are radiolucent. (p. 512). Culture of pus from the duct and aggressive antibiotic therapy (amoxicillin/clavulanate and metronidazole) for unclearable ducts. Stimulation of salivary flow by chewing or massage helps chronic recurring sialadenitis. Rarely, loculated pus collection within the gland necessitates incision and drainage; USS can localize collection. Once the acute symptoms have resolved, sialography is indicated to define duct structure and may prove therapeutic. Other treatments include irrigating the gland with antibiotics &/or steroids. Recurrent chronic sialadenitis is an indication for removal of the gland (p. 512). **Viral sialadenitis**, commonly mumps (↑ serum amylase and lipases), an acute, infectious viral disease which primarily affects the parotid. It is transmitted by direct contact with droplets of saliva and usually affects children and young adults with sudden onset of fever, pain, and parotid swelling. Classically, one gland is affected first, although bilateral swelling is the norm. In adults, the disease is more severe, with multisystem problems such as orchitis. Protection is now conferred by the measles, mumps, rubella vaccine. Rx: isolate patent for 7–10 days.

Rarely, sialadenitis can occur as a manifestation of allergy to various drugs, foodstuffs, or metals.

Sialolithiasis, p. 512.

Recurrent parotitis of childhood Unknown aetiology; congenital malformation of portions of ducts and infections ascending from mouth following dehydration. Ages 5–9; recurrent unilateral parotitis with malaise. Eased by antibiotics. Resolves by puberty. EBV implicated in aetiology, possibly by structural damage to ducts. Rx: antibiotics, duct irrigation.

Salivary duct and salivary gland fistulae Communications between the duct or gland and the oral mucosa or skin may occur post-traumatically or post-operatively. Duct repair or gland excision may be needed. Propantheline 15 mg tds before food can ↓ salivary flow and dry up small fistulae.

Mucocele, ranula, p. 414.

Salivary gland disease—2

Sialosis A non-inflammatory, non-neoplastic swelling of the major salivary glands, usually the parotids and usually bilateral. Of unknown aetiology, although linked with endocrine abnormalities, nutritional deficiencies, and alcohol abuse. Sialography is essentially normal. Histology is of serous acinar cell hypertrophy. Rx: aimed at any aetiological factors. Δ: exclusion of underlying organic disease by history, haematology, and biochemistry.

Sjögren syndrome (secondary Sjögren syndrome) The triad of xerostomia, keratoconjunctivitis sicca, and a connective tissue disorder, usually rheumatoid arthritis. When the connective tissue component is absent the condition is called **primary Sjögren syndrome (sicca syndrome)**. The aetiology is probably autoimmune and there is a 5% risk of malignant lymphomatous transformation of the affected gland. Δ: antinuclear antibodies (70% +ve), SSA (70% +ve), SSB (40% +ve). Rheumatoid factor (70% +ve), ESR (↑), immunoglobulins (↑), labial gland biopsy shows lymphocytic infiltrate. Parotid gland flow, sialography, schrimer test, and slit lamp exam are all advocated, but once a Δ is established all that can be done for the patient is symptomatic Rx and an awareness of complications. Synthetic saliva (p. 632), synthetic tears, meticulous OH, Rx of candida, and patient awareness of the risk of lymphomatous change. See also p. 760.

Salivary gland tumours 80% are benign; 80% occur in the parotid, and 80% of these are in the superficial lobe. The majority are **pleomorphic adenomas** which have a mixed cellular appearance on histopathology. Although benign, the cells lie within the capsule of the tumour and satellite cells may lie outwith the capsule, creating a tremendous propensity for recurrence if simply enucleated. Any tumour in the superficial lobe of the parotid should ∴ be removed by superficial parotidectomy, taking a safe margin of normal tissue (p. 512). **Lymphangiomas and haemangiomas** are the commonest tumours found in salivary glands in children. **Adenolymphoma** is found almost exclusively in the parotid, and **adenoid cystic carcinoma** is more commonly found in the minor than the major salivary glands. Tumours of the submandibular, sublingual, and minor salivary glands are more likely to be malignant than those found in the parotid. Pointers to malignant change in salivary gland tumours are: fixation to surrounding tissues, nerve involvement (particularly the facial nerve in parotid tumours), pain, rapid growth, and lymphadenopathy. For management, see p. 512.

Rare salivary tumours include mucoepidermoid carcinoma and acinic cell carcinoma, both of which can behave indolently or aggressively. Monomorphic adenomas are benign, with many histological varieties.

Miscellaneous Lymphoepithelial lesion (Miculicz disease) is essentially an aggressive form of the Sjögren syndrome without the eye or connective tissue component. **NB** Miculicz syndrome is salivary enlargement of known cause.

Frey syndrome, p. 757.

British Sjögren Syndrome Society, PO BOX 10867, Birmingham B16 02W; www.bssa.uk.net

Drug-induced lesions of the mouth

One way of thinking of these reactions is to divide them into local and systemic effects.

Local reactions

Chemical burns, e.g. from an aspirin tablet being held against the oral mucosa beside a painful tooth, are still seen and make one despair of the public at times. The burns are superficial necrosis of the epithelium and can appear as a transient white patch. Rx: re-education and removal of the irritant. The mucosa will spontaneously heal. Iatrogenic causes include trichloracetic acid and phenol. Also caused by accidental ingestion of corrosives (e.g. paraquat).

Interference with commensal flora Prolonged or repeated use of antibiotics, particularly topical antibiotics can lead to the overgrowth of resistant organisms, especially candida. Corticosteroids can cause a similar problem by immunosuppression.

Oral dyaesthesia A sore but normal-appearing tongue can be caused by certain drugs (e.g. captopril).

Systemic effects

Depressed marrow function There are a wide range of drugs which will depress any or all of the cell lines of the haemopoietic systems and these in turn can affect the oral mucosa, e.g. phenytoin. Long-term use can result in folate deficiency and macrocytic anaemia which can produce severe aphthous stomatitis. Chloramphenicol and certain analgesics can induce agranulocytosis, leading to severe oral ulceration. Chloramphenicol can also induce aplastic anaemia, which affects haemostasis, although spontaneous oral purpura and haemorrhage are a rare presentation.

Immunosuppression Steroids and other immunosuppressants predispose to viral and fungal infection.

Lichenoid eruption Classically associated with the use of gold in the Rx of rheumatoid arthritis (p. 546). NSAIDs, oral hypoglycaemics, and beta blockers are commoner offenders.

Erythema multiforme (Stevens–Johnson syndrome), p. 761.

Fixed drug eruptions Recurrent, sharply circumscribed lesions at the same site occurring on exposure to a specific drug. Extremely rare in the oral mucosa.

Exfoliative stomatitis Simply an oral manifestation of the very dangerous drug reaction known as exfoliative dermatitis, in which the skin and other membranes are shed. Again, gold has been implicated.

Gingival hyperplasia Common in patients on phenytoin, cyclosporin A, nifedipine, and certain other calcium channel-blockers; less commonly the OCP can have this effect. It is characterized by progressive fibrous hyperplasia and, while improved by OHI, will occur even in the presence of meticulous OH. Rx: gingival surgery may be needed.

Oral pigmentation   Black lines in the gingival sulcus are described as being a sign of heavy metal poisoning. Chlorhexidine causes a black or brown discoloration of the dorsum of the tongue, and some antibiotics can also do this. Tetracycline discoloration of teeth is well known.

Xerostomia,   p. 456.

Allergic reactions   Penicillin is a common offender.

There are a host of conditions affecting the oral mucosa which may be ascribed to the use of drugs. Recognition by history and patch testing of these is, of course, important, providing the drug can be withdrawn, but one has to pay attention to the reason the drug was given in the first place, and it may be that minor oral symptoms have to be tolerated when the drug is essential for the overall well-being of the patient.

Facial pain

Pain is an unpleasant sensory and emotional experience caused by actual or potential tissue damage, or described in terms of such damage. It is a complex and multifaceted symptom and several other sections of this book are relevant. The commonest source of pain in the region of the jaws and face is the tooth pulp. Pain not directly related to the teeth and jaws is dealt with here.

Trigeminal neuralgia Most common neurological cause of facial pain, it is an excruciating condition affecting mainly the >50s. It presents as a shooting 'electric shock' type of pain of rapid onset and short duration, which is often stimulated by touching a trigger point in the distribution of the trigeminal nerve. Patients may refuse to shave or wash the area which stimulates the pain although, strangely, they are rarely woken by it. In the early stages of the disease there may be a period of prodromal pain not conforming to the classical description and it may be difficult to arrive at a Δ; patients often have multiple extractions in an attempt to relieve the symptoms. It is thought to be a sensory form of epilepsy, although some cases are due to vascular pressure intracranially. Δ is by the history, and carbamazepine is useful both therapeutically and diagnostically, with an 80% response rate. Injection of LA can break pain cycles and be useful diagnostically. Cryotherapy can induce protracted analgesia, but sectioning the nerve rarely helps. For intractable cases, radiofrequency ganglionolysis or decompression of trigeminal nerve intracranially may be required.

Glossopharyngeal neuralgia A similar condition to trigeminal neuralgia, but less common. Affects the glossopharyngeal nerve, causing a sharp shooting pain on swallowing. There may be referred otalgia. Again, carbamazepine is the drug of choice.

▶ Patients under the age of 50 presenting with symptoms of cranial nerve neuralgia require full neurological examination and investigation, as these may be the presenting symptoms of an intracranial neoplasm, HIV, syphilis, or multiple sclerosis.

Temporal arteritis (cranial arteritis) A condition affecting older age groups. The pain is localized to the temporal and frontal regions and usually described as a severe ache, although it can be paroxysmal. The affected area is tender to touch. Major risk is involvement of retinal arteries, with sudden deterioration and loss of vision; underlying pathology is inflammatory arteritis. Tongue necrosis following lingual artery involvement has been described. Biopsy shows the arterial elastic issue to be fragmented with giant cells. Δ: pulseless temporal arteries, classical distribution of pain, and massively raised ESR. Rx: aim is to relieve pain and prevent blindness and involves systemic prednisolone, guided by symptoms and ESR.

Migraine, p. 549.

Periodic migrainous neuralgia (cluster headache) Similar aetiology to migraine but with different clinical presentation: periodic attacks of severe, unilateral pain, boring or burning in character, lasting 30–60min, located around the eye, associated with watering of eye on affected side; congestion of conjuctiva and nasal discharge common. Attacks often occur at a particular time of night (early morning 'alarm clock wakening'), and tend to be closely concentrated over a period of time, followed by a longer period of remission. Most sufferers describe alcohol intolerance. Rx: O_2 inhalation, NSAID drugs, ergotamine or sumatriptan, intranasal lidocaine. Pizotifen is used prophylactically.

Pain associated with herpes zoster, p. 436.

Glaucoma   Gives rise to severe unilateral pain centred above the eye, with a tense, stony hard globe. Due to raised intraocular pressure. Acute and chronic forms are recognized. The acute form presents with pain and responds to acetazolamide. Will need ophthalmological referral.

Myocardial infarction and angina   May on occasion radiate to the jaws.

Multiple sclerosis   May mimic trigeminal neuralgia or cause altered facial sensation. Eye pain (retrobulbar neuritis) is associated. Δ: depends upon finding multiple focal neurological lesions, disseminated in time and place.

Atypical facial pain   This constitutes a large proportion of patients presenting with facial pain. Classically, their symptoms are unrelated to anatomical distribution of nerves or any known pathological process, and these patients have often been through a number of specialist disciplines in an attempt to establish a Δ and gain relief. This Δ tends to be used as a catch-all for a large group of patients, with the connecting underlying supposition that the pain is of psychogenic origin. There may be a florid psychiatric history or undiagnosed depression; alternatively, the patient may simply be overreacting to an essentially minor discomfort or recently noticed anatomical variant as part of a general inability to cope with life. Pointers to a psychogenic aetiology include imprecise localization, often bilateral pain or 'all over the place'. Bizarre or grossly exaggerated descriptions of pain. Pain is described as being continuous for long periods with no change, and none of the usual relieving or exacerbating factors apply. Sleeping and eating are not obviously disturbed, despite continuous unbearable pain. Most analgesics are said to be unhelpful, although many will not have tried adequate analgesia. No objective signs are demonstrable and all investigations are essentially normal. After exclusion of any possible organic cause the introduction of an antidepressant, e.g. dothiepin, may (or may not) produce dramatic improvement in the pain.

Oral dysaesthesia   or burning mouth syndrome is an unpleasant abnormal sensation affecting the oral mucosa in the absence of clinically evident disease. Five times more common in women aged 40–50 yrs than other groups. Related to atypical facial pain. Δ: by exclusion of haematological, metabolic, nutritional, microbiological, allergic, and prosthetic causes. With experience the patient type often becomes obvious. Rx: dothiepin if sleep disturbance is prominent; paroxetine or fluoxetine if daytime stimulus is needed.

Bell's palsy   Caused by inflammation of VII in the stylomastoid canal. Although the main symptom is facial paralysis, pain in or around the ear, often radiating to the jaw, precedes or develops at the same time in ~50% of cases. Rx: steroids and antiviral (aciclovir) drugs improve chance for full recovery if Rx early (within 3 days of onset). If no Rx, 30% of patients will not completely recover.

Ramsey Hunt syndrome,   p. 760 Pain is associated with herpes zoster virus in the facial nerve. Systemic aciclovir and steroids improves recovery.[1]

1 Adour et al. 1996 *Ann Otol Rhinol Laryngol* **105** 371–8.

Oral manifestations of skin disease

Lichen planus A chronic inflammatory disease of adults involving skin and mucous membranes. It effects up to 2% of the general population. 50% of patients with skin lesions have oral lesions, whereas 25% have oral lesions alone. The oral lesions persist longer than the skin lesions. It affects females more commonly than males at the ratio of 3:2. It is an auto-immune condition mediated by a T lymphocyte attack on stratified squam-ous epithelia which leads to hyperkeratosis with erythema or striations. 'Lichenoid eruptions' are an unwanted reaction to some drugs. Usually the oral lesions are bilateral and posterior in the buccal mucosa; it is not seen on the palate but can, however, affect the tongue, lips, gingivae, and floor of mouth. The most common oral lesion is a lacey reticular pattern of hyper-kertotic epithelia seen bilaterally on the buccal mucosa. Other variants include coalesced plaque-like lesions. Six types are recognized: the reti-cular pattern just described, papular pattern, plaque-like pattern, erosive pattern, atrophic pattern, and bullous pattern. The skin lesions affect the flexor surfaces of the arms, and wrists and legs, and are particularly common on the shin as purple papules with fine white lines (Whickham's straie) overlying them. Histology shows hyperparakeratosis, with elongated rete ridges with a saw-tooth appearance, a prominent granular cell layer, acanthosis, and basal cell liquefaction. There is usually a dense band of lymphocytes directly beneath the epithelium. Lichen planus can last for months or years. It can always be distinguished histologically and usually clinically from leukoplakia. Lichen planus is essentially benign. Some contro-versy exists about the risk of malignant transformation; this risk has only really been identified in the *erosive* forms of lichen planus, and Rx of the erosive form is based around transforming it to the completely benign reticular pattern. Rx: distinction from leukoplakia, sytemic lupus erythe-matosus, or malignancy is needed; if there are lichenoid eruptions the implicated drugs should be identified and avoided if possible. If the condi-tion is symptomatic superinfection should be treated or prevented with chlorhexidine mouthwash. If severe atrophic or errosive components are present topical steroids may be used, such as triamincinolone in car-boxymethylcellulose paste, betamethazone pellets 1 mg in 10 ml of water used as a mouthrinse and expectorated in an increasing dose until symp-toms are resolved, systemic steroids, or topical tacrolimus. These should all be used in a specialist environment. Symptomatic reticular lichen planus can usually be safely managed with a low-dose topical steriod.

Dyskeratosis congenita A rare autosomal dominant condition, character-ized by oral leukoplakia, dystrophic changes of the nails, and hyperpigmen-tation of the skin; the oral lesion is prone to malignant change (p. 450).

Vesiculo-bullous lesions, p. 442.

Oral manifestations of connective tissue disease

Ehlers–Danlos syndrome rare inherited connective tissue disease char-acterized by hyperextensible skin, hypermobile joints, and fragile vessels due to mutations in collagen. This results in very easy bruising and bleeding of skin as well as hypermobility. Oral features include severe early onset periodontal disease, pulp stones, and occasional hypermobility of the TMJ. Bleeding during surgery, weak scars, sutures 'pulling through', and difficulty with root canal Rx are the main practical points. Some types of Ehlers– Danlos syndrome can lead to an ↑ susceptibility to infective endocarditis and significant heart damage due to mitral valve prolapse, and some types are prone to cerebrovascular accident due to weakness of intracranial blood vessels. Rx: aimed at the symptoms.

Rheumatoid arthritis (p. 546) Main associations are Sjögren syndrome and rheumatoid of the TMJ (10% cases), which may cause pain, swelling, and limitation of movement. Rarely, pannus formation within the joint may occur. Rx: as for systemic rheumatoid arthritis, which may include methotrexate or tumour necrosis factor alpha.

Systemic lupus erythematosus (SLE) A systemic multisystem disease of uncertain aetiology, although viruses, hormonal changes, and drug therapy have all been implicated. The association with the presence of antinuclear factor is more common in females. Gives rise to skin lesions, classical malar 'butterfly' rash, and oral mucosal lesions in 30%, which include ulceration and purpurae. Antinuclear antibodies are present. F > M. Arthritis and anaemia frequent.

Chronic discoid lupus erythematosus The lesions of this condition are limited to skin and mucosa. May present as disc-like white plaques in the mouth and can progress to SLE, although more likely to remain as a chronic and recurring disorder. Lip lesions in women may be premalignant. Rx: SLE—systemic steroids; DLE—topical steroids. Butterfly rash may be present. DLE can be distinguished from SLE by the presence of specific double-stranded DNA antinuclear antibody in serum. Rx: DLE recalcitrant lesions may respond to dapsone or thalidomide.

Systemic sclerosis A chronic disease characterized by diffuse sclerosis of connective tissues. F > M. It has an insidious onset and is often associated with Raynaud's phenomenon (painful reversible digital ischaemia on exposure to cold). Classically, the face has a waxy mask-like appearance. Eating becomes difficult due to immobility of underlying tissues, and dysphagia occurs due to oesophageal involvement. Autoantibodies are present. Circulating levels of E-selectin and thrombomodulin are useful markers in monitoring disease activity. Rx: combination of cyclophosphamide and steroids may help in early disease; penicillamine has always been used but has numerous unwanted effects.

Polyarteritis nodosa Characterized by inflammation and necrosis of small and medium-sized arteries; necrosis at any site may occur and is seen as ulceration in the mouth. Up to 60% of patients die in the first year; Rx with systemic steriods ↑ the 5 yr survival to 40%.

Dermatomyositis Inflammatory condition of skin and muscles; 15% are associated with internal malignancy. Tenderness, pain, and weakness of the tongue may be an early finding.

Reiter syndrome, p. 547.

Oral manifestations of gastrointestinal disease

Patterson–Brown–Kelly syndrome, p. 760

Coeliac disease This common form of intestinal malabsorption may present with oral ulceration as the only symptom in adults. Although children also present with ulceration, they are more likely to show weight loss, weakness, and failure to thrive. Other findings are glossitis, stomatitis, and angular cheilitis. Rx: haematological and gastrointestinal investigations are required, blood picture, and haematenic assay. ↑ malabsorption. Antibodies to gluten, reticulin, endomysium (antiendomysial Ab is marker for coeliac disease); small bowel biopsy required for definitive Δ. B$_{12}$, folate, iron ↓ ↓ should be corrected. Rx: gluten-free diet.

Ulcerative colitis (gluten-sensitive enteropathy) Rarely, pyostomatitis vegetans, a papilliferous, necrotic mucosal lesion can occur; more commonly ulcers indistinguishable from aphthae are seen. Gastrointestinal symptoms predominate. Arthritis, uveitis, and erythema nodosum also occur. Topical steroids and systemic sulfasalazine are used in Rx; low doses of thyoprine are effective in maintaining remission. Most of these patients are managed by gastrointestinal specialists.

Crohn's disease Chronic inflammatory disease affecting any part of the gut from mouth to anus. Primarily affects the terminal 1/3 of the ileum, although ~1% of cases will present with oral ulceration predating any other symptoms. These tend to affect the gingiva, buccal mucosa, and lips with purplish-red non-haemorrhagic swellings, linear long-standing ulcers, and granulations. Granulomatous cheilitis is probably a variant. Painful oral lesions seem to respond well to simple excision but Rx is aimed at the systemic disease.

Orofacial granulomatosis Clinically and histologically identical to oral manifestations of Crohn's disease. Δ of exclusion (Crohn's, sarcoid). Probable aetiology is as a hypersensitivity response to certain foods, additives such as benzoates, cinnaminides in toothpaste, etc. Δ is biopsy to demonstrate granulomata histically and exclusion of systemic disease p. 534. Rx: specific to the local problem; intralesional steroid. Most beneficial Rx is to identify and avoid the irritant factors. Patients who have generalized Crohn's or very severe orofacial granulomatosis may benefit from systemic Rx with sulfasalazine or TNF alpha.

Gardener syndrome, p. 758.

Peutz–Jegher syndrome, p. 760.

Cirrhosis Glossitis occurs in ~50% of patients. Sialosis is another association.

Oral manifestations of haematological disease

Anaemia The nutritional deficiencies associated with anaemia, iron, B$_{12}$, and folate, are all associated with **recurrent oral ulceration** (p. 440) and specific deficiencies may be present, even in the absence of a frank anaemia. **Atrophic glossitis** was formerly the commonest oral symptom of anaemia but is less often seen now. Red lines or patches on a sore, but normal-looking tongue, may indicate B$_{12}$ deficiency. **Candidosis** (p. 438) may be precipitated or exacerbated by anaemia, particularly iron deficiency, and **angular cheilitis** is a well-recognized association. The sore, clinically normal tongue (**burning tongue**) is sometimes a manifestation or even precursor of anaemia.

Patterson–Brown–Kelly syndrome,   p. 760.

Leukaemia This and other haematological malignancies are associated with a ↓ in resistance to infection. The mouth may be involved, either secondarily to this tendency to infection or as a direct consequence of infiltration of the oral tissues. The oral lesions of leukaemia are painful and can lead to difficulty in swallowing. Prevention of superinfection with chlorhexidine mouthwashes and aggressive appropriate Rx of infections which arise are of real help. There is an ↑ tendency to bleed manifested as fine petechial haemorrhages or bruising around the mouth, and the gingiva may bleed heavily in the presence of only negligible trauma. Management of the bleeding is aimed at the underlying disorder; local techniques include improving OH, avoiding extractions, and using local haemostatic methods (p. 390). Spontaneous gingival bleeding may be controlled by using impressions as a made-to-measure pressure dressing.

Cyclical neutropenia This condition may manifest as oral ulceration, acute exacerbations of periodontal disease, or NUG. As name suggests, recurs in 3–4 week cycles.

Myeloma Macroglossia is an occasional finding. Multiple osteolytic lesions in skull are a classic appearance. Rarely, similar lesions seen in jaws.

Purpura is due to platelet deficiency. Commonest as idiopathic thrombocytopenic purpura (ITP) in children. Palatal petechiae or bruising may be seen. Palatal petechiae are also seen in glandular fever, rubella, HIV, and recurrent vomiting.

Angina bullosa haemorrhagica Oral blood blisters; irritating but of no known significance (p. 444).

Oral manifestations of neurological disease

Examination of the cranial nerves: p. 548; general concepts of neurological disease: p. 550. Of the cranial nerves, the trigeminal and facial nerves contribute most to disorders affecting the mouth, face, and jaws.

Trigeminal nerve Ophthalmic lesions result in abnormal sensation in skin of the forehead, central nose, upper eyelid, and conjunctivae. *Maxillary* lesions affect skin of cheek, upper lip and side of nose, nasal mucosa, upper teeth and gingiva, palatal and labial mucosa. The palatal reflex may be lost. *Mandibular* lesions affect skin of lower face, lower teeth, gingivae, tongue, and floor of mouth. Lesions of the motor root manifest in the muscles of mastication. Taste sensation is *not* lost in such lesions, although other sensations from the tongue are. Testing is performed by having the patient close his eyes and report on sensations experienced, in comparison to each other, while the areas of superficial distribution of the nerve are stimulated by light touch (cotton wool) and pin-prick (probe or blunt needle). The motor branch is tested by moving the jaws against resistance. A blink should be elicited by stimulating the cornea with a wisp of cotton wool (corneal reflex).

Facial nerve is motor to the muscles of facial expression and stapedius, secretomotor to the submandibular and sublingual salivary glands, and relays taste from anterior $^2/_3$ of tongue via the chorda tympani. Tested by having the patient raise eyebrows, screw eyes shut, whistle, smile, and show their teeth. Upper and lower motor neurone lesions can be distinguished because the forehead has a degree of bilateral innervation and is relatively spared in upper motor neurone lesions. Taste is tested using sour, salt, sweet, and bitter solutions. If taste is intact, flow from the submandibular duct can be assessed by gustatory stimulation. Test hearing to assess stapedius.

Neurological causes of facial and oral pain, p. 462.

Neurological conditions causing altered sensation Intracranial: e.g. CVA, multiple sclerosis, polyarteritis, cerebral tumours, infection, trauma, sarcoidosis; *extracranial:* nasopharyngeal or antral carcinoma, trauma, osteomyelitis, Paget's disease, viral or bacterial infection, leukaemic infiltrate. Psychogenic causes include hyperventilation syndrome and hysteria.

Neurological causes of facial paralysis Upper motor neurone or lower motor neurone; of the former, strokes are the commonest. Combination lesions can be caused by amyotrophic lateral sclerosis of the cord. Lower motor neurone paralysis can be caused by Bell's palsy (p. 463), trauma, infiltration by malignant tumours, Ramsay Hunt syndrome, Guillain–Barré syndrome (post-viral polyneuritis, may even appear to be bilateral). Apparent paralysis may occur in myaesthenia gravis where abnormally ↑ fatigue of striated muscle causes ptosis and diplopia. Therapeutic paralysis may be induced for facial spasm, using botulinus toxin injected locally (as used for facial aesthetics!). Horner syndrome results in ptosis.

Neurological causes of abnormal muscle movement Tetanus is an obvious cause. Muscular dystrophy may present with ptosis and facial paralysis.

Hemifacial spasm and other tics may be caused by a tumour at the cerebello-pontine angle. Orofacial dyskinesia can be a manifestation of Parkinson's disease or an unwanted effect of major tranquillizers. Phenothiazines and metoclopramide are notorious for causing dystonic reactions in young women and children. Bizarre attacks of trismus due to masseteric spasm have been ascribed to metoclopramide.

Oral manifestations of HIV infection and AIDS

AIDS is the terminal stage of infection with the human immunodeficiency virus (HIV), which is recognized as undergoing a number of mutations. It is discussed in general terms on p. 558. The underlying severe immunodeficiency leads to a number of oral manifestations which, although not pathognomonic, should raise the possibility of HIV infection. They have been classified.[1]

Group I Strongly associated with HIV

Candidosis Seen in 60% of HIV patients as early manifestation (p. 438). Erythematous (early), hyperplastic, pseudomembraneous (late), and angular cheilitis in young people (most common oral feature of HIV).

Hairy leukoplakia Bilateral, white, non-removable corrugated lesions of the tongue, unaffected by antifungals but usually resolve with aciclovir or valacyclovir, and associated with EBV. It is a predictor of bad prognosis and possible development of lymphoma.

HIV gingivitis Unusually severe gingivitis for the general state of the mouth. Often characterized by linear gingival erythema, intense red band along gingival margin.

Acute ulcerative gingivitis (p. 222) Occurs in young, otherwise healthy mouths.

HIV periodontitis Severe localized destruction out of place with OH.

Kaposi's sarcoma (KS) Commonest malignancy among HIV patients. Rx: radiotherapy is effective. One or more erythematous/purplish macules or swelling, frequently on the palate. 50% occur intra- or perorally.

Non-Hodgkin's lymphoma Similar to the above. Less common.

Group II Less strongly associated with HIV

Atypical oropharyngeal ulceration
Idiopathic thrombocytopenic purpura
HIV associated salivary gland disease HIV children > adults. Similar to Sjögren syndrome.
Wide range of common viral infections

Group III Possible association with HIV

Wide range of rare bacterial and fungal infections
Cat scratch disease
Neurological abnormalities
Osteomyelitis/sinusitis/submandibular cellulitis
Squamous carcinoma
Clearly, the conditions in *Group III* are likely to be seen in patients who are HIV −ve at least as often as in patients who are HIV +ve.

1 S. Challacombe 1991 *BDJ* **73** 305.

Persistent generalized lymphadenopathy   Otherwise inexplicable lymph-adenopathy >1 cm persisting for 3 months, at two or more extrainguinal sites. Cervical nodes particularly commonly affected. May be prodromal or a manifestation of AIDS.

Rx for AIDS   AIDS is currently incurable, but then again so is life. Antiretroviral drugs prolong and improve quality of life in those with active AIDS. Rx with antiretroviral agents: AZT, didanosine (DDI), dideoxycyti-dine (DCC), HIV protease inhibitors, e.g. nevirapine or delavirdine, are effective in controlling the ↓ ↓ in CD4 cells. Early detection and Rx of opportunistic infections and neoplasms also has a major impact on quality of life.

Dental Rx for patients with AIDS   This group present two risks with regard to dental Rx.

1 To personnel carrying out the Rx. Affected patients carry an infectious disease with no known cure, which is transmitted by blood and blood products. As it is impossible to adequately identify all such patients, routine cross-infection control is now a necessity.

2 As these patients are immunocompromised, any Rx with a known risk of infective complications, e.g. extractions, should be covered with antiseptic and antimicrobial prophylaxis, and any surgery should be as atraumatic as possible. There may also be a slight tendency to bleeding in these patients, and local haemostatic measures (p. 390) may be needed.

Prophylaxis after contaminated needlestick injury, e.g. hollow point needlestick from AIDS patient. Combination therapy offers best chance of preventing HIV seroconversion.[2]

2 Consumers Association 1997 *Drugs and Therapeutics Bulletin* **39** 25.

Cervico-facial lymphadenopathy

You cannot palpate a normal lymph node, ∴ a palpable one must be abnormal. The most important distinction to make is whether this is part of the node's physiological response to infection or whether it is undergoing some pathological change. The finding of an enlarged node or nodes in children is relatively common and can be reasonably managed by watchful waiting. Undiagnosed cervical lymphadenopathy in adults mandates biopsy-establishing definitive Δ.

Investigations   Routine EO and IO examination (p. 12) to exclude the common causes: apical and periodontal abscesses, pericoronitis, tonsillitis, otitis, etc. The fundamentals are history and palpation.

History   Ask about pain or swelling in the mouth, throat, ears, face, or scalp. Was there any constitutional upset when the lump appeared? Has it been getting bigger progressively or has it fluctuated? Is it painful, and how long has it been present?

Palpation   Fully expose the neck and palpate from behind, with the patient's head bent slightly forward to relax the neck. Examine systematically, feeling the submental, facial, submandibular, parotid, auricular, occipital, the deep cervical chain, supraclavicular, and posterior triangle nodes. Differentiating between the submandibular salivary gland and node can be a problem, made simpler by palpating bimanually; the salivary gland can be felt moving between the external and internal fingers. Supraclavicular nodes are more liable to be due to occult tumour in the lung or upper gastrointestinal tract, whereas posterior triangle nodes are more liable to be haematological or scalp skin in origin.

If a node is palpable, note its texture, size, and site, and whether it is tender to touch or fixed to surrounding tissues.

Nodes which are acutely infected tend to be large, tender, soft, and freely mobile.

Chronically infected nodes are soft to firm and less liable to be tender.

Metastatic carcinoma in nodes tends to be hard and fixed.

Lymphomatous nodes are described as rubbery and have a peculiar firm texture.

Supplementary investigations   Examine axillary and inguinal nodes, liver, and spleen. Carry out a FBC to look for leukocytosis and a monospot test for glandular fever. Once infection is excluded it is essential to exclude, as far as possible, an occult primary malignancy of the head and neck; the best way to do this is by direct examination, flexible nasendoscopy, and CXR. If examination is limited, EUA.

Ultrasound-guided fine-needle aspiration cytology in specialist units is probably the gold standard minimalist investigation. MRI and CT scanning will confirm the presence, shape, and size of nodes and may reveal occult tumour. MRI/CT cannot, however, confirm the pathological process within the node.

If the Δ has still not been established it is reasonable to proceed to excision biopsy of the node, which should be cultured for mycobacteria as well as examined histologically. Find out how your pathology department likes the nodes sent; some want them fresh.

Common causes Dental abscesses, pericoronitis, tonsillitis, glandular fever, lymphoma, metastatic deposits, and leukaemia.

Rare causes Brucellosis, atypical mycobacteria, TB, AIDS, toxoplasmosis, actinomycosis, sarcoidosis, cat scratch fever, syphilis, drugs (e.g. phenytoin) mucocutaneous lymph node syndrome (Kawasaki disease) and Chron's disease. Other neck lumps: p. 518.

An approach to oral ulcers

Oral ulceration is probably the commonest oral mucosal disease seen; it may also be the most serious. It is important, ∴, to have an approach to the management of oral ulcers firmly established in your mind.

Duration How long has the ulcer been present?

▶ If > 3 weeks, referral for appropriate specialist investigation, including biopsy, is mandatory.

If of recent onset, ask whether it was preceded by blistering. Are the ulcers multiple? Is any other part of the body affected and have similar ulcers been experienced before? Then look at the site &/or distribution of the ulcer(s).

Blistering preceding the ulcer suggests a vesiculo-bullous condition (p. 442) such as herpetic gingivostomatitis. Blistering with lesions elsewhere in the body suggests erythema multiforme, or hand, foot, and mouth disease.

Distribution If limited to the gingivae, suggests AUG (p. 222). Unilateral distribution suggests herpes (p. 436). Under a denture or other appliance suggest traumatic ulceration.

Recurrence of the ulcers after apparent complete resolution is characteristic of recurrent aphthae (p. 440).

Pain Its presence or absence is not particularly useful diagnostically, although the character of the pain may be of value. Pain is often a late feature of oral carcinoma and the fact that an ulcer may be painless *never* excludes it from being a potential cancer.

For most ulcers of recent onset, and a few present for an indeterminant period, a trial of therapy is often a useful adjunct to Δ. This is especially useful in recurrent oral ulceration, viral conditions (where Rx is essentially symptomatic), and lesions probably caused by local trauma (Rx being removal of the source of trauma and review after 1 week).

Ulcers which need early diagnosis include:

Herpes zoster As early aggressive Rx with aciclovir may reduce post-herpetic neuralgia.

Erythema multiforme In order to avoid re-exposure to the antigen.

Erosive lichen planus As this may benefit from systemic steroids or other specialist Rx and will require specialist long-term follow-up.

Oral squamous cell carcinoma For obvious reasons.

Temporomandibular pain—dysfunction/facial arthromyalgia

The allocation of this section to a speciality chapter created problems in just the same way as the referral of the 'TMJ' patient to a specialist is fraught with confusion. We have selected this site because we feel it is important to look at these patients from a physician's approach rather than a dental or surgical one.

What is it? The problem being addressed is pain in the preauricular area and muscles of mastication with trismus, with or without evidence of internal derangement of the meniscus. Conditions which can otherwise be classified as facial pain syndromes or other forms of joint disease are excluded and can be found in the relevant pages (pp. 462, 502).

Prevalence Affects ~40% of the population at some time in their lives. F > M.

Aetiology Idiopathic. Multiple theories put forward regarding occlusion, trauma, stress, habits, joint hypermobility. To date, the concept of stress-induced parafunctional habits (bruxism, clenching) causing pain and spasm in the masticatory apparatus coupled with a ↓ pain threshold has seemed the most reasonable. This is compatible with the observed high association with back pain, headaches, and migraine. It does not explain the cause in those patients who can identify no different levels of stress in their lives nor does it help explain the high incidence of internal derangement of the meniscus. The discovery of a biochemical marker (tyramine sulfate in the urine) in non-depressed TMJ patients has suggested that these patients are somehow biochemically sensitive to both mediators of damage in the joint, such as neuropeptides, and centrally (via serotonin) resulting in a lowered ability to cope with the local discomfort. The neuropeptide release can explain both joint pain and internal derangement (see Diagram 1).[1]

Clinical features Pain, clicking, locking, crepitus, and trismus are the classical signs and symptoms. Some patients may be clinically depressed but most are not. Pain is elicited by palpation over the muscles of mastication &/or the preauricular region. Clicking commonly occurs at 2–3 mm of tooth separation on opening and sometimes closing. This is due to the meniscus being displaced anteriorly on translation of the head of the condyle and then returning to its usual position (the click). A lock is when it does not return.

Management Success has been claimed for a wide range of treatments, reflecting confusion over Δ and the multifactorial and self-limiting nature of the condition. Simple conservative Rx within the range of every dentist is successful in up to 80% of cases (see Diagram 2).

  1 Reassurance and explanation Advice as to the nature of the problem and its benign and frequently self-limiting course is all that many patients require. Do not create a problem where there is none! This is also the time to take a gentle but thorough social and family history to identify clinically depressed patients or those with significant stress.

1 M. Harris 1993 *BDJ* **174** 129.

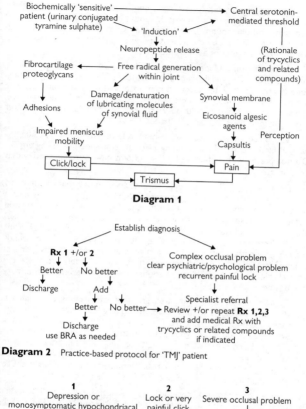

Diagram 1

Diagram 2 Practice-based protocol for 'TMJ' patient

Diagram 3 Specialist-based protocol (Once Rx 1,2,3 have been clearly exhausted and tricyclics instituted, residual problem is usually one of three).

2 Simple analgesia, rest, gentle heat, and remedial exercises Whether these are given by dentist, physiotherapist (in the form of short-wave diathermy and ultrasound) or ancillary staff is unimportant, as the crucial part is that carried out by the patient at home by taking the analgesics and performing the exercises as instructed.

3 Splint therapy Upper/lower, hard/soft have all been used with varying success. The initial aim of a splint is to: (a) show something is being done (placebo); (b) ↓ bruxism and joint load; and (c) ↑ the gap between condyle and fossa, whereby the disc may be freed. A simple, full-coverage upper or lower splint should be worn as often as possible, nights and evenings especially, and reassessed after 4–6 weeks.

These three simple measures should relieve symptoms in ~80% of patients and identify those needing referral to a specialist (Diagram 3). **Do not** persist with ineffective Rx if symptoms have not improved within 3 months.

4 Drug therapy There is a natural reluctance among many patients to take drugs, particularly those associated with psychiatry. There is also a misconceived reluctance among clinicians to use the tricyclics and related compounds. They are non-addictive and the commoner side-effects of weight gain, constipation, and dry mouth can be overcome. Benzodiazepines are not recommended but nortriptyline, dothiapine, and related compounds have been demonstrated to have analgesic and muscle relaxant effects independent of their antidepressant effect, and probably work via the central biochemical sensitivity identified by the presence of urinary conjugated tyramine sulfate.

5 Occlusal adjustment There are a group of patients where a significant occlusal problem exists. In these cases a hard diagnostic occlusal splint can be constructed for the mandible (Tanner) or for the maxilla (Michigan), and should be made to give multiple even contacts in centric relation and anterior guidance. The patient attempts to wear this full-time for up to 3 months. If pain is abolished while wearing the appliance, returns when it is removed, and is abolished on reinstitution, then occlusal adjustment by orthodontic, surgical, or restorative means is a reasonable option.

6 Surgery for internal derangement If pain can be abolished by other methods and the patient continues to be bothered by a painful click, particularly with recurrent locking, Rx aimed specifically at the meniscus is justified. The first line which may be useful diagnostically and improve pain due to capsulitis is arthroscopy. This is examination and irrigation of the upper joint space by a rigid endoscope, through which lysis and lavage of adhesions and synovial inflammatory mediators can be performed. Menisci damaged beyond the scope of arthroscopy can be repositioned at open arthrotomy. Consensus dictates that the minimum of interference to the articulatory surfaces and the avascular meniscus is carried out. Rarely, completely ruined joints will benefit from total joint replacement.

Maxillofacial surgery

In general, maxillofacial surgery is a postgraduate subject which has evolved from oral surgery, with foundations in medicine, dentistry, and surgery. It is included here as an introduction to students, an *aide-mémoire* for junior hospital staff, and a guide for those who will be referring patients.

Principal sources J. Watkinson 2000 *Head & Neck Surgery*, Butterworth-Heinemann. ACS 1997 *ATLS Core Course Manual*. M. Yaremchuk 1992 *Rigid Fixation of the Craniomaxillofacial Skeleton*, Butterworth-Heinemann. J. Shah 2003 *Oral Cancer*, Dunitz. R. Cawson 1997 *Pathology and Surgery of the Salivary Glands*, Isis Medical Media. Personal experience.

Advanced trauma life support—ATLS

ATLS is a system providing one safe way of resuscitating a trauma victim. It was first conceived in Nebraska, subsequently developed by the ACS, and has now reached international acceptance. It is not the only approach but it is one which works. It is highly recommended.

Trauma deaths have a trimodal distribution. The first peak is within seconds to minutes of injury. The second is within the first hour, the 'golden hour', and is the area of main concern. The third is days to weeks later but may reflect management within the golden hour.

The core concept behind ATLS is the **primary survey** with **simultaneous resuscitation**, followed by a **secondary survey** leading to definitive care.

Primary survey

This uses the mnemonic **ABCDE** on the basis of identifying and treating the most lethal injury first.

1 *Airway with cervical spine control* Establish a patent airway and protect the cervical spine from further injury. Chin lift, jaw thrust, oral airway, nasopharyngeal airway, intubation, surgical airway as needed, coupled with manual inline immobilization of cervical spine or rigid cervical collar, sandbags, and tape.
2 *Breathing and ventilation* Inspect, palpate, and auscultate the chest. Count respiratory rate. Give 100% O_2. Chest decompression by needle puncture in 2nd intercostal space mid-clavicular line if indicated for tension pneumothorax. Chest drain as indicated.
3 *Circulation with haemorrhage control* Assess level of consciousness, skin colour, pulse and BP, manual pressure control of extreme haemorrhage. Establish two large venous cannulae, take blood for X-match and baseline studies. Give 2 l of prewarmed Hartmann's solution. Establish ECG, seek help for operative control of bleeding if needed. Establish urinary catheter unless urethral transection is suspected, and oro- or nasogastric tube.
4 *Disability* (neuro-evaluation) Glasgow coma score. Pupillary response to light, visual acuity. Prevent hypotension and hypoxia.
5 *Exposure* Remove all clothing to allow full assessment of injuries. Ensure monitoring: respiratory rate, BP, pulse, arterial blood gases, pulse oximetry, and ECG. Prevent hypothermia.

If all these can be established and monitored parameters are normalized, the patient's chances of living are optimized.

X-rays At this stage obtain a chest and pelvis film in the resuscitation room. Cervical spine film may help but cervical spine should remain immobilized until fully assessed if mechanism of injury suggests spinal trauma.

Reassess the ABCs

If all is stable move to the **secondary survey**, which is a head-to-toe examination of the patient. It is at this stage *only* that specific non-immediately life-threatening conditions should be identified and dealt with in turn.

Maxillofacial injuries Other than those with a direct effect on the airway or cervical spine, or causing exsanguinating haemorrhage, should not be dealt with until the **ABCs** have been completed and this question should be asked of all referring doctors prior to accepting responsibility for a patient. Remember to exclude intracranial, visceral, and major orthopaedic injuries.

While ATLS is designed primarily for front-line physicians, modified courses for dental graduates are available, and recommended to anyone who may undertake care of the trauma patient.

Primary management of maxillofacial trauma

The first consideration is whether the patient has suffered polytrauma, which may have multiple and life-threatening ramifications, or, as is more commonly the case, trauma confined to the face. In the former the prime concern is keeping the patient alive, and the maxillofacial injuries can await Rx (p. 486). Remember that isolated facial injuries rarely cause sufficient bleeding to induce hypovolaemic shock. Ask yourself: Can they see?

Airway The brain can tolerate hypoxia for ~3 min. Most conscious patients can maintain a patent airway if the oropharynx is cleared. Give all traumatized patients maximal O_2 initially. Oral airways are not tolerated unless patient is unconscious. Nasopharyngeal airways are only of value if they can be inserted safely and kept patent. If the patient is unconscious and the airway is obstructed they should be intubated. If this is not possible, an emergency airway can be maintained by cricothyroid puncture with a wide-bore cannula. Long-term security of the airway can be achieved by surgical cricothyroidotomy as an emergency, or tracheostomy as a planned operation. Conscious patients with severe isolated facial trauma maintain their airway by sitting leaning forward; let them.

Cervical spine injuries Until these are excluded, the patient should be immobilized; must balance with need to remove from spine boards asap (painful, prevent pressure sores). Use common sense to decide between immobilization and sitting leaning forward.

Bleeding As above. Gunshot wounds and lacerated major vessels are exceptions which can cause extensive bleeding. Specific techniques to control naso- and oropharyngeal bleeding are: bilateral rubber mouth props to immobilize the maxilla; bilateral balloon catheters passed into the post-nasal space, inflated then pulled forward; and bilateral anterior nasal packs.

Scalp wounds Can exsanguinate children; control with pressure and heavy full thickness sutures.

Head injuries The main cause of death and disability in patients with isolated maxillofacial trauma. Assessment: p. 490. Do no further harm.

CSF leaks Facial and skull # can create dural tears, leading to CSF rhinorrhoea (from the nose) or otorrhoea (from the ear). Although controversial, prophylactic antibiotics are used by many. A combination penicillin in high dose is often used, despite the fact that conventional antibiotics do not cross the healthy blood–brain barrier in adequate levels, the rationale being that the blood–brain barrier is damaged in these cases. It was the concern that low levels of antibiotic in the CSF would only suppress *signs* of meningitis whilst selecting resistant organisms that prompted influential recommendations *against* prophylaxis.[1]

Tetanus immunity If in doubt give tetanus toxoid.

---

1 *Infection in Neurosurgery.* Working Party of the British Society for Antimicrobial Chemotherapy 1992 *Lancet* **344** 1547.

Analgesia May not be needed. Avoid opioids if possible as they interfere with neuro-observations. If needed, use diclofenac 75 mg IM bd or codeine phosphate 60 mg IM 4 hourly.

Patients to admit Any question of danger to the airway, skull #, history of unconsciousness, retrograde amnesia, bleeding, middle 1/3 #, mandibular # (except when very simple), malar # if +ve eye signs, children, and those with domestic or social problems. If in doubt *admit*. Place on, at least, initial hourly neurological observations (most will need 1/4 hourly obs initially). IV access and antibiotic. If not admitting, give the patient a head-injury card.

If teeth have been lost ensure they are not in the chest (CXR) or soft tissues.

X-rays, pp. 492, 494, 498 plate 7.

Assessing head injury

▶ All patients with recent facial trauma warranting hospital admission need at least initial assessment for head injury.

Change in the level of consciousness is the earliest and most valuable sign of head injury.

A combination of the following is generally used.

Glasgow coma scale (GCS)

Eyes open
- spontaneously   4
- to speech   3
- to pain   2
- do not open   1

Best verbal response
- orientated   5
- confused   4
- inappropriate   3
- incomprehensible   2
- none   1

Best motor response
- obeys commands   6
- localizes pain   5
- normal flexion   4
- abnormal flexion   3
- extension   2
- none   1

Pulse and BP ↓ pulse and ↑ BP is a late sign of ↑ intracranial pressure.

Pupils Measure size (1–8 mm) and reaction to light in both pupils.

Respiration ↓ rate is a sign of raised intracranial presure.

Limb movement
Indicate   normal
                mild weakness
                severe weakness
                extension
                no response
for arms and legs   (record right and left separately if there is a difference).

CT scan The definitive investigation. However, patients must *never* be transferred before correcting hypoxia and hypovolaemia.

Using GCS

Severe head injury &/or deterioration = call for help.

One accepted method of categorizing head-injured patients by severity using GCS is:[1]

Severe   <8

Moderate   9–12

Minor   13–15

In addition:
A severe head injury is present if the following are seen:
- Unequal pupils (except traumatic mydriasis).
- Unequal limb movement (except orthopaedic injury).

1 ACS 1997 *ATLS Core Course Manual.*

- Open head injury (i.e. compound to brain).
- Deterioration in measured parameters.
- Depressed skull #.

Subtle signs of deterioration include:
- Severe &/or worsening headache.
- Early unilateral pupillary dilatation.
- Early unilateral limb weakness.

A GCS of <6 in the absence of drugs has a dismal prognosis.

A change in GCS of 2 or more is significant. Beware changes in monitoring staff!

Optimizing outcome   You are preventing 2° brain injury:
- Oxygenate.
- Moderate hyperventilation to control P_{CO_2}.
- Control haemorrhage and optimize fluid balance.
- Contact neurosurgery and ask advice.
- Only use mannitol under expert advice.
- Do not use steroids at all.[2]

2 R. Bullock 1996 Guidelines for the management of severe head injury. *Eur J. Emerg Med* **3** 109.

Mandibular fractures

These are the commonest # of the facial skeleton. Most are the result of fights and road traffic accidents (the former appear to be increasing whereas the latter are decreasing as a result of seat belts, etc.). Rarely, they may be comminuted with hard and soft tissue loss, e.g. gunshot wounds.

Classification   The most useful is based on site of injury: dento-alveolar, condyle, coronoid, ramus, angle, body, symphyseal, or parasymphyseal. Further subclassification into unilateral, bilateral, multiple, or comminuted aids Rx planning. In common with all # they can be grouped into simple (closed linear #), compound (open to mouth or skin), pathological (# through an area weakened by other pathology), or comminuted; again, this influences Rx.

Muscle pull   Pull on # segments renders the # favourable or unfavourable depending on whether or not the # line resists displacement. This is of less importance than recognizing the # and its associated injuries.

Common #   Condylar neck # are commonest and range from easiest to most difficult. Often found with a # of the angle or canine region of the opposite side of the jaw. Rarely, bilateral condylar # is found with a symphyseal # 'guardsman's #' from falling on the point of the chin. Angle # usually occurs through wisdom-tooth socket, and body # commonly through canine socket.

Diagnosis   History of trauma. Ask if the patient can bite their teeth or dentures together in the manner which is normal to them. Inability to do this and a lingual mucosal haematoma is pathognomonic of a mandibular #. Look at the face; there is usually bruising and swelling over the # site and sometimes lacerations. If the # is displaced, there may be gagging on the posterior teeth and the mouth hangs open. The saliva is usually bloodstained. The patient may complain of paraesthesia in the distribution of the IDN. Gentle palpation over the mandible will reveal step deformities, bony crepitus, and tenderness. All have trismus.

Examination of the mouth   May reveal broken teeth or dentures which should be removed. Suction the mouth to clean away blood clots prior to examining both the buccal and lingual sulcus. Look for step deformities in the occlusion, and examine the teeth. Palpate for steps in the lingual and buccal sulcus. If Δ is uncertain it is sometimes worth trying to elicit abnormal mobility across the suspected # site, using gentle pressure. In cases where you are very unsure, place one hand over each angle of the mandible and exert gentle pressure; this will produce pain if there is a #, even if it is only a crack #. Never perform this if you have proved otherwise that there is a #.

X-rays   OPG and PA mandible are the essentials. Right and left lateral obliques if OPG is unobtainable. Rotated PA (helpful for # between the symphysis and canine region), IO periapicals, occlusal, high OPG, or reverse Townes for condyles, and CT are all second-line investigations which may help.

Preliminary Rx (p. 488) Most patients will be admitted to hospital, nursed sitting up and leaning forward as this is the most comfortable position. Barrel bandages are a waste of time. Keep nil by mouth and maintain hydration by IV crystalloid. Compound # need antibiotics. Assess need for analgesia; LA, temporary immobilization with circumdental wire (bridle wire), parenteral NSAIDs, or opioids may be needed.

Mid-face fractures

The mid-facial skeleton is a complex composite of fine fragile bones, which rarely # in isolation. It forms a detachable framework which protects the brain from trauma. Severe trauma can move the entire mid-face downwards and backwards along the base of the skull, lengthening the face and obstructing the airway (clot and swelling exacerbates this). Most *conscious* patients, however, can compensate for this. # of the cribiform plate of the ethmoids can lead to dural tears and CSF leak (p. 488).

Orbit The globe and optic nerve are well-protected by the bony buttress of the orbit. Most # lines pass around the optic foramen; however, swelling can cause proptosis. Late changes can include tethering and enophthalmos. *Retrobulbar haemorrhage* is an arterial bleed behind the globe following trauma. It presents as a painful, proptosed eye with decreasing visual acuity, and is a surgical emergency. The clot must be decompressed and evacuated. Medical management with mannitol 20% 2 g/kg, acetazolamide 500 mg and dexamethosone at least 1 mg/kg all IV may help while theatre is being arranged.

Bleeding Severe bleeding is rare, but severe mid-facial trauma may lacerate the 3rd part of the maxillary artery, resulting in profuse bleeding into the nasopharynx which requires anterior and posterior nasal packs and possibly direct ligation.

Classification Mainly based on the experimental work of Rene Le Fort. Le Fort I # detaches the tooth-bearing portion of the jaw via a # line from the anterior margin of the anterior nasal aperture running laterally and back to the lower 1/3 of the pterygoid plate. Le Fort II detaches the true mid-face in a pyramidal shape (see diagram). Le Fort III detaches the entire facial skeleton from the cranial base, as diagram.

Diagnosis Le Fort I may occur singly or associated with other facial #. The tooth-bearing portion of the upper jaw is mobile, unless impacted superiorly. There is bruising in the buccal sulcus bilaterally, disturbed occlusion, and posterior 'gagging' of the bite. Grasp the upper jaw between the thumb and forefinger anteriorly, place thumb and forefinger of other hand over the supraorbital ridges, and attempt to mobilize the upper jaw to assess mobility. Spring the maxillary teeth to detect a palatal split. Percussion of the upper teeth may also produce a 'cracked cup' sound. Le Fort II and III # produce similar clinical appearances; namely, gross oedema of soft tissues, bilateral black eyes (panda facies), subconjunctival haemorrhage, mobile mid-face, dish-face appearance, and extensive bruising of the soft palate. Look for a CSF leak and assess visual acuity. Le Fort II # may also show infra-orbital nerve paraesthesia and step deformity in the orbital rim. Peculiar to Le Fort III # are tenderness and separation of the frontozygomatic suture, deformity of zygomatic arches bilaterally, and mobility of entire facial skeleton.

X-rays Occipito-mental 10° and 30°, submento-vertex, lateral skull, postero-anterior skull **only** if C-spine is confirmed to be intact. Otherwise secure C-spine and await CT scan as the definitive imaging technique.

Preliminary Rx as pp. 486, 488; **definitive Rx**, p. 500.

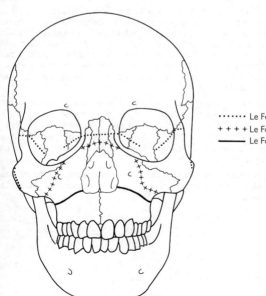

...... Le Fort III
+ + + + Le Fort II
——— Le Fort I

Nasal and malar fractures

Malar **(or zygoma) #**   A common and easily missed injury, usually the result of a blow with a blunt object (e.g. fist). The malar forms the cheek-bone and resembles a four-pointed star on occipito-mental X-ray. The 'star' points to the maxilla (orbital margin and lateral wall of antrum), frontal bone, and temporal bone. # can involve the arch alone or the whole malar, which may or may not be displaced. The nature of the displacement is of value in planning the Rx.

Diagnosis   From history, examination, and X-ray. Bruising around eye with subconjunctival haemorrhage (unilateral). Diplopia, a step deformity of the orbital rim, sometimes paraesthesia of the infra-orbital nerve, limitation of lateral excursion of the mandible on mouth opening, and unilateral epistaxis. There is often tenderness on palpation of the zygomatic buttress IO and usually some flattening of the cheek prominence.

Orbital floor #   Main signs are those of the malar # (or middle 1/3 # if that is the presenting injury). Late signs are enopthalmos and tethering of inferior rectus, causing diplopia in upwards gaze. Also known as orbital blow-out #; fat and muscle herniates through the thin orbital floor (a similar injury can occur to the medial wall). Classically, seen on X-ray as 'hanging drop sign' (radiolucent fat hanging into antrum). Confirm with coronal CT scan. Lateral wall &/or roof # are much less common.

Nasal #   Simple nasal trauma is seen by a number of different specialities and considered rather trivial. This is unfair to the patients, as long-term results of nasal # leave a lot to be desired. Nasal # are frequently associated with deviation or crumpling of the septum, obvious nasal deformity, epistaxis, and a degree of nasal obstruction. Rx: often consists of simply manipulating the nasal bones with the thumb and splinting. This leaves the septum untreated and contributes to poor long-term results, many needing rhinoplasty later.

Nasoethmoid #   Consists of nasal bones, frontal process of maxilla, lacrimal bones, orbital plate of ethmoid, and displacement of the medial canthus of the eye. These # require accurate reduction, stabilization, and fixation of the medial canthus. Δ: bilateral black eyes, obvious nasal deformity (particularly depression of the nasal bridge), septal deviation, epistaxis, and obstruction. Look for CSF leak.

Septal haematoma   A comparatively uncommon complication of nasal trauma which demands immediate evacuation as, if ignored, it can lead to septal necrosis.

Treatment of facial fractures

Essentially involves reduction, fixation, and immobilization of the # segments. In mandibular and maxillary #, this was traditionally achieved by IMF, i.e. immobilizing the jaws in occlusion. Nowadays, elastic traction is sometimes used to supplement internal fixation. Wisdom teeth, and grossly broken down or periodontally infected teeth in the # line should be removed. Otherwise, provision of antibiotics and adequate reduction and immobilizatiion with good follow-up (including endodontics as a 2° procedure) often allows preservation of teeth in the # line.

Open reduction and internal fixation (ORIF) of facial bone # has revolutionized Rx. # sites are exposed, usually via mucosal incisions, and reduced under direct vision; the teeth are placed in temporary IMF &/or a wire around the tooth on either side of the # (tension band or bridle wire) and small bone plates fixed by monocortical screws are placed to immobilize the reduction. IMF can then be released for recovery and elastics placed instead on the ward if needed. Very rarely interosseous wires replace plates, or IMF alone may be used. Resorbable plating systems are now coming onto the market but are yet to match titanium's reliability.

Edentulous mandible The absence of teeth in occlusion created problems when relying on IMF, and modified dentures called Gunning splints were used. This technique has been superseded by the use of bone plates in virtually all cases. Pencil-thin edentulous mandibles are best managed by thick (2.4 mm) plates with bicortical screws.

Condylar # Management depends on age and type of injury. <12 yrs: analgesia, soft diet, and intermaxillary elastic guidance (if needed) produces optimal results. >12 yrs: pain-free, pre-injury occlusion should be established (by elastic traction if need be), and the patient reassessed at 7 days. If spontaneous pain-free occlusion not possible at this stage: ORIF.[1]

Mid-face # Use one of the following methods:

   Internal fixation Interosseous wiring, plating, transfixation with Kirschner wires. Plating to recreate the pyriform and zygomatic buttress system is currently most widespread.

   External fixation E.g. Levant frame, box frame, which fix the mid-face to the cranium.

Malar # Are elevated by a temporal approach (Gillies) or bone hook percutaneously and supplemented by internal fixation with a range of plating techniques.

Nasal bones Are manipulated and splinted. Some benefit from mini-submucous resection of the septum.

Nasoethmoidal # Are openly reduced and wired or microplated to reposition the medial canthi and restore anatomy.

   Fractures in children Considerably rarer. Plates and pins tend to be avoided because of risk to unerupted teeth. Patients <10 yrs may require a

---

1 Faculty of Dental Surgery 1997 National clinical guidelines. *RCS Eng.*

form of Gunning splint which fits over the mixed dentition. # are usually firmly united within 3 weeks. Microplates can sometimes be used, or heavy resorbable sutures at the lower border of the mandible.

Post-op care Antibiotics and scrupulous OH are required. The main problems are presented by IMF, and these patients need to be 'specialed' post-operatively. IMF requires a liquidized diet of at least 2500 calories (2000 for F) and 3 l of fluid daily. Do not discharge until this can be maintained at home. ORIF requires a soft diet for up to 3 weeks.

Complications **Mandible** Infection, paraesthesia, damage to teeth, TMJ pain, malunion, delayed union, non-union, bony sequestration, plate and wire infection. **Maxilla** Post-op deformity, epiphora, diplopia, late enophthalmus, anosmia. Failure of union is very rare, although malunion is a problem with poor reduction or late referral. **Malar** Diplopia, retrobulbar haemorrhage, enophthalmos, paraesthesia. **Nasal** Deformity, nasal obstruction.

Composite tissue loss Increasing use of firearms in civilian life has led to more facial # presenting as composite defects of hard and soft tissue with tissue loss. These patients need to be stabilized, often with surgical debridement and external fixation prior to free-tissue transfer as part of definitive Rx.

Facial soft-tissue injuries

The face is highly visible and once cut no one can make the scar disappear. You can, however, give the patient the best possible scar by following certain principles.

Assessment ABCs, mechanism of injury, allergies, and PMH, need for tetanus and rabies prophylaxis. Wounds should be closed within 24 h.

Examination Type of patient, type of wound (cut, burst, flap, tissue loss), special anatomy, eye, eyelid, lip, V/VII, parotid/lacrimal duct.

Investigation X-ray for FB.

Plan treatment Clean simple wounds in cooperative patient are best closed under LA. Otherwise admit for GA in theatre.

Clean wound Irrigate clean wounds with saline or aqueous chlorhexidine. Bites or dirty wounds with ingrained FB need aggressive scrubbing with 50:50 water:betadine. Minimal or no excision of tissue for debridement. Explore all wounds for FB, #, nerve, duct, or vessel damage. Get haemostasis.

Wound closure In layers, mucosa, and muscle: resorbable 3/0–4/0; skin: monofilament 4/0–6/0. (Suturing: p. 392.) Avoid tension on skin edge.

Types of wound

Simple lacerations Close in layers with accurate anatomical apposition. Approximate, don't strangulate. Use minimum number of sutures to achieve intact wound with slight eversion.

Crush lacerations Skin has burst: minimal edge excision, deep closure, and light skin approximation. Tends to swell. Remove sutures at 3–4 days.

Slicing/shelving lacerations Convert to simple where possible by excision, as tends to 'trap door' otherwise. If excision would be excessive, tack down carefully.

Avulsion If flap, and seems viable: reposition and avoid haematoma. If complete: skin graft or local flap.

Penetrating injuries especially through platysma should be explored by senior surgeon in theatre.

Anatomical sites

Eye Exclude globe injury.

Ear Drain haematoma if present to avoid 'cauliflower'.

Septum Drain haematoma to prevent perforation/collapse.

Eyelid, pinna, eyebrow, and vermilion Require precise matching. Test pre-anaesthetic for facial and trigeminal nerve function.

Special wounds

Abrasions Heal spontaneously but must be cleaned thoroughly; dress with chloramphenicol ointment.

Bites Easily get infected. Use Co-amoxyclav,[1] clean very carefully, and close 1°. Small twist or finger drain helpful.

Burns Need specialist referral.

Tissue loss Nasal tip, pinna, and lip commonest. Skin graft or local flap repair is more likely to succeed than stitching severed part back on.

Gunshot wounds, p. 499.

◀ F. Moore 1997 *BMJ* **314** 88.

Surgery and the temporomandibular joint

TMPDS, p. 482.

Ankylosis May be true or false. **True ankylosis** is restriction of movement caused by a pathological joint condition, usually due to trauma (intracapsular # in childhood) or infection. Extreme limitation of movement and X-rays will confirm degree of bony union. In fibrous union, exercises are of value. In bony union, interpositional arthroplasty or condylectomy with reconstruction is needed. Post-op exercise is crucial. **False ankylosis** Restriction of movement imposed by extra-articular abnormalities is very rare. Rx depends upon cause. **Trismus** (limitation of movement due to spasm of muscles of mastication) may be confused with ankylosis but does not affect the joint. It is much more common and complicates many oral surgical procedures; may follow trauma or infection, or may be a manifestation of occult malignancy.

Trauma Condylar #, p. 492.

Intracapsular **#** Essentially a childhood injury (relatively shorter, thicker condylar neck) keep in function to prevent ankylosis. Condyle # are the subject of UK clinical guidelines (p. 498).

Dislocation Occurs in normal joints due to exceptional circumstances, or in lax joints where dislocation is recurrent. May be unilateral or bilateral. Condyle can be palpated anterior to articular eminence, X-rays confirm position, mouth is gagged open. Rx: immediate reduction; the vast majority can be performed with LA around the dislocated joint &/or sedation. Place thumbs over molar teeth and exert downward and backward pressure (if LA is used, less force is needed and thumbs can be placed in buccal sulcus, avoiding the risk of being bitten). Advise jaw support when yawning, etc.; this is usually enough, and avoids IMF. In chronically recurring dislocations, patients can be taught to self-reduce. Exercises are of limited benefit but may avoid surgery. Sclerosant injections are unpleasant and no longer used. Operations are legion; capsular plication, pins to augment articular eminence, Dautrey downfracture of zygomatic arch, obliteration of upper joint space, eminectomy, high condylectomy. No one operation has gained pre-eminence.

Condylar hyperplasia Rare. Rx: high condylectomy if active (bone scan, but interpretation variable and condylar replacement, e.g. with costochondral cartilage, is unpredictable) or wait for it to 'burnout', then definitive orthognathic surgery.

Tumours Rare. Rx: ablation, reconstruction, and radiotherapy if malignant.

Arthritides Rheumatoid, psoriatic, and gouty arthritides all manifest in the TMJ but in < 15% of patients with the systemic disease. The signs and symptoms are joint stiffness, pain, tenderness, and crepitus. Δ: knowledge of systemic disease and local signs. Rx: treat systemic condition. Symptomatic Rx of joint with appliances, physiotherapy, exercises, and intra-articular steroids. Main long-term problem is limitation of function.

Osteoarthrosis A distinct entity of the TMJ, with a different clinical course from that seen in other joints. Appears to be a degenerative condition of articular cartilage. Δ: crepitus, limitation, and pain on movement, tenderness over condyle, often with X-ray evidence of condylar erosions. Most have symptoms for ~1 yr which gradually ↓ over the next 2 yrs. X-rays show condylar remodelling to a flat smooth surface. Patients then enter a long period of remission. Rx is ∴ aimed at pain relief, using standard TMPDS measures (p. 482). Those remaining unresponsive may benefit from intra-articular steroids (p. 616), which probably accelerate natural remodelling. A small group will remain with pain 3–4 months after steroids, usually with X-ray abnormalities. They should be considered for high condylar shave or high condylectomy.

Surgery and TMPDS Approximately 20% of patients with TMPDS remain unresponsive to conservative Rx. They may benefit from arthrography or arthroscopy both as an investigation and a Rx (distension of the joint space-releasing adhesions). Surgery for pure TMPDS in patients unresponsive to the above may be of benefit (probably by cutting the nerve supply to the joint), although clicking can certainly be eliminated by meniscal plication &/or pterygoid myotomy, and irrevocably damaged menisci can be removed but require some form of interpositional reconstruction.

Major preprosthetic surgery

Minor procedures, p. 426; implantology, p. 428. The aim is to enable an edentulous patient to live comfortably with functioning dentures, ∴ surgery without liaison with an understanding and competent prosthodontist is pointless. All procedures for improving the denture-bearing area of the jaws are dependent on the use of a denture with a modified fitting surface (stent), which is placed at operation and must be worn virtually permanently for up to 8 weeks post-op, the fitting surface being modified at intervals with a soft acrylic lining material. There are many who would claim these procedures do not work, and indeed there is little scientific support for them.

▶ Warn all patients undergoing lower jaw procedures about post-op mental nerve damage.

Epithelial inlay (vestibuloplasty) Basically a skin graft to the alveolar surface of the jaw, creating a deeper sulcus. Important points: excise all areas of scarred or hyperplastic tissue, dissect off any strands of mentalis in the lower jaw, ensure preservation of the alveolar periosteum, ensure the stent extends to the new sulcus depth, and ensure the skin–mucosa junction lies on the labial surface.

Combination mucosal flap and epithelial inlay Usually suffices in the maxilla due to its ↑ potential for denture retention.

Mental nerve repositioning Mental nerve compression by a denture flange following alveolar resorption is a common problem, producing a sensation like an electric shock but with a background ache which ↑ during the day and ↓ overnight. Leaving the -/F out for several days ↓ the pain. The mental nerve is repositioned by creating a new foramen under its present position or laterally transposing the entire nerve into the soft tissues in grossly atrophic mandibles.

Alveolar augmentation Problems with osseous donor site morbidity and length of procedure in elderly patients put these operations out of favour. The use of 'sandwich' procedures (where the augmenting material is literally sandwiched between horizontally osteotomized jaw), coupled with effective bone substitutes and tunnelling procedures (p. 426), have made augmentation, even in the comparatively frail elderly, a far better proposition. Younger, fit patients with severe jaw atrophy or those with incipient or actual pathological # may still benefit from split rib grafting.

Vertical distraction osteogenesis A preprosthetic component to this well-accepted technique for 'growing' bone by osteotomizing and gradually moving bone apart (2 mm/day) will probably replace all major augmentation procedures.

Sinus lift ↑ popular procedure combined with simultaneous or delayed implants. After raising subperiosteal buccal flaps a window is created to expose antral lining. Lining of the floor and walls is elevated intact and this space is filled with bone from the iliac crest, tibia, or chin to provide retention for implants.

Transmandibular implant A box frame construction placed in the mandible from a submental incision. Reputed to ↑ bone deposition.

Clefts and craniofacial anomalies

▶ 20% of cases of congenital facial malformation are accompanied by a 2nd or 3rd systemic malformation.

Cleft lip and palate (see also p. 196)

▶ The aim is to replace anatomical structures in their correct position; the price is scarring, which will restrict growth to some degree. It is important to recognize that the stigmata of surgery is due to growth of the patient. At least as much deformity has been caused in the past by poor surgery as has been caused by the cleft.

Lip closure Two main philosophies: **'Plastic' approach** Performed neonatally or up to 3 months; flaps transgress skin boundaries and use supraperiosteal dissection. Gives good early aesthetic results (e.g. Millard). **'Functional' approach** All skin boundaries are respected; uses subperiosteal dissection. Immediate aesthetics are less good due to pout caused by muscle repair but ↑ function and growth potential (e.g. Delaire). In the UK a trend is emerging to blend the techniques of these philosophies.

Palatal closure Extensive surgery restricts maxillary growth, ∴ use minimal simple repair which recreates a functioning soft palate (e.g. Von Langenbeck or Delaire).

Alveolus Vomer flap to close anterior alveolus and gingivoperiosteoplasty are 1° procedures advocated by some and decried by others.

Ears Preschool audiology. Many will benefit from grommets.

Nasal deformity Perhaps the greatest surgical challenge. 1° functional lip/nose repair may alter this.

Secondary surgery Lip revision (simple or complex). Sometimes required preschool or at time of alveolar bone graft.

Alveolar bone graft, p. 197.

Speech, nasendoscopy, and pharyngoplasty All cleft palate patients have impaired speech. Fibre-optic nasendoscopy allows visualization of the palate during speech and aids assessment. Pharyngoplasty narrows the velopharyngeal opening to ↓ hypernasal speech. Successful palate repair ↓ need for pharyngoplasty.

Orthognathic surgery, p. 508.

Craniofacial anomalies

A broad group of conditions involving the cranio-maxillofacial region. A simple classification is:

Congenital

- Orbital malformations (hypertelorism, orbital dystopia)
- Craniosynostoses (premature fusion of cranial sutures)
- Craniofacial synostoses (Apert syndromes, Crouzon, pp. 756, 757)
- Encephaloceles
- Others (Treacher–Collins, hemifacial microsomia, hemifacial hypertrophy and atrophy)

Acquired

- Tumours (benign or malignant)
- Dysplasias (fibro-osseous)
- Neurofibromatosis
- Post-trauma deformity

These patients need craniofacial teams (minimum: craniofacial surgeon, neurosurgeon, and anaesthetist). Coronal flaps to deglove the face are the mainstay of access, followed by craniotomy and osteotomy as required. Main risks are cerebral oedema, infection, damage to optic nerves and vessels; and, in neonates and children, paediatric fluid balance.

Orthognathic surgery

This is the surgery of facial skeletal deformity and merges with cleft and craniofacial surgery. Prime indications are functional: speech, eating. Secondary indications are aesthetic.

▶ Patients may not see these as quite such separate issues. Their reasons and motivation for seeking surgery must be understood and the limitations of surgery made absolutely clear before embarking on protracted and complex Rx.

Diagnosis and treatment planning, p. 194.

Mandibular procedures

Involve ramus, body, alveolus, or chin.

Intra-oral vertical subsigmoid osteotomy   Used to push back the mandible. EO approach used when suitable equipment for IO not available. The IO procedure is straightforward, performed via an extended third-molar type incision. Bone cuts are made with a right-angled oscillating saw from sigmoid notch to lower border. Technique is very instrument-dependent.

Sagital split osteotomy   Can move mandible backwards or forwards. IO incision similar to above. Bone cuts made from above lingula, across retromolar region, down buccal aspect to lower border. Split sagitally with osteotome followed by spreaders. Main complication is paraesthesia of IDN.

Inverted L- and C-shaped osteotomy   Usually EO approach. Rarely used; can lengthen ramus if used with bone graft.

Body ostectomy   Shortens body of mandible. Need to gain space orthodontically or remove tooth. Watch mental nerve.

Subapical osteotomy   Used to move dento-alveolar segments. Technically more difficult than it looks. Risk to tooth vitality.

Genioplasty   The tip of the chin can be moved pretty much anywhere; the secret is to keep a sliding contact with bone and a muscle pedicle. Fixation should be kept away from areas of muscle activity as this leads to bone resorption.

Maxillary procedures

Segmental   Can be single-tooth, or bone and tooth blocks, e.g. Wassmund procedure, which involves tunnelling incisions in buccal sulcus and palate to move premaxilla. Problems are finding space for bone cuts and avoiding damaging teeth.

Le Fort I   Mainstay procedure. Standard approach is the 'down-fracture' with horseshoe buccal incision, bone cuts at Le Fort I level, and segment pedicled on the palate. The freed maxilla can be moved up, down, or forward. In cleft palate cases, concern over the adequacy of the palatal blood supply has led to some surgeons using tunnelled buccal incisions to make the bone cuts, thus preserving some of the buccal blood supply to the maxilla. Fixation is a problem when using this technique.

Le Fort II   Usually used for mid-face advancement. Bilateral canthal and vestibular incisions allow bone cuts at the Le Fort II level.

Le Fort III   Really a subcranial craniofacial operation using a coronal flap plus vestibular and orbital incisions to move the entire mid-face and malar complex.

Malar osteotomy   Used for post-traumatic defects. Approach via coronal incisions. Risk to infra-orbital nerve from maxillary bone cut.

Rhinoplasty   The correction of isolated nasal deformity. Usually done intranasally, supplemented by tiny incisions over the nasal bones to allow bone cuts. 'Open rhinoplasty', which involves degloving the nasal skeleton via a collumella incision, is becoming popular.

Stability   ↑ use of mini-plates in the fixation of the osteotomized segments has ↓ the reliance on bone grafts. Pre-surgical orthodontics (p. 194) makes a significant contribution to ↓ rate of relapse. IMF &/or elastic traction remains vital for long-term success. Good dental interdigitation, and planning movements within the capacity of the soft tissues, are probably the best antirelapse measures.[1]

1 D. Tuinzing 1993 *Surgical Orthodontics*, VU University Press.

Salivary gland tumours

Diseases (see also p. 456, 458)

Classified by WHO into epithelial tumours, non-epithelial tumours, and unclassified tumours.

Common benign tumours **Pleomorphic adenoma**, p. 458. **Monomorphic adenoma** Adenolymphoma (Warthin's tumour) affects M > F; rare <50 yrs. Bilateral in 10%. Feels soft and cystic. Benign, very unlikely to recur despite being multifocal.

Carcinomas Rare. **Adenoid cystic carcinoma** Characteristic 'Swiss cheese' appearance histologically. Spreads locally, particularly along perineural spaces. Can be compatible with long-term survival despite propensity for 2° in lungs, although rarely cured. **Adenocarcinomas** There are a wide range of these malignant tumours, ranging from the highly aggressive to the relatively indolent, e.g. polymorphous low grade adenocarcinoma. It is essential that adequate histological Δ is made early (expert head and neck pathologist needed). Other carcinomas are rare, but may arise in a pre-existing pleomorphic adenoma or *de novo*. 5 yr survival ~30%.

Other epithelial tumours Include *acinic cell tumour* and *mucoepidermoid tumour*. Both have variable, unpredictable behaviour, can recur locally, and metastasize, and can occur at any age. On average, both compatible with ~80% survival.

Non-epithelial tumours Include haemangioma, lymphangioma, and neurofibroma. Account for 50% of salivary tumours in children.

Unclassified group Includes lymphomas, secondaries, lipomas, and chemodectomas.

Parotid History and examination are the prime diagnostic tools. Long history, no pain, and no facial nerve involvement suggest benign tumour. Facial palsy, pain, and rapid growth suggest malignancy. The feel of many tumours are characteristic. CT, FNAC, USS, MRI may help; however, Rx almost always involves parotidectomy and most investigations simply delay this.

Submandibular Less common tumours. Pleomorphic adenoma remains most common. Malignant tumours account for up to 30%. Rx of most is gland excision via a skin crease in the neck. Modified neck dissection for malignant or recurrent tumours.

Sublingual and minor glands >50% of tumours are malignant (mostly adenoid cystic) and require extensive surgery and reconstruction similar to floor of mouth cancer.

Surgery of the salivary glands

Surgery of the major salivary glands is primarily for tumours, obstruction, and, less commonly, inflammatory conditions. The minor glands are most commonly removed for mucoceles (p. 414) and more rarely for tumours. With the exception of lymphomas *all* salivary gland tumours should have surgery initially, patient permitting.

Parotidectomy Principles are complete excision of tumour with margin of healthy tissue and preservation of facial nerve. Clinically benign tumours in superficial lobe have superficial parotidectomy; and in deep lobe, total conservative parotidectomy. Malignant tumours require radical excision &/or radiotherapy. Whether or not to sacrifice the facial nerve adjacent to malignant parotid tumour is complex decision. Many would accept: *nerve clinically affected*, pre-op, sacrifice, and reconstruct; *nerve clinically intact*, pre-op, preserve, and rely on post-op radiotherapy.

Salivary duct calculi History is of recurrent pain and swelling in the obstructed gland, particularly before and during meals. Plain X-rays (lower occlusal for submandibular, cheek for parotid) reveal radio-opaque calculi, but do not exclude the radiolucent calculi and mucous plugs. Sialography reveals a stricture or obstruction. Commonest in the submandibular duct. Rx: *submandibular duct* for calculi lying anterior in duct—remove by passing a suture behind the calculus to prevent it slipping further down the duct, dissect the duct from an IO approach, and lift out stone; either marsupialize the duct or reconstruct. Posterior calculi—excise gland and duct. Rx: *parotid duct*—expose duct via IO approach for anterior stones or via a small skin flap onto a probe in the duct for more posterior calculi. Otherwise, selective superficial parotidectomy is the only safe approach. Laser lithotripsy is available in some centres for proximal calculi in patients wishing to avoid gland excision.

Recurrent sialadenitis Severe recurrent infection of the parotid or submandibular glands leads to dilatation and ballooning of the ducts and alveoli called sialectasis. Sialography is the investigation of choice and often therapeutic, inducing long remissions between episodes of infection. *Conservative* Rx: irrigation of gland with tetracycline solution. When remission periods are short or intolerable, or the patient requires *definitive* Rx: submandibular gland excision or total conservative parotidectomy with removal of 90% of the duct. Interventional sialography with specialized balloon/basket catheters is now being used to dilate or retrieve obstructions but has not replaced open surgery.

Surgery for drooling In severe cases it is possible to re-site the parotid ducts into the hypopharynx &/or perform bilateral submandibular gland excision to control drooling without impairing lubrication for swallowing and oral health (Wilkes procedure). A more physiological approach is to reposition submandibular ducts and excise sublingual glands, as these are major source of pooled saliva *at rest*. Intraglandular botulinum toxin can help.

Mucoceles, p. 414.

Facial skin cancer

Skin cancer, p. 552.

The common facial skin cancers are BCC, SCC, and malignant melanoma. They may be preceded by actinic keratosis, carcinoma-*in-situ*, or lentigo maligna.

The 'best buy' Rx is usually excision with repair by 1° closure, skin graft, or local flap.

Margins A margin of normal skin around the cancer of 5 mm for BCC, 10 mm for SCC, and 10–15 mm for melanoma.

Techniques Mark out the periphery of the tumour, line of excision, and any flap repair *before* injecting LA (if used). Cut at 90° to skin through dermis and excise at level of fat layer. *Always* obtain good haemostasis (bipolar diathermy). Mark specimen to orientate for pathologist.

Repair

1° closure Try to design excision in natural crease or resting skin tension line. Excise in an ellipse, undermine both sides, and close by halfing the length of the wound. Use deep sutures to minimize tension. Excise any 'dog ears'.

Wedge excision Allows 1° closure of lip, eyelid, and helix.

Split skin grafts Are thin and take well, but tend to shrink and are a poor colour match. Taken with a Humby/Watson knife or a dermatome they leave a raw donor site. Useful for scalp defects.

No skin graft will take on bare bone, tendon, or cartilage. Grafts will fail if they move, develop haematoma, or become infected, as this prevents plasmatic imbibition and capillary ingrowth.

Full thickness skin grafts Thicker and more robust, they do not take as easily. They are taken with a scalpel and donor site is closed 1°. Better colour match.

Grafts are sutured to periphery of wound and immobilized with a bolster of antiseptic cotton or sponge and tie-over sutures for 7–10 days. The thicker the graft, the longer to take.

Local flaps

Have their own blood supply and work by a combination of geometry and widespread undermining.

Flap is marked out at same time as excision before LA. Held in new position by deep and skin sutures. Do not use pressure dressings. Haematoma is biggest cause of failure in adequately designed flaps: take sutures out to ↓ pressure and ↑flap circulation with delayed resuture.

Common local flaps

Transposition flap Simple switch over of skin.

Rhomboid flap Very useful; relies on lax skin at donor site.

Bilobed flap Transfers circles 80% and 60% to created defect.

Subcutaneous advancement flap A teardrop of skin is advanced on a subcutaneous fat pedicle.

Oral cancer

Aetiology, epidemiology, Δ, and staging, p. 452; neck lumps, p. 518; salivary tumours, p. 510.

Various parameters affect the choice of Rx for patients with oral cancer; not least among these, but often forgotten, are the patients themselves, their general health, understanding of their disease, geographical location, and social and domestic commitments. Classically, broad Rx principles are based on tumour staging, using TNM classification, p. 452, and the patient's fitness for surgery (this tends to imply that if they can't cope with surgery they can cope with travelling for radiotherapy, which is not always the case). In many instances of oral cancer, combined surgery and radiotherapy constitutes optimal Rx.

Suggested management plan (this will vary according to the surgeon concerned)

1 Establish provisional Δ. History, examination, and get to know patient. FBC, ESR, U&Es, LFTs (including albumin), bone biochemistry, VDRL, blood group, CXR, ECG, OPG.

2 Arrange tissue Δ. By biopsy—usually under LA. Flexible nasendoscopy, head, neck, thorax, imaging (CT/MRI). This is to exclude synchronous 1° tumour in upper aerodigestive tract (present in, at most, 15% of cases). Palpate the neck for nodes. Stage tumour (TNM).

3 Unless patient has made it very obvious they do not want to know the Δ, first inform them, then relatives, fully.

- T1–N0 Surgery or radiotherapy (often brachytherapy—radioactive implants) offer equal cure rate.
- Tumour close to bone having radiotherapy: safest to remove associated teeth to prevent osteoradionecrosis.
- T2 and T3 > 50% of patients will have occult metastases; consider: to watch and wait; prophylactic radiotherapy (works for occult but not for obvious bulky nodes); or prophylactic selective neck dissection. Later usually best.
- For large tumours, close or +ve margins, and extracapsular spread, radiotherapy given post-op.
- Vastly ↑ access is obtained for resection by osteotomizing the mandible (position plate beforehand).
- Anterior floor of mouth cancer may spread to bilateral lymph nodes; bilateral selective neck dissection can be simultaneous and is usual.
- Presence or absence of extracapsular spread in cervical lymph nodes is strongest prognostic indicator.

Simultaneous chemotherapy and radiotherapy can have a dramatic effect on poorly differentiated SCCs, especially those originating from post-nasal space, tonsil, and tongue base.

5-year survival 90% for T1–N0, but 30% for T2/3–N1 and worse for T4; however, this does *not* mean that extensive combination therapy and reconstruction is pointless in those with advanced oral cancers. Death comes in many ways, and a fungating uncontrolled cancer of the head and neck is one of the less pleasant. Attempted surgical 'cure' which alleviates local disease and symptoms and allows the patient a few more years of life and a gradual demise due to carcinomatosis or another disease is still worthwhile from all viewpoints. (Palliative surgery with curative intent.)

Chemotherapy   There is, as yet, no proven role for cytotoxics in oral cancer, other than in combination with radiotherapy or in palliation.

Neck lumps

▶ Do not leave chronic cervical lymphadenopathy undiagnosed.
▶ A 1° head and neck malignancy must be excluded before biopsy.

Children are an exception; inflammation is common and tumour is rare, so a watch and wait policy is reasonable.

Diagnosis Listen to the story, look at the patient and lump. Palpate it. If needed, carry out a full head and neck examination. Most diagnoses will be made by then.

Investigation Ultrasound, aspiration cytology, biopsy.

Causes Think (a) anatomy, (b) pathology, (c) oddity.

Skin Lesions lie superficially.

Sebaceous cyst Look for punctum; is within skin. Excise.

Lipoma Soft, often yellowish. Excise.

Sublingual dermoid cyst Lies in floor of mouth, often under mylohyoid. Arises from trapped epithelium during embryonic fusion; contains keratin. Rx: total excision.

Lymph nodes Deep to platysma. Try to diagnose *before* biopsy. Opening of malignant nodes ↓ survival (p. 516).

Infection (p. 478) Nodes are large and tender. Causes: viral (e.g. glandular fever, HIV), bacterial (e.g. mycobacterial (which can calcify), actinomycosis), or reactive to other head and neck infection.

Malignancy Either metastatic from head and neck 1° (hard, rock-like nodes) or lymphoma/leukaemia (large rubbery), p. 478. FNAC unhelpful in lymphoma; biopsy needed.

Glandular Think anatomically.

Salivary (p. 510) Submandibular/lower pole of parotid: abscess, sialadenitis, obstruction, sarcoidosis, Sjögren syndrome. Sublingual: ranula, tumour.

Thyroid Benign and malignant tumours, goitre, thyroglossal cyst (may lie anywhere between foramen caecum of tongue and thyroid, tract goes behind, around, or through hyoid bone, moves with swallowing).

Arterial Don't biopsy!

Carotid aneurysm (pulsatile).

Carotid body tumour Found around carotid bifurcation. Usually firm, not hormonally active, 5% malignant. Rx: excise if symptomatic.

Schwannoma/neurofibroma All major nerves in neck can develop painless masses. Rx: subadvential excision, preserving healthy fibres if possible.

Pharynx

Diverticulum (or pharyngeal pouch) Fills on swallowing. Evert endoscopically or excise.

Larynx

   Laryngocele   Rare. Mainly M > 60. 80% unilateral. Excise.

Sternomastoid

   'Sternomastoid tumour'   (congenital ischaemic fibrosis causing torticollis).

   True muscle tumours   Rare.

Bone

   Cervical rib, prominent hyoid bone

Infections (see also p. 408) Ludwig's angina, submasseteric abscess, retropharyngeal abscess, parapharyngeal cellulitis, collar stud abscess (TB), infected cysts or pouches.

Oddities

Branchial cyst   Either a remnant from 2nd and 3rd branchial arches or degeneration of lymphoid tissue. Is an epithelial lined cyst which presents as a deep-seated swelling lying anterior to sternomastoid at or above the level of the hyoid. Prone to infection. Rx: total excision.

Branchial fistula   A fistula from the tonsillar fossa to the skin overlying anterior lower 1/3 of sternomastoid. Present at birth; discharges intermittently. Rx: total excision of tract.

Cystic hygroma   Presents in infancy and is a form of lymphangioma which appears as endothelium-lined multilocular cysts containing lymph. May be found anywhere in head–neck but classically behind lower end of sternomastoid. May suddenly ↑ in size if bled into or ruptured. Rx: total excision (in practice, excise as much as possible) as soon as child is fit for operation. Cystic areas may be sclerosed using modified streptococcal antigen (DK432).

Flaps and grafts

A **graft** is transferred tissue dependent on the recipient site capillaries for its survival. A **flap** is transferred tissue independent, at least initially, of the recipient site capillaries for survival.

It is the possibility of functional reconstruction of the head and neck in conjunction with the potential for cure that justifies the mutilation of radical surgery for oral cancer; however, head and neck reconstruction is used in other aspects of maxillofacial surgery, particularly trauma.

Mucosal grafts, p. 244. **Mucosal flaps**, p. 245.

Skin grafts May be split thickness or full thickness. Split thickness (taken by knife or dermatome from thigh or inner arm) take quickly and become wettable in the mouth. They are 'quilted' in place with sutures. Full thickness (supraclavicular, post-auricular, or abdominal) provide a mediocre colour match when repairing skin defects of the face. Full thickness donor sites are closed 1°.

Free bone grafts From rib, iliac crest, or calvarium. Rib, which is partially split at 1 cm intervals, can be bent to conform to the shape of the mandible. Iliac crest supplies cortical or cancellous bone and can be cut to a template, but ↑ risk of DVT. Various synthetic mesh containers as a mould for cancellous bone exist.

Nasolabial flap Random pattern pedicle flap based above and lateral to the upper lip; useful local flap. Requires division ~3 weeks later.

Tongue flaps Random pattern pedicle flap for lip and palate repair. Requires division and inset 3 weeks later.

Forehead flap Based on anterior branch of superficial temporal artery; very safe flap, rarely used because of the poor donor site defect. Requires division later.

Masseter muscle flap Limited in size; can be used intra-orally.

Temperoparietal fuscia flap Pedicle or free flap based on superficial temporal vessels. Long flexible reconstruction. Difficult to raise.

Temporalis flap Inferiorly based on deep temporal branches of maxillary artery. Limited use due to size and tendency to fibrose.

Deltopectoral flap Based on perforating internal mammary vessels. Thin skin suitable for skin or mucosa repair. Usually divided and inset after 3 weeks.

Pectoralis major myocutaneous flap Also described with bone, but the bone is really a free rib graft. Based on acromiothoracic axis. Usually tunnelled after neck dissection. Very bulky flap; covers carotids after radical neck dissection. Workhorse head and neck pedicle flap.

Latissimus dorsi myocutaneous flap Very bulky flap based on thoracodorsal vessels. Needs to be tunnelled through axilla if pedicled. More commonly used as a free flap.

Free tissue transfer by microvascular re-anastomosis has been the biggest advance in reconstruction. The following are useful and commonly used flaps.

Radial forearm flap   A fasciocutaneous flap based on the radial artery. The skin available is thin and supple and can conform to the complex anatomy of the mouth (skin is often hairless, which is a big bonus). A thin segment of up to 10 cm of radius can also be transferred for bony reconstruction.

Deep circumflex iliac artery flap   Based on the deep circumflex iliac artery. This flap has potential for sufficient bone transfer to reconstruct the entire mandible. Internal oblique muscle usually transferred for soft tissue—good where non-mobile soft tissue repair needed. Skin transfer possible but less useful.

Free fibula flap   25 cm of fibula can be excised within a muscle cuff supplied by the peroneal vessels. Excellent length and thickness of bone for mandibular reconstruction. Skin transfer for mobile soft tissue available.

Free rectus abdominus   Bulky skin/muscle flap based on inferior epigastric vessels. Useful for massive facial defects but often limited by fat volume.

Anterolateral thigh free flap   Recently popularized soft tissue flap from thigh (descending branch of lateral circumflex femoral artery. Skin thickness can limit usefulness infra-orally.

Subscapular system flaps   Several skin, fat, and bone flaps can be harvested from these vessels; disadvantage is need to turn patient perioperatively.

Craniofacial implants   Prosthetic eyes, ears, and noses can be securely fixed to the facial skeleton with implants using techniques similar to oral implants. Probably the best available ear reconstruction.

Medicine relevant to dentistry

Principal sources   C. Scully 1998 *Medical Problems in Dentistry*,
Wright. M. Longmore 2002 *Oxford Handbook of Clinical Medicine*,
OUP. Various 1995 *Procedures in Practice*, *BMJ*. HMSO *Prescribers
Journal*. Medicine online BNF 44.

NB All drug doses relate to fit adult patients $\cong$70kg in weight.
Always check doses for children, the elderly, and those with
other medical conditions.

Anaemia

Anaemia is a ↓ in the level of circulating haemoglobin to below the normal reference range for a patient's age and sex. It indicates an underlying problem and, as such, the cause of the anaemia should be diagnosed *before* instituting Rx.

▶ Never rush into transfusing patients presenting with a chronic anaemia. Perform basic blood investigations before giving iron or transfusing. Elective surgery in patients with an Hb <10 g/dl is rarely appropriate.

Clinical features of anaemia are notoriously unreliable, but beloved of examiners and include: general fatigue, heart failure, angina on effort, pallor (look at conjunctivae and palmar creases, but unreliable), brittle nails &/or spoon-shaped nails (koilonychia), oral discomfort &/or ulceration, glossitis, and classically angular cheilitis.

Syndromes, p. 760.

Types of anaemia

Microcytic (MCV < 78fl) Iron-deficiency anaemia is by far the commonest cause. Causes: chronic blood loss (gastrointestinal or menstrual), inadequate diet. FBC and biochemistry show microcytic, hypochromic anaemia with a low serum iron and a high total iron binding capacity (TIBC). ↑ RBC zinc protoporphyrin is a fast and sensitive early test. Thalassaemia and sideroblastic anaemia are rare causes of microcytosis.

Normocytic Commonly, anaemia of chronic disease. Other causes: pregnancy, haemolytic anaemia, and aplastic anaemia. Once pregnancy is excluded, the patient needs investigation by an expert. The TIBC is usually ↓.

Macrocytic (MCV > 100 fl) Low B_{12} &/or low folate are the common causes. B_{12} is ↓ in pernicious anaemia (deficit of intrinsic factor), alcohol abuse, small gut disease, and chronic exposure to nitrous oxide. Low folate is usually dietary, but may be caused by illness (e.g. coeliac disease, skin disease) or drugs such as phenytoin, methotrexate, trimethoprim, and cotrimoxazole.

Management In all cases the cause must be sought; this may necessitate referral to a haematologist. Drugs used in iron deficiency: ferrous sulfate 200 mg tds. Transfusion of packed cells covered with frusemide 40 mg PO if elderly or ↓ cardiac function, indicated rarely for severe microcytic anaemia. Lifelong IM hydroxycobalamin 1 mg 3-monthly is used to treat B_{12} deficiency, and folic acid 5 mg od for folate deficiency.

▶ Never use folate alone to treat 'macrocytosis' unless it is proven to be the only deficiency. **NB** Folic acid is **not** the same as folinic acid.

Note on sickle cell anaemia A homozygous hereditary condition causing red cells to 'sickle' when exposed to low O_2 tensions, resulting in infarctions of bone and brain. In sickle cell trait (heterozygous form) the cells are less fragile and sickle only in severe hypoxia. Management: perform haemoglobin electrophoresis (or Sickledex if result needed urgently) on all Afro-Caribbean (and consider Mediteranean, Middle Eastern, and Indian) patients planned for GA.

Haematological malignancy

Leukaemias are a neoplastic proliferation of white blood cells. Acute leukaemias are characterized by the release of primitive blast cells into the peripheral blood and account for 50% of childhood malignancy. Acute lymphoblastic leukaemia, the commonest childhood leukaemia, now has up to 90% cure rate in favourable cases. May present as gingival hypertrophy and bleeding. Acute myeloblastic leukaemia is the commonest acute leukaemia of adults, but although an 80% remission rate is possible this is rarely maintained. Chronic leukaemias have cells that retain most of the appearance of normal white cells. Chronic lymphocytic leukaemia is the commonest and has a 5 yr survival of >50%. Chronic myeloid leukaemia is characterized by the presence of the Philadelphia chromosome, a fact beloved by examiners. Affects the >40s. Rx: interferon and &/or BMT or stem cell transplantation. Remissions are common, although a terminal blast crisis usually supervenes at some stage.

Myeloproliferative disorders are proliferation of non-leukocyte marrow cells, with a wide range of behaviour and presentation, including anaemia, bleeding, and infections.

Monoclonal gammopathies such as multiple myeloma are B-lymphocyte disorders characterized by production of a specific immunoglobulin by plasma cells. Multiple myeloma is also a differential Δ of lytic lesions of bone, particularly the skull. Δ: monoclonal paraprotein band on plasma electrophoresis, Bence–Jones proteins in urine.

Lymphomas A group of solid tumours arising in lymphoid tissue; divided into Hodgkin's or non-Hodgkin's lymphomas, with the latter carrying a poorer prognosis. Lymphoma should always be considered in the differential Δ of neck swellings.

Cytotoxic chemotherapy Has been the mainstay of Rx for these diseases, with supplemental radiotherapy for masses or prior to bone marrow transplant. It is essential to remember that any patient receiving these drugs will be both immunocompromised and liable to bleed.

Hints In haematological malignancy, anaemia, bleeding, and infection are the overwhelming risks. Look for and treat anaemia. Avoid aspirin, other NSAIDs, trauma, and IM injections. Prevent sepsis, and if it occurs treat very aggressively with the locally recommended broad-spectrum antibacterials and antifungals, e.g. azlocillin 5 g and gentamicin 80 mg IV tds plus fluconazole up to 100 mg daily. Liase with haematologist urgently.

Amyloidosis Characterized by deposits of fibrillar eosinophilic hyaline material in a wide range of organs and tissues. Two types: 1° *amyloidosis* (AL amyloid), a plasma cell dyscrasia. Signs and symptoms include peripheral neuropathy, renal involvement, cardiomyopathy, xerostomia, and macroglossia. Rx: immunosuppression (rarely helps). 2° *amyloidosis* (AA amyloid). It reflects an underlying chronic disease: infection, rheumatoid, neoplasia. May respond to Rx of underlying disease. Δ: biopsy of rectum or gingivae—stain with Congo red.

Other haematological disorders

For the practical management of a bleeding patient, see p. 390.

Bleeding disorders

Platelet disorders May present as nosebleeds, purpura, or post-extraction bleeding. Remember that aspirin is the most common acquired cause, its effect being irreversible for 1 week. Other causes include diseases such as Von Willebrand's disease; immune thrombocytopenic purpura (ITP); virally associated (especially HIV) thrombocytopenic purpura; thrombocytopenia secondary to leukaemia; cytotoxic drugs; or unwanted effects of drugs, notably aspirin and chloramphenicol. Management: ensure platelet levels of $> 50 \times 10^9/l$, preferably $75 \times 10^9/l$ for anything more than simple extraction or LA. If actively bleeding, use a combination of local measures (p. 390), tranexamic acid, and platelet transfusion. Platelet transfusions are short-lived and if used prophylactically must be given immediately prior to or during surgery. Liase closely with the lab. The quality of preparation varies by locality. Tranexamic acid mouthwash may ↓ oral bleeding.

Coagulation defects Present as prolonged wound bleeding &/or haemarthroses. Causes include the haemophilias, anticoagulants, liver disease, and von Willebrand's disease.

Others Less common causes include: hereditary haemorrhagic telangectasia, aplastic anaemia, chronic renal failure, myeloma, SLE, disseminated intravascular coagulation, and isolated deficiency of clotting factors.

Haemophilia A (factor VIII deficiency) The commonest clotting defect. Inherited as a sex-linked recessive, it affects males predominantly, although female haemophiliacs can occur. All daughters of affected males are potential carriers. Usually presents in childhood as haemarthroses. Bleeding from the mouth is common. Following trauma, bleeding appears to stop, but an intractable general ooze starts after an hour or so. Severity of bleeding is dependent on the level of factor VIII activity and degree of trauma.

Haemophilia B (factor IX deficiency) Clinically identical to haemophilia A; also known as Christmas disease.

Von Willebrand's disease A combined platelet and factor VIII disorder affecting males and females. Mucosal purpurae are common, haemarthroses less so. Wide range of severity. May improve with age &/or pregnancy.

Management The haemophilias and Von Willebrand's disease should always be managed at specialist centres. Check the patient's warning card for the contact telephone number.

Anticoagulants

Heparin Given IV or high-dose SC for therapeutic anticoagulation. Its effect wears off in ~8 h although it can be reversed by protamine sulfate in an emergency. Measure in activated partial thromboplastin time (APTT).

Warfarin Given orally; effects take 48h to be seen. Normal therapeutic range is an International Normalized Ratio (INR) of 2–4. Simple extractions are usually safe at a level within therupeutic range. Avoid attempts to reverse warfarin with vitamin K unless *in extremis*. Use fresh frozen plasma if needed, but consider why the patient is anticoagulated in the first place.

Cardiovascular disease

This is the commonest cause of death in the UK.

Clinical conditions

Hypertension is a consistently raised BP (>160 systolic, >90 diastolic >3 months) and is a risk factor for ischaemic heart disease, cerebrovascular accidents, and renal failure. Up to 95% of hypertension has no definable cause: essential hypertension. 5% is secondary to another disease such as renal dysfunction or endocrine disorders.

Ischaemic heart disease is a ↓ of the blood supply to part of the heart by narrowing of the coronary arteries, usually by atheroma, causing the pain of angina pectoris. If occluded, an MI occurs (p. 564).

Heart failure is the end result of a variety of conditions, not all of them cardiovascular. Basically, the heart is unable to meet the circulatory needs of the body. In right heart failure, dependent oedema and venous engorgement are prominent. In left heart failure, breathlessness is the principal sign. The two often coexist. There is an ever-present risk of precipitating heart failure, even in treated patients, by ↑ the demands on the heart, e.g. by fluid overload or excessive exertion.

Hypovolaemic shock is collapse of the peripheral circulation due to a sudden ↓ in the circulating volume. If this is not corrected there can be failure of perfusion of the vital organs, resulting in heart failure, renal failure, and unconsciousness ending in death.

Murmurs are disturbances of blood flow which are audible through a stethoscope. They may be functional or signify structural disorders of the heart. Echocardiography will differentiate. They are of great relevance to dentists as their presence warns of the potential for colonization of damaged valves by blood-borne bacteria. Such a bacteraemia is often caused by dental procedures. Instrumentation liable to do this should be covered by antibiotic prophylaxis (p. 598). Colonization of the valves may lead to a potentially fatal illness: IE.

Dental implications

IE prophylaxis as above. Patients with a PMH of rheumatic fever are very likely to have some damage to a heart valve, usually the mitral valve. They should receive antibiotic prophylaxis unless valvular damage is excluded by a cardiologist. The risk of precipitating heart failure or MI in patients with compromised cardiovascular systems is ever-present. Prevent by avoiding GA, especially within 6 months of an MI, using adequate LA with sedation if necessary, and avoid excessive adrenaline loads. Consider potential drug interactions (p. 634) and remember some of these patients will be anticoagulated.

Exclusion of septic foci may be requested in patients at high risk from bacteraemia, e.g. heart transplant recipients, those with prosthetic valves or valvular damage, or those with a history of IE. It is prudent to err on the side of caution with these individuals and some will need dental clearances.

Respiratory disease

Disease of the chest is an everyday problem in developed countries. The principal symptoms are cough, which may or may not be productive of sputum, dyspnoea (breathlessness), and wheeze. The coughing of blood (haemoptysis) mandates that malignancy be excluded.

Clinical conditions

Upper respiratory tract infections Include the common cold, sinusitis, and pharyngitis/tonsillitis (which may be viral or bacterial), laryngotracheitis, and acute epiglottitis. *All* are C/I to elective general anaesthesia in the acute phase. Sinusitis (p. 422). Penicillin is the drug of choice for a strepto-coccal sore throat. Avoid amoxicillin and ampicillin, as glandular fever may mimic this condition and these drugs will produce a rash, of varying severity, in such a patient. Epiglottitis is an emergency, and the larynx should NEVER be examined unless expert facilities for emergency intubation are to hand.

Lower respiratory tract infections Both viral and bacterial lower tract infections are debilitating and constitute a C/I to GA for elective surgery. Bear in mind TB and atypical bacteria, e.g. legionella, mycoplasma, and coxiella. Open TB is highly infectious and cross-infection precautions are mandatory (p. 748).

Chronic obstructive pulmonary disease (COPD) A very common condition usually caused by a combination of bronchitis (excessive mucus produc-tion, persistent productive cough >3 months per year for 3 yrs) and emphysema (dilation and destruction of air spaces distal to the terminal bronchioles). Smoking is the prime cause and must be stopped for Rx to be of any value. Be aware of possible systemic steroid use.

Asthma Reversible bronchoconstriction causes wheezing and dyspnoea. Up to 8% of the population are affected; there is often an allergic compo-nent. Patients complain of the chest feeling tight. May be precipitated by NSAIDs. Penicillin and aspirin allergies are more common. Management of acute asthma, p. 578.

Cystic fibrosis An inherited disorder whereby viscosity of mucus is ↑. Patients suffer pancreatic exocrine insufficiency and recurrent chest infec-tions. Δ: by history and sweat sodium measurement.

Bronchial carcinoma Causes 27% of cancer deaths. Principal cause is smoking. ↑ incidence in females. Symptoms are persistent cough, haemo-ptysis, and recurrent infections. 2 yr survival is only 10%. Mesothelioma is an industrial disease caused by asbestos exposure.

Sarcoidosis Most commonly presents as hilar lymphadenopathy in young adults. Oral lesions can occur. Erythema nodosum common.

Dental implications

Avoid GA. Use analgesics and sedatives with caution; opioids and sedatives ↓ respiratory drive, NSAIDs may exacerbate asthma. Advise your patients to stop smoking (and if you are a smoker, stop). Refer if suspicious, especially in the presence of confirmed haemoptysis.

Gastrointestinal disease

The mouth and its mucosal disorders and disorders of the salivary glands are covered in Chapter 9.

Oesophagus Presents symptoms which can be confused with those originating from the mouth, the most important being *dysphagia*. Difficulty in swallowing may be caused by conditions within the mouth (e.g. ulceration), pharynx (e.g. FB), benign or malignant conditions within oesophagus, compression by surrounding structures (e.g. mediastinal lymph nodes), or neurological causes. It is a symptom which should be taken seriously and investigated by at least CXR, barium swallow, &/or endoscopy. Reflux oesophagitis is a common cause of dyspepsia, sore throat, cough, and bad taste.

Peptic ulceration and gastric carcinoma (duodenal malignancy rare)   May present with epigastric pain, vomiting, haematemesis, or melaena.

Peptic ulceration   Commonly due to infection with *Helicobacter pylori* and usually responds to *H. pylori* eradication therapy (combination of proton pump inhibitor/broad spectrum antibiotic/anaerobicidal, i.e. metronidazole). Other causes include stress ulceration in critically ill or major surgical patients, and elderly people on NSAIDs. Prophylaxis with sucralfate, a mucosal protectant, is more appropriate than H2 antagonists as the gastric pH barrier is maintained. Symptomatic relief of dyspepsia without significant ulceration is with antacids and alginates. Persisting epigastric pain or other symptoms *must* be investigated as gastric carcinoma requires early surgery and carries a poor prognosis. => Endoscopic investigation of patients > 40 with persisting epigastric symptoms is mandatory.

Non-malignant, *Helicobacter*-negative ulceration (oesophagitis, gastritis, duodenitis) clears with 1 month of proton pump inhibitor Rx (e.g. omeprazole 10–20 mg od) and can often be maintained with H2 antagonists (ranitidine or cimetidine).

Small bowel   This has a multitude of associated disorders which tend to present in a similar manner; namely, malabsorption syndromes, diarrhoea, steatorrhoea, abdominal pain, anaemia, and chronic deficiencies. Coeliac disease and Crohn's disease are the best known conditions. Coeliac disease is a hypersensitivity response of the small bowel to gluten and treated by strict avoidance. A number of oral complaints are related, typically 'cobblestoning' of the mucosa. Crohn's disease may affect any part of the gastrointestinal tract but has a preference for the ileo-caecal area. It is a chronic granulomatous disease affecting the full thickness of the mucosa and may result in fistula formation. Ulcerative colitis is often mistaken for Crohn's disease initially, but affects the colorectum only. Treatment with systemic steroids and other immunosuppresants is common.

Large bowel   Diverticular disease is a condition with multiple outpouching of large bowel mucosa which can become inflamed, causing diverticulitis. The irritable bowel syndrome is a condition associated with ↑ colonic tone, causing recurrent abdominal pain; there may be some psychogenic overlay.

Colonic cancer is common in older patients; it may present as rectal bleeding, a change in bowel habit, intestinal obstruction, tenesmus (wanting to defecate but producing nothing), abdominal pain, or anaemia. It is treated surgically, with up to 90% 5 yr survival if diagnosed early (Duke's A). Familial polyposis coli is associated with the Gardener syndrome (p. 758). Antibiotic-induced colitis results from overgrowth of toxigenic *Clostridium difficile* after use of antibiotics, commonly ampicillin and clindamycin. It responds to *oral* vancomycin or metronidazole.

The pancreas   Malignancy has the worst prognosis of any cancer and most Rx is essentially palliative.

    Acute pancreatitis   Often a manifestation of alcohol abuse. Aetiology is not entirely clear. Causes acute abdominal pain. Amylase levels are a guide but not infallible. Patients need aggressive rehydration, maintenance of electrolyte balance, and analgesia, in high-dependency or ICU setting.

Hepatic disease

The main problems presented by patients with liver disease are: the potential for increased bleeding, inability to metabolize and excrete many commonly used drugs, and the possibility that they can transmit hepatitis B, C &/or D (Hep A and E are spread by faecal–oral route). The liver is also a site of metastatic spread of malignant tumours. Patients in liver failure needing surgery, especially under GA, are a high-risk group who should have specialist advice on their management.

Jaundice The prime symptom of liver disease. It is a widespread yellow discoloration of the skin (best seen in good light, in the sclera), caused by the inability of the liver to process bilirubin, the breakdown product of haemoglobin. This occurs either because it is presented with an over-whelming amount of bilirubin to conjugate (e.g. haemolytic anaemia), or it is unable to excrete bile (cholestatic jaundice). Cholestatic jaundice in turn may be either intrahepatic or extrahepatic. **Intrahepatic cholestasis** represents hepatocyte damage; this is reflected by ↑ aspartate transaminase levels on liver function tests, and results in impaired bile excretion, as indicated by ↑ plasma bilirubin. Causes include alcohol and other drugs, toxins, bacterial and viral infections. A degree of hepatitis is present with these causes, whereas primary biliary cirrhosis and anabolic steroids cause a specific intrahepatic cholestasis without hepatitis. **Extrahepatic cholestasis** is caused by obstruction to the excretion of bile in the common bile duct by gallstones, tumour, clot, or stricture. Carcinoma of the head of the pancreas, or adjacent lymph nodes, may also compress the duct, and must be excluded.

Surgery in patients with liver disease
- Ascertain a Δ for the cause. Do hepatitis serology. Cross-infection precautions (p. 748).
- Do coagulation screen. May need correction with vitamin K or fresh-frozen plasma.
- **Always** warn the anaesthetist, as it will affect the choice of anaesthetic agents.
- If a jaundiced patient must undergo surgery correct fluid and electrolyte balance, and ensure a good peri-operative urine output by aggressive IV hydration with 5% dextrose and mannitol diuresis to avoid hepato-renal syndrome (see OHCM).
- Do not use IV saline in patients in fulminant hepatic failure, as there is a high risk of inducing encephalopathy.

Liver disease patients in dental practice
- Know which disease you are dealing with. If Hep B or C employ strict cross-infection control (p. 748).
- Be cautious in prescribing drugs (consult the BNF/DPF) and with administering LA.
- **Do not** administer GAs.
- Take additional local precautions against post-op bleeding following simple extractions (p. 390). A clotting screen should be obtained for anything more advanced, and in all patients with severe liver disease.

Renal disorders

The commonest urinary tract problems, infections, are of relevance only to those who manage in-patients. Rarer conditions such as renal failure and transplantation are, surprisingly, of more general relevance because these patients are at ↑ risk from infection, bleeding, and iatrogenic drug overdose during routine Rx.

Urine This is tested in all in-patients. 'Multistix' will test for glycosuria (diabetes, pregnancy, infection), proteinuria (diabetes, infection, nephrotic syndrome), ketones (diabetic ketoacidosis), haematuria (infection, tumour), and bile as bilirubin and urobilinogen (cholestatic jaundice).

Urinary tract infections A common cause of toxic confusion in elderly in-patients, especially females. Send a mid-stream urine (MSU) for culture and sensitivity, then start trimethoprim 200 mg bd PO or ampicillin 250 mg qds PO and ensure a high fluid intake. Minimal investigations of renal function are U&Es, creatinine, and ionized Ca^{2+}.

Nephrotic syndrome A syndrome of proteinuria (>3.6 g/day), hypoalbuminaemia, and generalized oedema. Facial oedema is often prominent. Glomerulonephritis is the major precipitating cause and investigations should be carried out by a physician with an interest in renal medicine.

Acute renal failure (ARF) A medical emergency causing a rapid rise in serum creatinine, urea and K^+. It may follow surgery or major trauma and is usually marked by a failure to PU. *Remember* the commonest causes of failing to PU post-op are under-infusion of fluids and urinary retention. Rx: ↑ IV fluid input and catheterize (p. 592). If ARF is suspected get urgent U&Es, ECG, and blood gases. Obtain aid from a physician. Control of hyperkalaemia, fluid balance, acidosis, and hypertension are the immediate necessities.

Chronic renal failure Basically the onset of uraemia after gradual, but progressive renal damage, commonly caused by glomerulonephritis (inflammation of the glomeruli following immune complex deposits), pyelonephritis (small scarred kidneys due to childhood infection, irradiation, or poisoning), or adult polycystic disease (congenital cysts within Bowman's capsule). It has protean manifestations, starting with nocturia and anorexia, progressing through hypertension and anaemia to multi-system failure. Continuous ambulatory peritoneal dialysis, haemodialysis, and transplants are the mainstays of Rx.

Main problems relevant to dentistry
- ↑ risk of infection, worsened by immunosuppression.
- ↑ bleeding tendency.
- ↓ ability to excrete drugs.
- Veins are sacrosanct; **never** use their A-V fistula.
- Bone lesions of the jaws (renal osteodystophy, 2° hyperparathyroidism).
- Generalized growth impairment in children.
- Potential carriage of Hep B, HIV.

Renal transplantation An increasingly common final Rx of renal failure, and when successful renal function may reach near normal levels. Kidneys are, however, immunosuppressed and at greatly ↑ risk from infection.

They may share the problems associated with chronic renal failure depending on the level of function of the transplant.

Hints

- Take precautions against cross-infection (p. 748).
- Treat all infections aggressively and consider prophylaxis.
- Use additional haemostatic measures (p. 390).
- Be cautious with prescribing drugs (p. 610).
- Never subject these patients to out patient GA.
- Remember veins are precious.
- Try to perform Rx just after dialysis if possible.

Endocrine disease

Addison's disease   1° hypoadrenocorticism. Atrophy of the adrenal cortices causes failure of cortisol and aldosterone secretion. 2° hypoadrenocorticism is far commoner, due to steroid therapy or ACTH deficiency (p. 602). All need steroid cover.

Conn syndrome   Primary hyperaldosteronism causes hypokalaemia and hypernatraemia with hypertension.

Cushing's disease and Cushing syndrome   These are due to excess corticosteroid production. The disease refers to 2° adrenal hyperplasia due to ↑ ACTH, whereas the syndrome is a 1° condition, usually due to therapeutic administration of synthetic steroid or adenoma. Classical features are obesity (moon face, buffalo hump) sparing the limbs, osteoporosis, skin thinning, and hypertension.

Diabetes insipidus   Production of copious dilute urine due to ↓ ADH secretion or renal insensitivity to ADH. May occur temporarily after head injury.

Diabetes mellitus   Persistent hyperglycaemia due to a relative deficiency of insulin (p. 576).

Gigantism/acromegaly   Excess production of growth hormone, before and after fusion of the epiphyses, respectively.

Goitre   A large thyroid gland, of whatever cause.

Hyperthyroidism   Symptoms of heat intolerance, weight loss, and sweating occur. Signs are tachycardia (may have atrial fibrillation), lid lag, exopthalmos, and tremor. Commonest cause is Graves' disease (p. 758). Functioning adenomas are another cause.

Hypothyroidism   Can be 1° due to thyroid disease, or 2° to hypothalamic or pituitary dysfunction. 1° disease is often an autoimmune condition. Symptoms are poor tolerance of cold, loss of hair, weight gain, loss of appetite, and poor memory. Signs are bradycardia and a hoarse voice.

Hyperparathyroidism   1° is caused by an adenoma. 2° is a response to low plasma Ca^{2+}, e.g. in renal failure, and 3° follows on from 2° when the parathyroids continue ↑ production, even if Ca^{2+} is normalized.

Hypoparathyroidism   Usually 2° to thyroidectomy, when parathyroid glands inadvertently removed. Plasma Ca^{2+} ↓, resulting in tetany. Chvosteck's sign is +ve if spasm of facial muscles occurs after tapping over the facial nerve.

Hypopituitarism   Can lead to 2° hypothyroidism or 2° hypoadrenocorticism.

Inappropriate ADH secretion   Caused by certain tumours (e.g. bronchial carcinoma), head injury, and some drugs. Hyponatraemia, overhydration, and confusion occur.

Lingual thyroid   May be the only functioning thyroid the patient has; do not excise lightly. Do pre-op isotope scan.

Phaeochromocytoma   A very rare tumour of the adrenal medulla, secreting adrenaline and noradrenaline. Symptoms are recurring palpitations and headache with sweating. Simultaneous hypertension with a return to baseline on settling of symptoms, is a good marker.

Pituitary tumours   May erode the pituitary fossa (seen on lateral skull X-ray) and can cause blindness via optic chiasma compression.

Endocrine-related problems

▶ Always ask yourself 'Is she, or can she be, pregnant?'

Pregnancy A C/I to elective GA, the vast majority of drugs (p. 610), and non-essential radiography (the most vulnerable period being in the first 3 months). Elective Rx is best performed in the mid-trimester.

Menopause The end of a woman's reproductive life and her periods. It is often associated with hot flushes and other relatively minor physical problems. Emotional disturbances may coexist, and the incidence of psychiatric disorders increases at this time.

Related problems

Suxamethonium sensitivity Around 1:3000 people have an inherited defect of plasma cholinesterase. These families are absolutely normal in every respect except in their ability to metabolize suxamethonium. This leaves them unable to destroy the drug which, normally wearing off in 2–4 min, produces prolonged muscle paralysis. This paralysis requires ventilatory support until the drug wears off, which, in the homozygote, may take as long as 24 h.

Malignant hyperpyrexia A rare, potentially lethal reaction to, usually, an anaesthetic agent. Characterized by ↑ pulse, muscle rigidity, and ↑ temperature. Dantrolene sodium and cooling may be life-saving.

Rare endocrine tumours

Glucagonoma Secretes glucagon causing hyperglycaemia.

Insulinomas Secrete insulin. Causes sporadic hypoglycaemic episodes.

Gastrinomas Secrete gastrin causing duodenal ulcers and diarrhoea (Zollinger–Ellison syndrome).

Multiple endocrine neoplasia (MEN) syndromes A rare group of endocrine tumours. MEN IIb is medullary thyroid cancer, phaeochromocytoma, and oral mucosal neuromas.

Bone disease

Pathology of the bones of the facial skeleton is covered in Chapter 8.

Osteogenesis imperfecta (brittle bone disease) An autosomal dominant type 1 collagen defect. Multiple # following slight trauma with rapid but distorted healing is characteristic. Associated with blue sclera, deafness, and dentinogenesis imperfecta (p. 73). The jaws are *not* particularly prone to # following extractions.

Osteopetrosis (marble bone disease) There is an ↑ in bone density and brittleness, and a ↓ in blood supply. Prone to infection which is difficult to eradicate. Bone pain, #, and compression neuropathies may occur. Anaemia can complicate severe disease. Facial characteristics are frontal bossing and hypertelorism.

Achondroplasia An inherited defect in cartilaginous bone formation, usually autosomal dominant. Causes a 'circus dwarf' appearance with skull bossing; many have no other problems.

Cleidocranial dysostosis An inherited defect of membraneous bone formation, usually autosomal dominant. Skull and clavicles are affected. Multiple unerupted teeth with retention of 1° dentition is characteristic.

Disorders of bone metabolism

Rickets/osteomalacia Failure of bone mineralization in, respectively, children and adults. Can be caused by deficiency, failure of synthesis, malabsorption, or impaired metabolism of Vitamin D, and also hypophosphataemia or ↑ Ca^{2+} requirement in pregnancy.

Osteoporosis A lack of both bone matrix and mineralization. Important causes are steroid therapy, post-menopausal hormone changes, immobilization, and endocrine abnormalities. HRT in post-menopausal women appears helpful. Results in ↑ incidence of #, especially femoral neck and wrist.

Fibrous dysplasia Replacement of a part of a bone or bones by fibrous tissue with associated swelling. It usually starts in childhood and ceases with completion of skeletal growth. Termed monostotic if one bone is affected, polyostotic if > one bone, and Albright syndrome if associated with precocious puberty and *café au lait* areas of skin hyperpigmentation.

Cherubism A bilateral variant of fibrous dysplasia.

Paget's disease of bone A common disorder of the elderly, where the normal, orderly replacement of bone is disrupted and replaced by a chaotic structure of new bone, causing enlargement and deformity. The hands and feet are spared. Complications include bone pain and cranial nerve compression, or, more rarely, high output cardiac failure or osteosarcoma.

Diseases of connective tissue, muscle, and joints

Connective tissue diseases

These are mainly vasculitidies (inflammation of vessels).

Cranial arteritis (temporal arteritis) Giant cell vasculitis of the craniofacial region. Presenting symptom is unilateral throbbing headache. Signs are high ESR with a tender, pulseless artery. Major complication of temporal arteritis is optic nerve ischaemia causing blindness, so start high-dose steroids (60 mg prednisolone PO od) and monitor using ESR. Biopsy confirms.

Polymyalgia rheumatica More generalized vasculitis affecting proximal axial muscles. Accounts for 25% of cases of cranial arteritis. Responds to steroids; gradual improvement with time.

Disease of muscles

Muscular dystrophy A collection of inherited diseases characterized by muscle degeneration. Most are fatal in early adulthood.

Myotonic disorders Distinguished by delayed muscle relaxation after contraction. They are genetically determined in a complex fashion.

Polymyositis A generalized immune-mediated inflammatory disorder of muscle. If a characteristic rash is present the condition is known as **dermatomyositis** and has an association with occult malignancy.

Joint disease

Osteoarthritis 1° degeneration of articular cartilage, cervical and lumbar spine, hip and knee joints, commonly affected or 2° to trauma or other joint disease, resulting in pain and stiffness. Osteophyte formation and subchondral bone cysts, which collapse leading to deformity, are characteristic. Physiotherapy, weight loss, and analgesia are the mainstays of Rx. Joint replacement is definitive Rx.

Rheumatoid arthritis Immunologically mediated disease where joint pain and damage are the most prominent symptoms. Morning pain and stiffness in the hands and feet, usually symmetrical, is characteristic. There may be systemic upset and anaemia. Ulnar deviation of the fingers is pathognomonic. Rx includes NSAIDs, steroids, and physiotherapy. Second line or disease-modifying antirheumatic drugs (DMARDs) may favourably influence outcome at expense of unwanted effects, e.g. penicillamine, antimalarials, immunosuppressants. Dry eyes and mouth may be associated with rheumatoid arthritis (Sjögren syndrome, p. 458). TMJ symptoms are rare in rheumatoid arthritis, although up to 15% of patients have radiographic changes in the joint.

Juvenile rheumatoid arthritis (Still's disease) Rarer form of the disease affecting children. It can be much more severe than the adult condition and can cause TMJ ankylosis.

Psoriatic arthritis Associated with the skin condition and affects the spine and pelvis. It is milder than rheumatoid arthritis and has no serological abnormalities. The TMJ can be affected, but symptoms are usually mild despite some isolated case reports to the contrary.

Gout   Urates are deposited in joints, causing sudden severe joint pain, often in the great toe. Affected joints are red, swollen, and very tender. Gout 2° to drugs, radiotherapy, or haematological disease is commoner than that caused by an inborne error of metabolism.

Ankylosing spondylitis   Affects the spine, usually in young men. Inflammation involves the insertion of ligaments and tendons. It is associated with HLA-B27. Later, kyphotic deformity and increased risk of cervical fractures.

Reiter syndrome   Seronegative arthritis, urethritis, and conjunctivitis, usually in response to an infection. Oral lesions are often present. Genital and intestinal variants.

Perthes' disease   Osteochondritis of the femoral head in, mainly, boys aged 3–11 yrs. No systemic implications.

Neurological disorders

Cranial nerves

1 **Olfactory** Sense of smell is rarely tested, although damage is quite common following head &/or mid-face trauma.

2 **Optic** Examine the pupils for both direct and consensual reflex; assess the visual fields; check visual acuity and examine the fundus with an opthalmoscope (p. 12).

3 **Oculomotor** The motor supply to the extra-ocular muscles *except* lateral rectus and superior oblique. It supplies the ciliary muscle, the constrictor of the pupil, and levator palpebrae superioris. A defect ∴ causes impairment of upward, downward, and inward movement of the eye, leading to diplopia, drooping of the upper eyelid (ptosis), and absent direct and consensual reflexes.

4 **Trochlear** Supplies superior oblique, paralysis of which causes diplopia; worst on looking downward and inward.

5 **Trigeminal** The major sensory nerve to the face, oral, nasal, conjunctival, and sinus mucosa, and part of the tympanic membrane. It is motor to the muscles of mastication. Sensory abnormalities are mapped out using gentle touch and pin-prick. Motor weakness is best assessed on jaw opening and excursion.

6 **Abducens** Supplies lateral rectus. A defect causes paralysis of abduction of the eye.

7 **Facial** Motor to the muscles of facial expression. Supplies taste from the anterior 2/3 of tongue (via chorda tympani) and is secretomotor to the lacrimal, sublingual, and submandibular glands. It innervates the stapedius muscle in the middle ear. The lower face is innervated by the contralateral motor cortex, whereas the upper face has bilateral innervation. Assess by demonstrating facial movements.

8 **Vestibulocochlear** Is sensory for balance and hearing. Deafness, vertigo, and tinnitus are the main symptoms.

9 **Glossopharyngeal** Supplies sensation and taste from the posterior 1/3 of the tongue, motor to stylopharyngeus, and secretomotor to the parotid. Lesions impair the gag reflex in conjunction with

10 **Vagus** Has a motor input to the palatal, pharyngeal, and laryngeal muscles. Impaired gag reflex, hoarseness, and deviation of the soft palate to the unaffected side are seen if damaged. The vagus has a huge parasympathetic output to the viscera of the thorax and abdomen.

11 **Accessory** Is motor to sternomastoid and trapezius, causing weakness on shoulder shrugging and on turning the head away from the affected side.

12 **Hypoglossal** Motor supply to the tongue. Lesions cause dysarthria (impaired speech) and deviation towards the affected side on protrusion.

Headache

The vast majority of headaches are benign; the secret is to pick out those which are not. Read on.

Tension headache Commonest type. Due to muscle tension in occipitofrontalis. Usually worse as the day progresses; may feel 'band-like'. Responds to reassurance, anxiolytics, and analgesics.

Migraine A distinct entity characterized by a preceding visual aura (fortification spectra). Severe, usually unilateral headache with photophobia, nausea, and vomiting. Thought to be due to cerebral vasoconstriction, followed by reflex vasodilation (the latter is the cause of the pain). 5HT agonists, e.g. rizatripan (C/I: ischaemic heart disease, cerebrovascular disease) abolish an attack if used early, and pizotifen is used prophylactically. F > M, the oral contraceptive being a contributing factor. There are many variants of classical migraine.

Migrainous neuralgia Rarer than migraine and causes localized pain, usually around the eye, with associated nasal stuffiness. M > F. There is a typical time of onset, often in early morning, which recurs for several weeks: 'clustering'. Alcohol is a common precipitant. 5HT agonists to treat and 5HT antagonists (e.g. pizotifen) for prophylaxis.

Raised intracranial pressure A cause of headache demanding urgent further investigation. Pointers are headache, worse on waking, irritation, ↓ level of consciousness, vomiting, sluggish or absent pupillary reflexes, bulging of the optic disc (papilloedema). *Rising BP and slowing pulse* are late premorbid signs of ↑ ICP.

Medication misuse headache Affects up to 1:50. Presents as daily headache due to excessive or regular use of OTC analgesics (especially codeine-containing) and some antimigraine preparations. Pain pathways may be altered and after withdrawal of the drug the headache may be slow to resolve.

Rare and wonderful headaches Ice-cream headache, post-coital headache, needle-through-eye headache, and many other distinctive and benign headaches are described.

More neurological disorders

CNS infections

Bacterial meningitis Must be considered in the differential Δ of headache with photophobia and neck stiffness. Organisms are *Haemophilus influenzae*, *Neisseria meningitidis* (meningococcus), *N. gonorrhoeae*, and *Streptococcus pneumoniae*. In children, the meningococcus is especially important and classically associated with a non-blanching purpuric rash. This is one of the very few indications for instituting immediate blind antibiotic therapy (parenteral penicillin).

Viral meningitis Usually mild and self-limiting. Distinguished from bacterial meningitis by lumbar puncture.

Herpetic encephalitis A rare manifestation of infection with the herpes simplex virus. Can be distinguished from drunkenness or dementia by history and rapid onset. Parenteral aciclovir can be curative.

CNS tumours Most brain tumours are 2° deposits. Although both benign and malignant primary tumours are found, they are rare. Despite this, they are the commonest cause of cancer death in children after leukaemia.

Epilepsy An episodic outflow from the brain causing disturbances of consciousness, motor, and sensory function. Most causes are idiopathic but those with onset in adult life must be investigated for local or general cerebral disease. Major or *grand mal* epilepsy is characterized by an aura and loss of consciousness, and followed by tonic and clonic phases. Incontinence is a good guide to a genuine seizure. The fit rarely lasts > 5 min, if it does the patient has entered status epilepticus (p. 574).

Petit mal (absence attacks) Are epileptic attacks usually confined to children, taking the form of a short absence when movement, speech, and attention cease.

Temporal lobe epilepsy Characterized by hallucinations of the special senses.

Localized (Jacksonian) epilepsy Affects limbs in isolation. Patients with established epilepsy (once any treatable cause has been excluded) must be maintained on adequate levels of antiepileptic drugs.

Febrile convulsions Fits, usually in children > 5 yrs old, 2° to pyrexia.

Cerebrovascular accidents (strokes) A very common cause of death in the elderly. A stroke is basically death of part of the brain following cerebral ischaemia, either due to bleeding into the brain or occlusion of vessels. It is often clinically difficult to distinguish these different types of stroke. CT scanning is of value when Rx is to be attempted to decide if infarct or haemorrhage, but wait 24 h after symptoms to allow infarct to become visible on scan. Cerebral angiography defines the source of subarachnoid bleeds.

Multiple sclerosis A disorder characterized by demyelination in multiple 'plaques' throughout the CNS. Symptoms are multiple and disseminated in both time and place. It is the commonest neurological disease of young adults. MRI helps in Δ but is not specific. No current cure; hyperbaric therapy and interferon remain controversial. Progress, although relentless, is widely variable.

Myasthenia gravis   Muscle weakness due to inadequate response to, or levels of, acetylcholine. Extra-occular muscles are often first affected. Diagnosed using the 'tensilon' test.

Parkinson's disease   A disease affecting the basal ganglia associated with a ↓ in the local levels of dopamine. Characterized by a 'pill-rolling' tremor, 'cog-wheel' rigidity, and bradykinesis with a shuffling gait.

Skin neoplasms

▶ The skin of the face is the commonest site of curable skin cancers, so look and think (p. 514).

BCC (epithelioma, rodent ulcer) An indolent skin cancer which very rarely metastasizes. If it kills it does so by local destruction. Chronic exposure to sunlight is a major aetiological factor. There are various forms, the commonest being an ulcerated nodule with raised pearly margins and a telangiectatic surface. Rx: excision (micrographic or conventional), radiotherapy (especially electron beam), cryotherapy, curretage, and electrodessication.

SCC of the skin is surprisingly indolent in comparison to SCC of mucosa. Presents as an ulcerated lesion with raised edges. Keratin horns may be present, and it may arise in areas of previously sun-damaged skin or in gravitational leg ulcers. Surgical excision or radiotherapy are Rx of choice.

Malignant melanoma This condition is being increasingly diagnosed, with a doubling of the incidence in the last 20 yrs. The prognosis is dependent primarily on the depth of the tumour (Breslow thickness), as the thicker the lesion the poorer the prognosis. Early metastasis is common. Sunlight is a major aetiological factor, possibly due to burning at early age. Suspect if a pigmented lesion rapidly enlarges, bleeds, ulcerates, shows 'satellite' lesions or changes colour. Prompt referral for specialist management is needed.

Naevi Areas of skin containing a disproportionate number of melanocytes.

Lentigo simplex A freckle.

Dysplastic naevi Premalignant lesions often found in patients with malignant melanoma. They should be excised and patients advised to use high-factor sunscreens.

Lentigo maligna A premalignant pigmented lesion of the elderly.

Carcinoma-in-situ (Bowen's disease) Presents as a scaly, red plaque. It is basically a squamous carcinoma which has not yet penetrated beyond the basal layer.

Actinic keratosis Persistently sun-damaged areas of skin in which cancer may arise.

Kaposi's sarcoma A purple, vascular, multifocal malignant tumour typically seen in AIDS and other immunocompromised patients. Also seen intraorally.

Metastatic deposits to the skin occur most frequently from breast, kidney, and lung, but skin secondaries from oral cancer are being seen increasingly.

Dermatology

Psoriasis A common, relapsing proliferative inflammatory skin disease. Appears as a red plaque with silvery scale, chiefly on extensor skin of knees and elbows, although any area can be affected. Can be associated with systemic disease, particularly arthropathy (p. 546). Rx is mainly topical: steroids, coal tar, dithranol &/or UVB radiation, or psoralen-sensitized UVA radiation (PUVA). Rarely, methotrexate can be used.

Eczema Also called dermatitis. Has several variants according to aetiology.

Atopic eczema Starts in the 1st year of life with a red symmetrical scaly rash. Emulsifying ointments help prevent fissuring, although steroids are sometimes needed. Up to 90% grow out of it by age 12.

Exogenous eczema Can be produced in anyone exposed to a sufficient irritant. The hands are the usual target, with blistering, erythema, and cracking of skin.

Allergic contact eczema A genuine allergic response, e.g. to nickel.

Seborrhoeic eczema A fungal infection mainly affecting the scalp ('cradle cap') in neonates.

Skin infections Fungal infections are particularly common, causing angular cheilitis, athlete's foot, paronychia, vaginitis, etc. Furuncles are staphylococcal boils. Erysipelas is a streptococcal cellulitis. Viruses cause herpes zoster and simplex infections, molluscum contagiosum, and warts.

Infestations of the skin brings a shudder to most people, but they are also a hazard of working closely with patients! Head lice respond to malathion. Flea bites, as well as being unpleasant, can spread plague, among other serious diseases. Scabies is an infestation with a mite which creates a characteristic itchy burrow in the finger webs.

Acne Acne vulgaris is characterized by the blackhead (comedone), and is an inflammatory condition caused by increased sebum secretion. Hormone-dependent, although superinfection with the acne bacillus is a contributing factor. Tends to scar. After proprietary lotions, low-dose tetracyclines help. Dianette, a combined oral contraceptive, is a useful alternative in women. The teratogenic retinoid, isoretinoin, is particularly useful in severe and late onset acne unresponsive to other Rx.

The skin and internal disease

The skin, like the mouth, acts as an outside indicator for many internal diseases.

Erythema nodosum Painful, red, nodular lumps on the shins.

Erythema multiforme Circular target lesions.

Erythema marginatum Vanishing and recurring pink rings. These are all non-specific markers for a variety of diseases.

Vitiligo An autoimmune hypopigmentation, associated with other autoimmune conditions.

Pyoderma gangrenosum Blue-edged ulcers, especially on the legs; associated with ulcerative colitis and Crohn's disease.

Granuloma annulare Subcutaneous circular thickening and **necrobiosis lipoidica** (yellow plaques on the shins) are associated with diabetes.

Dermatitis herpetiformis Vesicular rash of knees, elbows, and scalp. Associated with coeliac disease.

Pretibial myxoedema Red swellings above the ankle. Associated with hyperthyroidism.

Skin diseases associated with malignancy are **acanthosis nigricans** (rough, pigmented, thickened areas of skin in axilla or groin) and **thrombophlebitis migrams** (tender nodules within blood vessels which move from site to site).

Psychiatry

One way of getting to grips with a new subject—and to virtually all dentists psychiatry as opposed to psychology is new—is to categorize. The major adult psychiatric diagnoses are listed in order of severity. This is known as the 'hierarchy of diagnosis'.

Organic brain syndromes

Acute organic reaction (delirium, toxic confusion)   Clouding of consciousness and disorientation in time and place are major symptoms. Mood-swings are common, and visual hallucinations, rare in other psychiatric conditions, can be present.

▶ There is an underlying, frequently treatable cause to this condition (infection, hypoxia, drugs, dehydration, alcohol withdrawal, etc.). Rx: find the cause and correct it, using sedation until the cause is identified and Rx has taken effect.

Chronic organic reaction (dementia)   A global intellectual deterioration highlighted by a worsening short-term memory. *Never* label someone as demented until all other possible causes, including depression, have been excluded by a psychiatrist. Alzheimer's disease and multi-infarct dementia are the commonest causes. There is no cure, although effective support services can improve the quality of life considerably. Anticholinesterase inhibitors, e.g. donepezil, may slow the rate of cognitive decline.

Mental disabilities, p. 52.

Psychosis

Contact with reality is lost and normal mental processes do not function. There is loss of insight. If an organic condition is excluded, the Δ is one of three.

Schizophrenia   A disorder where the victims live in an incomprehensible world full of vivid personal significance. First-rank symptoms are a good guide to Δ: delusions, thought insertion, broadcasting and withdrawal, passivity feelings, visual and auditory hallucinations.

Affective disorders   Mania, hypomania, manic-depressive psychosis, and depression. Mania and hypomania are characterized by euphoria, hyper-activity, overvalued ideas or grandiose delusions, and pressure of speech. They differ only in degree. Cyclical mania and depression is known as bipolar affective disorder. Rx is with major tranquillizers and prophylaxis with lithium carbonate.

Depression   May be either psychotic or neurotic. Markers of major depressive illness are anhedonia (failure to find pleasure in things which once did please), anorexia, especially with weight loss, early morning wakening, tearfulness, inability to concentrate, feelings of guilt and worth-lessness, and suicidal ideation.

Paranoid states   are psychoses where paranoid symptoms predominate and, despite lack of insight, other diagnoses do not apply.

▶ The commonly abused drugs can all mimic or precipitate psychotic states, as can giving birth—puerperal psychosis.

Neuroses

A neurosis is a maladaptive psychological symptom in the absence of organic or psychotic causes of the symptom and after exclusion of a psychopathic personality. Insight is present.

Anxiety neurosis frequently coexists with depression. These patients often have physical symptoms for which there is no physical explanation.

Obsessional neurosis Intrusive thoughts or ideas which the subject recognizes as coming from within themselves, but resents and is unable to stop. May be associated with *compulsive behaviour* where repeated purposeless activity is carried out due to an inexplicable feeling that it must be done.

Phobia is the generation of fear or anxiety out of proportion to the stimulus. Numerous stimuli exist, including dentists.

Anorexia nervosa/bulimia nervosa

The development of weight reduction as an overvalued idea. Associated with weight ↓ of > 25% of ideal body weight and obsessive food avoidance. Commonest in females, it is also associated with amenorrhea. Has a significant mortality rate; binge-eating followed by vomiting &/or laxative abuse can occur. Bingeing without weight loss is bulimia nervosa. Dental effects, p. 310.

Personality disorders

These are not illnesses but extremes of normal personality traits, e.g. obsessional, histrionic, schizoid (cold, introspective). The most important is the psychopathic (sociopathic) individual who has no concept of affection, shame, or guilt, and is characterized by antisocial behaviour. They are often superficially personable, highly manipulative, and totally irresponsible. They have insight and are responsible for their own actions (bad not mad).

The immunocompromised patient

There are a group of individuals who present special problems because of defects in, or suppression of, their immune system. The condition with the highest profile among these is AIDS.

The chief effect of being immunocompromised is an ↑ susceptibility to infection, often due to opportunistic organisms. Anything which changes the host environment in favour of opportunistic pathogens (e.g. surgery, broad-spectrum antibiotics) can lead to potentially fatal infection with rare or otherwise innocuous organisms.

Drugs which suppress the immune response: corticosteroids, cyclosporin A, azathioprin, cytotoxics, etc., are now in common use therapeutically. Cross-infection, p. 748. Aggressive Rx of infections and antimicrobial prophylaxis are needed, p. 598.

Congenital immunodeficiency states There are at least 18 of these. The commonest is selective IgA deficiency, which affects ~1:600; it has a wide spectrum of severity but may remain asymptomatic.

Acquired immunodeficiency

Autoimmune disease, e.g. SLE, rheumatoid arthritis, carry a minor ↑ risk of infection.

Chronic renal failure (p. 538)   Moderately ↑ risk.

Deficiency states, e.g. anaemia. Carry a minor ↑ risk.

Diabetes mellitus is common and carries a moderate ↑ risk of infection.

Infections Severe viral infections, TB, AIDS (specific defect).

Neoplasia All haematological malignancies severely ↑ risk of infection.

AIDS

An increasingly common disease caused by the HIV (HIV-1, HIV-2). CD4 T lymphocyte defect ensues with failure of (mostly) cell-mediated immunity. Although HIV exposure produces antibody response, the virus remains infective in the presence of antibody; it must ∴ be regarded as a marker of infectivity. Absence of HIV antibody *does not*, however, guarantee that that person is not infected with HIV. HIV antibody +ve patients are at risk of developing AIDS, usually after a prolonged latent period during which CD4 cells ↓ in number. AIDS-related complex, which includes cervical lymphadenopathy, oropharyngeal candidiasis, and 'hairy leukoplakia', is precursor to full-blown AIDS. Infections characteristic of AIDS are *Pneumocystis carinii* pneumonia and disseminated mycobacterial infection. Kaposi's sarcoma is the tumour most often associated with the condition. The mode of transmission, for those visiting from another planet, is (traumatic) anal or vaginal sex, or as a recipient of contaminated blood or blood products, or mother to fetus transmission. The main risk groups, in the developed world, are ∴ male homosexuals (although transmission through the heterosexual population is ↑), IV drug abusers. Transfusion recipients and haemophiliacs, who were at risk prior to screening of blood products, now have a minimal risk.

In the developing world, heterosexual spread is common and mother to fetus transmission is creating a huge ↑ in HIV +ve children. Antenatal testing for HIV is crucial as is avoiding breast-feeding. Zidovudine (AZT) therapy and delivery by Caesarean section dramatically ↓ vertical transmission.[1] While there is no cure or vaccination, numerous symptom-reducing and life-prolonging Rx are available, with mixed results. Combination therapy, especially triple therapy including a protease inhibitor, can prolong survival and delay disease progression.[2] Psychological and social support are the most helpful options after preventive advice. Prophylaxis consists of screening blood products, and avoidance of unprotected sexual activities and shared needles. Oral manifestations of AIDS, p. 476. Practical procedures for control of cross-infection, p. 748.

Prophylaxis after needlestick injury   depends on estimation of the likely HIV exposure risk. Triple therapy guidelines in the USA. Local implementation via G-U consultant in UK.

1 Editor *BMJ* 1998 **316**.
2 *Drugs and Therapeutics Bulletin*, 1997 **35** 28.

Useful emergency kit

Every practice should possess apparatus for delivering O_2, or at least air. In addition, the facility to deliver nitrous oxide and O_2 mixture, e.g. via an anaesthetic or relative analgesia machine, can be invaluable.

The following should be readily available:

- Oral airway, preferably with a bag system, e.g. ambu-bag.
- High-vacuum suction.
- Disposable syringes (2, 5, and 10 ml), needles (19 and 21 G), and a tourniquet. Butterfly needles and IV canulae are great assets to those familiar with their use.
- Alcohol wipes.

Drugs

- Adrenalin, 1:1000 solution (1 mg adrenalin in 1 ml saline).
- Hydrocortisone (as sodium succinate or sodium phosphate) (100 mg and water for injection).
- Benzodiazepine, lorazepam (4 mg ampoules), or midazolam (10 mg ampoules).
- Glucose, as dextrose 20% or 50% solution and an oral glucose solution.
- Chlorpheniramine 20 mg injection.
- Flumazenil 100 >g/ml 5 ml ampoule.
- Glucagon 1 mg injection.

The above *really* is a minimum for any professional performing invasive Rx. Ideally, all public areas, let alone dental practices, should have access to an automatic defibrillator as this is the most valuable single piece of equipment in a cardiac arrest (p. 570). Additional useful equipment include Clinistix/"BM" sticks, glyceryl trinitrate spray, salbutamol inhaler, one-way valve face mask, glucagon 1 mg **IM** injection, atropine 3 mg single-shot injection, IV fluids (crystalloid is cheaper and can be warmed). In hospital, check your 'crash cart' and be amazed at its contents.

▶ If you buy something learn how to use it!

Fainting

Fainting (vaso-vagal syncope) is innocuous providing it is recognized. It is easily the most common cause of sudden loss of consciousness, with up to 2% of patients fainting before or during dental Rx. The possibility of vaso vagal syncope while under GA, and hence failure to recognize the condition and correct cerebral hypoxia, is the major reason for recommending the supine position.

Predisposing factors are pain, anxiety, fatigue, relative hyperthermia, and fasting. Characteristic signs and symptoms are: a feeling of dizziness and nausea; pale, cold, and clammy skin; a slow, thin, thready pulse which rebounds to become rapid, and loss of consciousness with collapse, if unsupported.

A faint may mimic far more serious conditions, most of which can be excluded by a familiarity with the patient's PMH. These include strokes, corticosteroid insufficiency, drug reactions and interactions, epileptic fit, heart block, hypoglycaemia, and MI.

Prevention
- Avoid predisposing factors.
- Treat patients in the supine position unless specifically contraindicated (e.g. heart failure, pulmonary oedema).

Management
- Lower the head to the level of, or below, the heart. Best achieved by laying the patient flat with legs slightly elevated.
- Loosen clothing (in the presence of a witness!).
- Monitor pulse. If recovery does not occur rapidly, then reconsider the Δ.
- Determine the precipitant and avoid in the future.
- If bradycardia persists with no evidence of recovery to rapid full pulse, try tiny dose of atropine (100 µg IV). Dose may be repeated up to 600 µg.

Acute chest pain

Severe, acute chest pain is usually the result of ischaemia of the myocardium. The principal differential Δ is between angina and MI. Both exhibit severe retrosternal pain described as heavy, crushing, or band-like. It is classically preceded by effort, emotion, or excitement, and may rediate to the arms, neck, jaw, and, occasionally, the back or abdomen. Angina is usually rapidly relieved by rest and glyceryl trinitrate (0.5 mg) given sublingually, or GTN spray (400 µg per spray), which most patients with a history of angina carry with them.

Failure of these methods to relieve the pain, and coexisting sweating, breathlessness, nausea, vomiting, or loss of consciousness with a weak or irregular pulse, suggest an infarct.

Management depends on your immediate environment, but always ensure the patient is placed in a supported *upright* position if conscious, as the supine position increases pulmonary oedema and hence breathlessness.

Management

In dental practice   Summon help (ambulance). Administer analgesia; the most appropriate form available here will be nitrous oxide/O_2 mixture (50% O_2). Don't panic. Be prepared should cardiac arrest supervene. Give aspirin 150–300 mg PO. Tell ambulance staff what you have done.

In hospital   Nurse upright. Give O_2. Establish IV access and give an opioid analgesic if available (2.5–5 mg of diamorphine is most useful). Get ECG, U&Es. Summon help; in units integrated into general or teaching hospitals this may best be achieved by contacting the medical on-call team via the switchboard urgently, as thrombolysis, if appropriate improves outcome.

Cardiorespiratory arrest

▶ Don't await 'expertise'. **ACT**.

Ninety percent of deaths from cardiac arrest occurring outside hospital are due to ventricular fibrillation (VF). This is also the commonest arrest pattern seen in hospital. It is potentially reversible by prompt (<90 sec) defibrillation. The commonest underlying cause is ischaemic heart disease but other causes may exist, especially in younger people. Acute asthma, anaesthesia, drug overdose, electrocution, immersion, or hypothermia often precipitate pulseless electrical activity (PEA) arrests. These are treatable conditions and potentially reversible.

In certain instances properly performed cardiopulmonary resuscitation (CPR) can sustain life for up to an hour while a precipitating condition is being treated.

Diagnosis and management These proceed simultaneously.

Approach and assess Protect yourself! Do not become another casualty, whether in the street, practice, or hospital environment. Gently 'shake and shout' to assess the person's level of consciousness. If there is no response shout for help (and ask whoever goes for help to come back to tell you help is coming). **Then**:

- In *witnessed* or monitored arrests a single sharp blow over the heart (precordial thump) is worthwhile.
- *Airway* Carry out a chin lift or jaw thrust, and clear oropharynx. Remove loose dentures, but retain if they are well fitting (it gives a better mouth seal).
- *Breathing* Look, listen, and feel for breathing for up to 10 sec (if hypothermia suspected, up to 1 min). If the person is breathing, place in recovery position. If not, **Get help, even if this means leaving the patient yourself to do it**. Then give 2 *effective breaths* (chest moves). Make up to 5 attempts to achieve this. After doing this (even if it is unsuccessful) move to:
- *Circulation* Feel for a carotid pulse. If it is present, provide 10 breaths per minute, checking the pulse for 10 sec every 10 breaths. **If no pulse** commence chest compression, at the middle of the lower half of the sternum, depressing 4–5 cm **100** times per minute.
- Remember, statistically the patient's best chance at survival once absence of breathing is confirmed is defibrillation, therefore getting early help may be the most useful thing you can do. Children and victims of trauma or drowning are exceptions and may benefit from 1 min of resuscitation before you leave to get help.

Adult basic life support

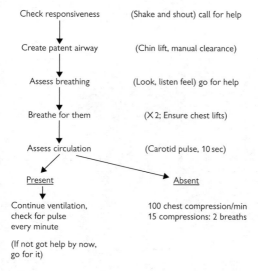

Check responsiveness   (Shake and shout) call for help

Create patent airway   (Chin lift, manual clearance)

Assess breathing   (Look, listen feel) go for help

Breathe for them   (X 2; Ensure chest lifts)

Assess circulation   (Carotid pulse, 10 sec)

<u>Present</u>   <u>Absent</u>

Continue ventilation,   100 chest compression/min
check for pulse   15 compressions: 2 breaths
every minute

(If not got help by now,
go for it)

Rates of compression/ventilation:
- Ventilation only (good cardiac output) 10–15 breaths/min.
- CPR, single and two rescuer: 15 compressions to 2 ventilations.
- Aim for 100 compressions/min.

For those working in an environment where facilities for advanced life support (defibrillation, intubation/ventilation) exist, the 2002 UK Resuscitation Council Guidelines (based on ILCOR advisory statement and support by the European Resuscitation Council) are reproduced.

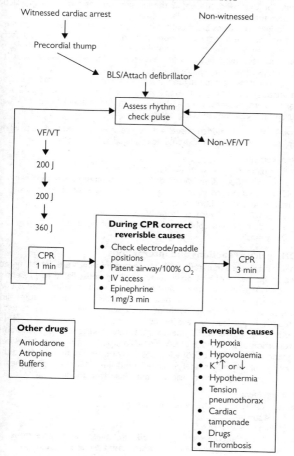

Algorithm for advanced cardiac life support
Resuscitation Council UK ILS Course Manual 2002

Witnessed cardiac arrest

Non-witnessed

Precordial thump

BLS/Attach defibrillator

Assess rhythm
check pulse

Non-VF/VT

VF/VT

200 J

200 J

360 J

CPR
1 min

**During CPR correct
reverisble causes**
- Check electrode/paddle
  positions
- Patent airway/100% O_2
- IV access
- Epinephrine
  1 mg/3 min

CPR
3 min

Other drugs

Amiodarone
Atropine
Buffers

Reversible causes
- Hypoxia
- Hypovolaemia
- $K^+\uparrow$ or $\downarrow$
- Hypothermia
- Tension
  pneumothorax
- Cardiac
  tamponade
- Drugs
- Thrombosis

Anaphylactic shock and other drug reactions

Penicillins are the commonest offender, but it is worth remembering that there is a 10% cross-over in allergic response between penicillins and cephalosporins.

An anaphylactic reaction is not an all-or-nothing response, and grades of severity are seen. Generally, the reaction starts a few minutes after a parenteral injection, and not immediately as does a simple faint. Some caution should be exercised, though, as the quicker the onset of an anaphylactic reaction the more severe it is likely to be.

Principal symptoms are facial flushing, itching, numbness, cold extremities, nausea, and sometimes abdominal pain. Signs include wheezing, facial swelling and rash, and cold clammy skin with a thin thready pulse. Loss of consciousness may occur, with extreme pallor which progresses to cyanosis as respiratory failure develops.

It can be difficult to distinguish anaphylaxis from acute asthma in, e.g., an asthmatic given an NSAID they are allergic to. Don't panic, just go through management for acute asthma, then start on management for anaphylaxis. Adrenaline is a bronchodilator anyway.

Angio-oedema is sudden onset, with severe face and neck allergic swelling. The airway is at risk and ∴ should be managed as for anaphylaxis.

Management
- Place patient supine with legs raised, if possible.
- 0.5 ml of 1:1000 adrenaline IM or SC. Repeat after 15 min, then every 15 min until improved. Do not give IV in this concentration as it will induce ventricular fibrillation.
- Up to 500 mg of hydrocortisone IV.
- Up to 20 mg of chlorpheniramine slowly IV (if available).
- O_2 by mask.

Other drug reactions and interactions

While there are a multitude of drug interactions which the dental surgeon should be aware of as a prescriber, the drugs most liable to present an emergency problem to the dentist are those which we administer as LAs.

Although it is possible to achieve toxic levels of lignocaine, adrenaline, prilocaine, or felypressin without intravascular injection, this generally requires a particularly cavalier attitude to the administration of LA. Commonly, this effect is due to intravascular injection of a substantial proportion of a cartridge of LA. Confusion, peri-oral tingling, drowsiness, agitation, fits, or loss of consciousness may occur. Do not use more than 10×2.2 ml cartridges of lignocaine/adrenaline (440 mg lignocaine). In practice, you will rarely consider coming near this amount.

Management
- Stop procedure! (They won't be numb.)
- Place supine.
- Maintain airway, give O_2.
- Await spontaneous recovery (in ~30 min) unless tragically a serious event such as MI supervenes, in which case treat as indicated.

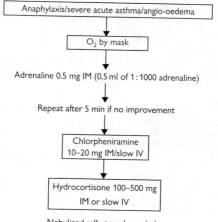

Treatment for anaphylaxis algorithm
Resuscitation Council UK ILS Course Manual 2002

Anaphylaxis/severe acute asthma/angio-oedema

O_2 by mask

Adrenaline 0.5 mg IM (0.5 ml of 1 : 1000 adrenaline)

Repeat after 5 min if no improvement

Chlorpheniramine
10–20 mg IM/slow IV

Hydrocortisone 100–500 mg
IM or slow IV

Nebulized salbutamol may help

IV fluids can supplement anti-shock Rx

In children <12 years reduce drug dose

6–12   0.25 mg adrenaline
        5–10 mg chlorpheniramine   half
        100 mg hydrocortisone

1–6   0.12 mg adrenaline
        5–10 mg chlorpheniramine   half
        100 mg hydrocortisone

<6/12   0.05 mg adrenaline   half again

Collapse in a patient with a history of corticosteroid use

The use of corticosteroids therapeutically or otherwise for whatever cause may suppress the adrenal response to stress. The longer the course of Rx and the higher the dose used the more likely this is to occur.

The prime aim is to prevent the occurrence of stress-induced collapse ∴, if patients have received steroids in the past year or are on steroids at present, cover any stressful procedure, anaesthetic, infection, or episode of trauma with 100 mg hydrocortisone IM 30 min prior to elective stress. It is a fallacy to believe you are ↓ risk of steroid unwanted effects by trying to avoid giving prophylactic steroids. Doubling the oral dose may work but is rather hit and miss. Calculating an 'exact' dose is unnecessarily complicated and risks people 'forgetting'. Stick to sticking them with 100 mg hydrocortisone IM unless you have a very valid reason to change.

In patients presenting acutely, treat immediately. If collapse occurs in such a patient, Δ is established by pallor, rapid, thin pulse with a profound and sudden ↓ in BP, and loss of consciousness.

Management
• Place in supine position. Maintain airway. Give O_2. Obtain IV access.
• Up to 500 mg hydrocortisone IV immediately.
• Ensure help (i.e. an ambulance) is requested.
• Exclude other causes of collapse.

Fits

The majority of epileptic fits do not require active intervention as the patient will usually recover spontaneously. All that is needed is sensible positioning to prevent the patient from damaging himself. Fits may be precipitated in a known epileptic by starvation, flickering lights, certain drugs such as methohexitone, tricyclics or alcohol, or menstruation. They may also follow a deep faint.

Diagnosis Many epileptics have a preceding aura followed by sudden loss of consciousness with a rigid extended appearance and generalized jerking movements. Frequently, they are incontinent of urine and may bite their tongue. There is a slow recovery with the patient feeling sleepy and dazed. There may be a *cause* for the fitting: trauma, tumour, and alcohol withdrawal are common. There are numerous others, any adult should have a first fit fully investigated.

▶ Should the fitting be repeated, the patient has entered the state of status epilepticus. This is an emergency and requires urgent control.

Management In a simple major fit the patient should be placed in the recovery position when practicable and allowed to recover. If they enter status epilepticus, IV lorazepam 4 mg or IV diazepam 10–20 mg (in 5 mg boluses, 2 min between boluses) (preferably as a lipid emulsion—diazemuls) usually aborts the fit; beware respiratory depression. Assess cardiorespiratory function; clear and maintain airway, and give O_2 if available. It is worthwhile considering placing an IV cannula or a butterfly in any epileptic patient with less than perfect control, as stress is an important precipitant. Status epilepticus should not be allowed to continue for more than 20 min as the mortality rate (up to 30%) and chance of permanent brain damage ↑ with the length of attack.

Management in hospital After giving IV benzodiazepines and maintaining an airway, give an IV bolus of up to 50 ml of 20–50% glucose unless certain blood glucose (BM stick) is > 5 mmol/l. Establish a 0.9% saline infusion and repeat the benzodiazepines if necessary. If the fits are not controlled it may be necessary to use a phenytoin infusion or induce anaesthesia with thiopentone, an inhalational agent, and ventilate. Before this stage is reached help should have been requested.

Hypoglycaemia

Hypoglycaemia is the diabetic emergency most likely to present to the dentist. It is an acute and dangerous complication of diabetes and may result from a missed meal, excess insulin, or increased calorific need due to exercise or stress. Most diabetics are expert in detecting the onset of hypoglycaemia themselves; however, a small number may lose this ability, particularly if changed from porcine to human insulin. Recognition of this state is essential and an acutely collapsed diabetic should be assumed hypoglycaemic until proven otherwise, e.g. by "BM" sticks or blood-glucose levels.

Diagnosis Disorientation, irritability, increasing drowsiness, excitability, or aggression in a known diabetic suggest hypoglycaemia. They often appear to be drunk.

Treatment

- If conscious, give glucose orally in any available form.
- If unconscious, protect airway, place in recovery position, establish IV access and give up to 50 ml of 20–50% dextrose. If available, 1 mg of glucagon IM may be used. Ensure help is requested.

Acute asthma

An acute asthmatic attack may be induced in a patient predisposed to bronchospasm by exposure to an allergen, infection, cold, exercise, or anxiety. Characteristically, the patient will complain of a tight chest and shortness of breath. Examination will reveal breathlessness, with wide-spread expiratory wheezing. The accessory muscles of respiration may be used to support breathing. If the patient is unable to talk, you are dealing with a potentially fatal episode.

Management   Make use of the patient's own anti-asthmatic drugs, such as salbutamol inhalers. Ideally, this should be administered in the form of a nebulizer using 24% O_2 and nebulized salbutamol. A do-it-yourself nebulizer can be fabricated from the patient's own inhaler pushed through the base of a paper cup. Repeated depressions of inhaler plunger will create an aerosol inside the cup which the patient can inhale. This will relieve most reversible airways obstruction. Steroids should be administered either as oral prednisolone, if the patient carries these with them, or as IV hydrocortisone up to 200 mg IV. This combination of salbutamol, steroids, and O_2 will often completely resolve an attack; however, in individuals who do not respond, an urgent hospital admission is required. Patients who are only partially responsive must have underlying irritants such as a chest infection either excluded or treated.

▶ Be aware of the possibility of anaphylaxis mimicking acute asthma. Remember adrenaline 0.5 ml 1:1000 SC.

Management in dental practice
- Keep the patient upright.
- Administer salbutamol either by inhaler or by DIY nebulizer.
- Give O_2.
- Give steroids.

If a complete response takes place it is reasonable to allow the patient to return home. If there is any doubt arrange for the patient to be seen at the nearest emergency department.

Management in hospital
- Nurse patient upright.
- Give nebulized salbutamol 5 mg (with O_2) up to 2 hourly.
- Give nebulized ipratropium 500 µg (with O_2).
- Establish IV access and give up to 200 mg hydrocortisone IV or prednisolone 40 mg PO.
- Monitor peak expiratory flow, arterial blood gases, and pulse oximetry.
- Obtain a CXR; exclude infection, pneumothorax.
- If incomplete response, obtain expert help rather than embarking on alternative Rx such as aminophyline.

Inhaled foreign bodies

The combination of delicate instruments and the supine position of patients for many dental procedures inevitably ↑ the risk of a patient inhaling a FB. Two basic scenarios are likely, depending on whether or not the item impacts in the upper or lower airway.

Upper airway   This will stimulate the cough reflex, which may be sufficient to clear the obstruction. A choking subject should be bent forward to aid coughing. If the obstruction is complete or there are signs of cyanosis in:

1 *Conscious patient* Support chest with one hand, strike between the scapulae with the heel of your other hand. Repeat up to 5 times if needed. If this fails carry out abdominal thrusts (Heimlich) by encircling victim with your arms from behind and deliver sharp upward and inward squeeze to create sudden expulsion of air. Repeat up to 5 times. Alternate 5 back blows with the 5 abdominal thrusts.
2 *Unconscious patient* Finger sweep to try to remove foreign body. Abdominal thrusts with victim supine.[1]

If all else fails cricothyroid puncture may preserve life if the obstruction lies above this level.

Lower airway   As only a segment of the lungs will be occluded this presents a less acute problem. It is also easier to miss. Classically, this involves a tooth or tooth fragment slipping from the forceps and being inhaled. With the patient in a semi-upright position the object ends up in the right posterior basal lobe. Should this happen, inform the patient and arrange to have a CXR taken ASAP. If the offending item is in the lungs, removal by a chest physician by fibre-optic bronchoscopy is indicated, as this is inevitably followed by collapse and infection distal to the obstruction. Rarely, lobectomy may be needed. See plate 7.

1 Resuscitation Council (UK) 2002 *Immediate Life Support Course Manual.*

If in doubt

When presented with a suddenly collapsed patient the first thing to assess is your own response. Don't panic.[1] You are only of value to the patient if you can function rationally. If presented with a case of sudden loss of consciousness, in the absence of an obvious Δ, the following steps should be followed.

- **Maintain the airway** and provide O_2 if available.
- **Place in supine position**. If the patient has simply fainted they will recover virtually immediately.
- **Are they breathing?** If not begin artificial respiration, p. 566.
- **Feel for the pulse**. If it is absent, there has been a cardiac arrest (p. 566). If it is present:
- Establish IV access and give up to 20 ml 20–50% dextrose IV.
- Give hydrocortisone up to 200 mg IV.
- If unable to get access, use glucagon 1 mg IM.

These measures will usually resolve most cases of sudden, non-traumatic loss of consciousness.

If the patient is acutely distressed and breathless they should be treated in an upright position and given O_2 while you try to differentiate between an acute asthmatic attack, anaphylaxis, and heart failure, and treat as indicated.

Always ensure that someone has requested assistance in the form of an ambulance or, if in hospital, that the appropriate staff have been contacted. If at all possible, try to speak to the receiving doctor *yourself*.

Immediately after resolution of an emergency there tends to be a period of numb inactivity amongst the staff involved. Use this period to review your management of the situation and carefully document what happened. If the patient has been transferred to hospital or another department a brief, legible account of proceedings must accompany them. Include drugs used, their dosages, and when they were given. Try to ensure that a friend or relation of the patient is aware of the situation.

1 Thank you Douglas Adams!

Management of the dental in-patient

The vast majority of in-patients will experience considerable anxiety on being admitted for operation, including about those procedures which are in themselves 'routine'. In addition, as dentists have little training in medical clerking and ward work, there is a substantial risk of compounding an already stressful situation by being overly stressed yourself. Minimize this by preparation. Learn about the ward(s) you will work on before taking up a post. Never be afraid to ask nursing staff if you are unsure, and try to know a day in advance what cases are coming in.

Pre-operation

All patients attending as in-patients for operation must (a) be examined and 'clerked', and (b) have consented to surgery. In addition, many will require a variety of pre-op investigations; these vary widely from consultant to consultant, so get to know the local variations. Common investigations and their indications are listed below. Sampling techniques, p. 586; samples, p. 16.

(a) Clerking This basically consists of taking a complete medical and dental history from the patient, including any drugs which they are taking at present (which you must remember to continue while in hospital by writing up in the drug 'kardex'), a family history for inherited disease, and a social history for problems related to smoking, alcohol, drug abuse, and ability to cope at home post-op. This is followed by a systematic clinical examination (p. 10). Any special investigations are then arranged, and the results of these should be seen before the patient goes to theatre. Any problems uncovered should be relayed to the anaesthetist, who is the only person capable of saying whether or not the patient is 'fit for anaesthesia'. Any required pre-, peri-, or post-op drugs are written up, p. 610.

(b) Consent All patients undergoing GA or sedation must give written, informed consent. It is advised that patients receiving interventions under LA also do so. Every hospital has its own surgical consent form which you complete. After having the procedure and its likely potential risks explained, the patient also signs. It is essential that you are happy in your own mind that you understand what the operation entails: if in doubt ask your senior. Obtain consent only for procedures with which you are familiar. No one should wake up with scars or a tracheostomy without being previously warned.

Investigations (p. 16)

Full blood count Elderly patients. Any suspicion of anaemia.

Sickle cell test All Afro-Caribbeans for GA. Consider also those of Mediteranean, Arabic, or Indian origin. There may be a local policy but usually not. Ask your anaesthetist.

Urea and electrolytes All patients needing IV fluids, on diuretics, diabetics, or with renal disease. Have a low threshold for doing this test.

Coagulation screen All major surgery, any past history of bleeding disorders, liver disease, or history of ↑ alcohol, anticoagulants.

Liver function tests Liver disease, alcohol, major surgery.

Group and save/cross-match   Major surgery, trauma, shock, anaemia.

ECG   Heart disease, all major surgery, most patients >50.

CXR   Trauma, active chest disease, possible metastases.

Hepatitis B and C, and HIV markers   Varies; usually at-risk groups only; pretest counselling now considered mandatory. Check local hospital policy.

Post-operation

Immediately post-op, patients are resuscitated in a recovery room adjacent to theatre, with a nurse monitoring cardiorespiratory function. Once recovered, unless they are to be monitored in the ICU/HDU they will be returned to the ward. In all patients, ensure a patent airway and consider:

Analgesia   may take the form of LA (should be given post-anaesthetic/ pre-surgery), oral or parenteral NSAIDs, or oral or parenteral opioids. Immediately post-op, analgesia is best given parenterally. Antiemetics such as cyclizine 50 mg oral, IM, or IV, or ondansetron 4 mg IM or IV should be given if nausea or vomiting is present.

Antimicrobials   are given in accordance with the selected regimen (p. 598). Certain patients may benefit from corticosteroids pre- and post-op to ↓ oedema; regimens vary.

Nutrition   is a problem principally for patients undergoing major head and neck cancer surgery (p. 516), but it is worthwhile reminding nursing staff to order soft diets for all oral surgery patients who can feed by mouth and to have liquidizers available for patients in IMF.

Fluid balance   is covered on p. 588. Special consideration needs to be given to patients in IMF and those with tracheostomies. Although the use of immediate post-op IMF is rare it is still required, and post-op elastic IMF is common. These patients need to be specially attended by a nurse looking after that patient only, for the first 12–24 h ('specialed'). Lighting, suction, and the ability to place the patient head-down if they vomit, is mandatory. Other techniques include tongue suture, nasogastic intubation, prolonged retention of a nasopharyngeal airway, elective prolonged intubation, and tracheostomy. Avoiding this situation, see p. 498. Tracheostomy is a great aid to secure airway management, but enormously inconvenient for patients and has its own complications. If indicated it is essential to care for the tube by suction and humidification to ensure patency.

Venepuncture and arterial puncture

Venepuncture   To become proficient in the skills of venepuncture you must practise the art in all its forms. To develop the skill of placing IV cannulae, cultivate a sympathetic anaesthetist, as anaesthetized patients are venodilated and will not feel pain! When carrying out cannulations and arterial punctures on patients in the ward, a drop or two of 2% plain lignocaine deposited SC with a fine needle will aid both your peace of mind and the patient's comfort.

Tools of the trade   Tourniquet, alcohol wipes, cotton wool. Green (21G) needles and butterflies are commonly used. Many hospitals have adopted sealed 'vacutainer' systems which are convenient but fiddly to use. Learn the basics first, then your hospital's system. Sometimes finer needles or butterflies are needed, e.g. blue (23G). Patients who are difficult to cannulate can have fluids and certain drugs through fine (20G) or even 22G IV cannulae; most have 18G. Shocked patients or those needing blood should have at least a 16G and preferably a 14G cannula inserted. Note that gauges and colours are not consistent between needles and cannulae.

Sites of puncture

For sampling   First choice is the cubital fossa. Inspect and palpate; veins you can feel are better than those you can only see. Insert the needle at a 30–40° angle to the skin and along the line of the vein. If no veins are found in the cubital fossa try the back of the hand with a butterfly and use a similar approach. The veins of the dorsum of the foot are a last resort before the femoral vein lying just medial to the femoral artery in the groin.

For infusion   Single bolus injections; use a 21G butterfly in a vein on the back of the hand.

- For IV fluids or multiple IV injections place a 18G IV cannula in a straight segment of vein in the forearm, hand, or just proximal to 'anatomical snuffbox'. Try to avoid crossing a joint as the cannula tissues more quickly if subjected to repeated movements. When inserting the cannula ensure the skin overlying the vein is fixed by finger pressure; pierce the skin, and move the stillete along the line of the vein until it enters the vein and blood flows into the cannula. As soon as you enter the vein, pull the stillete back into the cannula to minimize the risk of going through the vein. Insert the full length of the cannula into the vein and secure. Keep patent with heparinized saline.

Arterial puncture   Whenever possible, obtain an arterial sampling syringe. Use LA unless patient anaesthetized. The syringe and needle must be flushed with heparin. Use radial, brachial, or femoral arteries. Palpate, prepare area with alcohol wipe, and insert needle at 30–60° to skin. When the needle enters the artery, blood pulsates into the syringe. Only 1–2 ml are needed. Remove needle and place in a bag with ice, contact the biochemist, and treat as an urgent specimen. The puncture site needs to be firmly pressed on for 2–3 min to prevent formation of a painful haematoma.

Intravenous fluids

Principles The maintenance of daily fluid requirements plus replacement of any abnormal loss by infusion of (usually) isotonic solutions. Normal requirements are ~2.5–3 l in 24 h. This is lost via urine (normal renal function needs an absolute minimum of 30 ml/h, but aim for 60 ml/h), faecal loss, and sweating. Where possible replace with oral fluids; IV fluids are a second best.

Common IV regimens 1 l normal saline (0.9%) and 2 l 5% dextrose in 24 h, or 3 l dextrose/saline solution in 24 h. Add 20 mmol potassium chloride per litre after 36 h, unless U&Es suggest otherwise. Hartmann's solution is more expensive but most physiological crystalloid (aka Ringer's lactate).

Increase the above in the presence of abnormal losses, burns, fever, dehydration, polyuria, and in the event of haemorrhage or shock.

Special needs
1 For burns, start with Hartmann's and be guided by the Burns Centre.
2 For fever, use saline.
3 For dehydration or polyuria, use 5% dextrose, unless hyponatraemic. Exception is ketoacidosis: use saline.
4 Haemorrhage demands replacement whole blood if available; packed cells are second best, and shock needs blood, crystalloid challenge, and control of haemorrhage. Be guided by the pulse, BP, urine output, haemoglobin, the haematocrit, and the U&Es.

↓ the above in heart failure, and avoid saline. Shock and dehydration are rare complications of maxillofacial trauma or any other condition principally presenting to the dentist; ∴ in their presence consider damage to other body systems and seek appropriate advice.

Polyuria Post-op, is usually due to over-transfusion. Review anaesthetic notes, and if this is the case simply catheterize and observe.

Oliguria Post-op, is usually due to under-transfusion or dehydration pre- or perioperatively. First, palpate abdomen for ↑ bladder and listen to chest to exclude pulmonary oedema. Then catheterize the patient to exclude urinary retention and allow close monitoring of fluid balance. Then ↑ rate of infusion of fluid (**max** 1 l/h) **unless** the patient is in heart failure or bleeding. The former needs specialist advice, the latter needs blood or an operation. In an otherwise healthy post-op patient, if this does not produce a minimum of 30 ml/h of urine, a diuretic (20–40 mg frusemide PO/IV) may be tried. Take care when using fluid challenges, as if failure to PU is renal it is possible to fluid overload the patient quickly. Review the fluid balance, U&Es, over several days for an overview.

Blood transfusion

▶ Group and save: you won't get blood; group and cross-match: you will get blood in ~1 hr; type specific group: you will get blood urgently.

Blood may be required for patients in an acute (e.g. traumatized) situation, electively (e.g. peri-operatively) during major surgery, or to correct a chronic anaemia (p. 524). In practice, the former two are much more commonly encountered by junior dental staff.

Whole blood is indicated in patients who have lost >20% blood volume, exhibit signs of hypovolaemic shock, or in whom this appears inevitable.

▶ Remember maxillofacial injuries *alone* only rarely result in this degree of blood loss (p. 488).

Always take blood for grouping in severely traumatized patients, and proceed to cross-match as indicated by the clinical signs. Always use cross-matched blood, except in utter extremis when O Rhesus −ve blood can be used. Massive transfusions create problems with hyperkalaemia, thrombocytopenia, and low levels of clotting factors; ∴ in patients with severe haemorrhage, simultaneous fresh frozen plasma (4–6 units) and platelets (6 units) will be needed. Most labs only provide packed cells.

Autologous blood is blood donated by a patient prior to elective surgery for use only on themselves. It avoids risks of cross-infection but requires a specially interested haematology department, so check locally. Autotransfusion is sometimes used in vascular surgery.

Packed cells are used for the correction of anaemia if too severe for correction with iron, or if needed prior to urgent surgery. This ↓ the fluid load to the patient, but elderly individuals and those in heart failure should have their transfusion covered with 40 mg frusemide PO or IV.

Useful tips
- Cross-match one patient at a time and be sure you are familiar with local procedures.
- Nurse will perform regular observations of temperature, pulse, respiration, and urine output during transfusion—look at them!
- Don't use a giving set which has contained dextrose, as the blood will clog.
- Except in shock, transfuse slowly (1 unit over 2–4 h; >4 h the cannulae start to clog).
- 1 unit of blood raises the Hb by 1 g/dl = 3% haematocrit.

Complications
- ABO incompatibility. Causes anaphylaxis; manage accordingly (p. 570).
- Cross-infection.
- Heart failure can be induced by over-rapid transfusion.
- Milder allergic transfusion reactions are the commonest problem; Rx by slowing the transfusion. If progressive or temperature >40°C stop transfusion and inform lab to check cross-matching. IV hydrocortisone 100 mg and chlorpheniramine 10 mg are useful standbys.
- Citrate toxicity is a hazard of very large transfusions and can be countered by 10 ml of calcium gluconate with alternate units.

Catheterization

This is not a topic normally covered by the dental syllabus, but the dental graduate may find him or herself confronted with a patient needing urethral catheterization if working on an oral and maxillofacial surgical ward. The only procedure they are likely to need to be able to perform is temporary urethral catheterization. This is indicated for urinary retention (almost always post-op), for precise measurement of fluid balance, or, rarely, to avoid use of bedpan or bottle. Avoid catheterization if a history of pelvic trauma is present, as an expert is needed. Catheters are associated with a high incidence of UTIs, and presence of a UTI is a relative C/I.

Equipment Most wards have their own; ask for it and ensure you have an assistant available. It should contain a tube of local anaesthetic gel, a dish with some aqueous chlorhexidine, swabs, a waterproof sheet with a hole in the middle, sterile gloves, a 10 ml syringe filled with sterile water, and a drainage bag. In most cases a 14–16 French gauge Foley catheter will suffice. Use a silicone catheter if you anticipate it being *in situ* for more than a few days.

Procedure Explain what you are going to do and why. If catheterizing for post-op fluid balance, do it in the anaesthetic room after intubation (ask the anaesthetist first!). The operating theatre is the best place to learn. The procedure can be made both aseptic and aesthetic by wearing two pairs of disposable gloves; one pair is discarded after achieving analgesia, which is done by instillation of lignocaine gel (also acts as a lubricant). Find the urethral opening and, using the nozzle supplied, squeeze in the contents of the tube. In the female, finding the opening is the only significant problem and most women are catheterized by female nursing staff. In the male, it is necessary to massage the gel along the length of the penis and leave *in situ* for several minutes before progressing. Once analgesia is obtained, the female urethra is easily catheterized; if you have been unable to find the meatus to instil LA you should not proceed but get help. In the male, hold the penis upright and insert the tip of the catheter; pass it gently down the urethra until it reaches the penoscrotal junction, pull the penis down so that it lies between the patient's thighs, thereby straightening out the curves of the urethra, and advance the tip into the bladder until urine flows.

Once urine flows, the catheter balloon can be inflated with sterile water. In the conscious patient it should be painless; if not, deflate the balloon and reposition the catheter. In the anaesthetized patient, insert the catheter all the way, inflate, then pull back. Connect the drainage bag and remember to replace the foreskin over the glans to avoid a paraphimosis.

▶ If, in the presence of adequate analgesia, you are unable to pass the catheter **do not** persist, but get expert assistance.

Enteral and parenteral feeding

The main role for this type of feeding, as far as dental staff are concerned, is in the care of debilitated patients and those undergoing surgery for head and neck cancers. In view of the latter, it is worthwhile having a basic understanding of the subject.

Enteral feeding is providing liquid, low-residue foods either **1** by mouth, or **2** more commonly, by fine-bore nasogastric tube. A range of proprietary products are available for these feeds. Be guided by the local dietitian, who has expertise in this area which you will lack. The major problem is osmotic diarrhoea, which can be ↓ by starting with dilute solutions.

Fine-bore nasogastric tubes are the mainstay in enteral nutrition for patients undergoing major oropharyngeal surgery. In many institutions, nurses are not allowed to pass these tubes, although they are allowed to pass standard nasogastric tubes for aspirating stomach contents. You can ∴ find yourself asked to pass such a tube by someone who is more proficient but forbidden to do so.

Technique Wear gloves. Explain the procedure to the patient and have them at 50–60° upright with neck in neutral position. Place a small amount of lignocaine gel in the chosen nostril after ensuring it is patent. Keep a small drink of water handy. Select a tube; check the guidewire is lubricated and does not protrude. If a tracheostomy tube is present the cuff should be deflated to allow passage of the tube. Lubricate the tube and introduce it into the nostril; pass it horizontally along the nasal floor. There is usually a little resistance as the tube reaches the nasopharynx; press past this and ask the patient to swallow (use the water if this helps). The tube should now pass easily down the oesophagus, entering the stomach at 40 cm. Secure the tube to the forehead with sticky tape and only now remove the guidewire, being careful to shield the patient's eyes. Inject air into the tube and listen for bubbling over the stomach. Confirm position with a CXR. (Some systems require leaving a radiopaque guidewire in prior to X-ray: check the tube you are using.)

Problems

- *Nasal patency* Select the least narrow nostril, use a lubricant, and, if necessary, a smaller tube and topical vasoconstrictor.
- *Gagging/vomiting* Press ahead; all sphincters are open.
- *Tube coiling into mouth* Cooling the tube makes it more rigid and often helps. As a last resort, topical anaesthesia and direct visualization with a laryngoscope or nasendoscope, while an assistant passes the tube, may be necessary.
- *Tube pulled out by patient* If they must have the tube, consider a septal suture or stitch to soft tissue of the nose.

Parenteral feeding Extremely hazardous and expensive. It requires central venous line and considerable expertise if your patient is to survive. Avoid if at all possible.

PEG Feeding tube placed directly in stomach through abdominal wall at endoscopy.

RIG Ultrasound version of PEG. Needs NGT in place to inflate stomach

Pain control

LA (p. 640); RA (p. 646); IV sedation (p. 648); cryoanalgesia (p. 412); and TENS (p. 643).

Pain control aims to relieve symptoms while identifying and removing the cause; the exception is when the cause is not treatable, as in terminal care. Then, the approach is to deal with the symptoms to enable the patient to have a quality to the end of their life.

Acute and post-op pain May often be well controlled by LA (p. 640), but it is often necessary to use systemic analgesics. Useful analgesics in this situation include paracetamol (1000 mg PO/PR 4 hourly) and ibuprofen (400–600 mg 8 hourly). Both these can be combined with codeine (8–30 mg). Also, NSAIDs such as diclofenac (50 mg PO 8 hourly or 75 mg IM perioperatively, followed by one further dose of 75 mg IM). These drugs are all simple analgesics and, with the exception of paracetamol, have the advantage of an anti-inflammatory action which is at least as important as their central analgesic effect. In *post-op* pain, opioid analgesics are helpful when used parenterally and short-term. Morphine 10 mg 3–4 hourly combined with an antiemetic such as metoclopramide (10 mg IM/IV) is useful in the immediate post-op period. PCA systems (see below) after major surgery are commonly used. They are set up and maintained by the anaesthetists.

Pain following maxillofacial trauma is a problem, as these patients must be assessed neurologically for evidence of head injury which C/I opioids. The addition of codeine phosphate (60 mg IM) to a NSAID is often effective and does not significantly interfere with neurological observations. Alternatively, PR or IM diclofenac sodium may suffice. There is often a hospital acute pain team who will be happy to advise in difficult cases.

Facial pain not of dental or iatrogenic origin is covered on p. 462. These conditions often require the use of co-analgesics such as antidepressants, antiepileptics, and anxiolytics.

Pain control in terminal disease An important subject in its own right. Points to note include: aim for continuous control using oral analgesia; use regular, not on demand, analgesia titrated to the individual; diagnose the cause of each pain and prescribe appropriately (e.g. steroids for liver secondaries or ↑ intracranial pressure, NSAIDs &/or radiotherapy for bone metastases, co-analgesics for nerve root pain, etc.). Remember that psychological dependence is very rare in advanced cancer patients using long-term opioids, and analgesic tolerance slow to develop. When starting patients on opioid analgesia, always consider using an antiemetic (p. 620) and a laxative. OH may be incredibly difficult for patients with oral cancer or following head and neck surgery. Use of chlorhexidine gluconate (corsodyl) and metronidazole (200 mg bd) ↓ the smell associated with wound infection or tumour fungation even when there is no prospect of eliminating it entirely. Patients rarely develop the disulfiram reaction to metronidazole on this regimen that occurs with higher doses.

Pre-emptive analgesia Surgery is painful. Providing LA (consider the long-acting agent bupivacaine/levopivacaine) or systemic analgesia before surgery begins may ↓ overall requirements for analgesia.

Patient-controlled analgesia   The optimal technique for severe post-op pain. Small machine delivers a bolus (1–2 mg morphine) when patient presses a button. Can be repeated as needed.

Two variables: **1** bolus dose; **2** 'lock out time' time during which machine will not respond (allows time for opioid to achieve maximum effect and prevents overdosage).

Prophylaxis

Prophylaxis is the prevention of an occurrence. Prophylaxis used to prevent the occurrence of bacterial infection is quite different from treating an established infection. There are two broad categories of patients requiring antibiotic prophylaxis: **1** those who have it to prevent a minor local bacteraemia causing a serious infection out of all proportion to the procedure, e.g. people at risk from IE, or the immunocompromised; those who receive it to prevent local septic complications of the procedure, e.g. wisdom-tooth removal.

Principles of prophylaxis The regimen should be short, high dose, and appropriate to the potential infecting organisms. The aim is to prevent pathogens establishing themselves in surgically traumatized or otherwise at-risk tissues,∴ the antimicrobial must be in those tissues prior to damage or exposure to the pathogen. It must not, however, be present too long before this, as there is then a risk of pathogen resistance and damage to commensal organisms. The regimen should∴ start immediately pre-op (i.e. <6 h) or perioperatively (e.g. with anaesthetic induction) and should be continued for 24–48 h maximum. When practicable select an antimicrobial as specific to the common pathogens for that procedure as possible except in the immunocompromised, where broad-spectrum prophylaxis is appropriate.

Examples
- *IE prophylaxis* (BSAC 2004).
- Use of chlorhexidine mouthwash for 5 min. Also recommended before dental procedure.

Ordinary risk Valvular disease with murmur, past rheumatic fever, coarctation, prosthetic valve (but not previous endocaditis).

LA – 3 g amoxicillin PO 1 h pre-op.
- Penicillin-allergic or course within last month: 600 mg clindamycin PO 1 h pre-op.

GA – 1 g amoxicillin. IV/IM at induction: 500 mg PO 6h later, *or*
- 3 g amoxicillin PO 4 h pre-op and ASAP after procedure.
- Penicillin-allergic: as high risk. Children 5–10 1/2 adult dose, < 5 1/4 adult dose.

'High risk' Treat in hospital LA or GA (e.g. past IE)

Amoxicillin 1 g plus gentamicin 120 mg.	IV/IM with amoxicillin 500 mg PO 6 h later.

Penicillin-allergic or course within last month.

Teicoplanin 400 mg plus gentamicin 120 mg	IV, *or*

Clindamycin 300 mg IV with 150 mg PO 6 h later, *or*

vancomycin 1 g plus gentamicin 120 mg.	IV separately. Vancomycin is infused over 100 min.

NB Amoxicillin IM *hurts*: mix with 2.5 ml of 1% plain lignocain. Vancomycin makes people feel terrible: they often faint; teicoplanin slightly better. Pacemakers, coronary artery bypass grafts, and hip replacements *do not* need prophylaxis.[1]

- *Immunocompromised* (e.g. severe leukopenia) 5 g azlocillin plus 120 mg gentamicin IV pre-op. Repeat qds for 24 h.
- *Dento-alveolar surgery* Simple extractions need not be covered but third-molar surgery often is. Regimens: metronidazole 400 mg PO (500 mg IV) pre-op followed by 400 mg tds for 24 h, amoxicillin 1 g PO/IV followed by 500 mg tds for 24 h.

Prophylactic anticoagulation Prevention of DVT&/or pulmonary embolus in susceptible patients (e.g. women on the pill, prolonged surgery, iliac crest grafts) can be achieved using 5000 units heparin SC bd. TED antiembolism stockings will also ↓ DVT. Low molecular weight heparins given SC od are now favoured. There are many different types. Check which one your hospital favours. Rx of pulmonary embolus, p. 604.

---

1 Working Party of the British Society for Antimicrobial Chemotherapy, as quoted in up-to-date BNF.

Management of the diabetic patient undergoing surgery

▶ Many hospitals have a diabetic team who will advise on the management of these patients. Find out if this happens in your locality and make use of them.

Guidelines

- Know the type and severity of the diabetes you are dealing with.
- Inform the anaesthetist (and diabetic team if available).
- Remember these patients are more likely to have occult heart disease, renal impairment, and ↓ resistance to infection, so get an ECG, U&Es, and use antibiotics prophylactically.
- If nursing staff are experienced with blood glucose estimation using "BM" sticks or similar, 2–4 hourly "BM"s will suffice for monitoring control. Otherwise pre-, peri-, and post-op blood glucose estimation is needed.
- If in doubt and you are on your own (although you never should be) use a GKI (see below).
- Always have diabetics first on the operating list, in the morning if possible. Admit to hospital the day before surgery if insulin regime is to be used.

Management: non-insulin-dependent

If anything other than a minor, short procedure, treat as insulin-dependent. If random blood glucose is >15 mmol/l treat as insulin-dependent.

Patients being treated under LA, or LA and sedation should maintain their carbohydrate intake and any oral hypoglycaemic drugs as normal. Plan surgery to fit their regular mealtimes. Have carbohydrate readily to hand if needed, and ensure adequate post-op analgesia, as pain or trismus can easily interfere with their usual intake. Remember antibiotic prophylaxis.

Patients for GA Halve the dose of oral hypoglycaemic 24 h prior to surgery and omit on day of surgery. Do "BM"s or blood glucose pre- and post-op (if >15 go to GKI). Halve normal dose of oral hypoglycaemic until able to take normal diet, then back to normal dose. Keep an eye on the K concentration (U&Es pre- and post-op) and keep well hydrated.

Management: insulin-dependent

Admit 24–48 h pre-op to optimize control. If glycaemic control poor involve diabetic team *early*. Examine the patient carefully. Get an ECG, FBC, U&Es, and random blood glucose. Look for heart and respiratory disease, leucocytosis indicating infection, anaemia, hypo- or hyperkalaemia, and renal impairment. If these are acceptable, normal insulin/carbohydrate intake up to and including evening meal the day before surgery. Omit long acting insulin on the day before surgery. Starve following this, and place on an IV infusion of *glucose* (dextrose 5–10% 500 ml), *potassium* (10 mmol K injected into bag of dextrose) infused via a controlled rate device over 5 h i.e. 100 ml/hr. This is infused via three-way tap into a peripheral cannula. Simultaneously, *insulin* (short acting e.g. actrapid) is infused via a pump through the three-way tap into the same cannula at a rate indicated by the sliding scale. The insulin is normally made up as 49 ml N saline with

IU of actrapid giving 50 mls = 50 IU insulin, but always check your local
urses' policy.

The original GKI had a fixed amount of insulin injected into the 500 ml of
extrose but the flexibility of sliding scale delivery has made this technique
e most frequently used.

liding scale

M	Insulin IU/h
22	8
–22	6
–18	4
–14	3 Target zone
-10	2
-6	1
2	Stop and give glucose/dextrose

he scale details will vary according to the type of fingerprick glucose tests
ailable in your locality; numbers are *not* absolute but the principle will
ways work. Choice of crystalloid is variable; 10% dextrose ↑carbohyd-
te and anabolism but tends to tissue veins quickly.

Once the patient can eat and drink, resume normal insulin regimen and
scontinue infusion as BMs normalize.

Management of patients requiring steroid supplementation

Principle These patients are unable to respond to the stress of surgery due to depletion or absence of their endogenous corticosteroid response.

Groups Patients with Addison's disease, patients prescribed corticosteroids for modulation of the immune system, and steroid abusers from various 'sports'.

Addison's disease The rarest of these groups but requires the most aggressive supplementation as sufferers are entirely reliant on prescribed steroids. Minor surgery can safely be covered with IM hydrocortisone sodium succinate 100 mg qds the day of surgery. Major surgery should be covered for 3 days using the same regimen. IV administration is kinder over the longer period.

Patients prescribed steroids Do you know why they are on these drugs? Consider the underlying disease and whether it has any bearing on your Rx plan; e.g. a patient receiving steroids as part of a cytotoxic regimen will also be at risk from bleeding and infection. In an uncomplicated case before minor surgery, all that is needed is a single IM injection of hydrocortisone 100 mg 30 min prior to the procedure. Alternatives are an IV injection immediately pre-op followed by double the normal oral dose of steroid. Or relying on the patient to take a double dose on the day of the operation, normal dose plus 50% the day after, and normal plus 25% on the third day, thereafter returning to their usual dose. Those undergoing major surgery should have the IM/IV regimen over 24 h or longer.

Steroid abusers Unfortunately these are a real and ↑ problem.[1] Although these drugs are taken for their androgenic effect, few 'sportspersons' have access to appropriate advice or drugs and many users will have a degree of suppressed steroid response. It is probably safest to cover procedures using the IM regimen as for those on prescribed steroids, although this could be considered overkill. Remember the risk of shared needles.

1 HMSO, *Drugs and Therapeutics Bulletin*, January 2004.

Common post-operative problems

General

Pain Use appropriate analgesia (p. 614).

Pyrexia A small physiological ↑ in temperature occurs post-op. Othe causes: atelectasis, infection (wound, chest, urine), DVT, incompatibl transfusion, allergic reactions.

Nausea and vomiting Antiemetics, e.g. IM/IV cyclizine 50 mg. Prochlorperazin 12.5 mg or metoclopramide 10 mg. Ondansetron for the recalcitrant (4 m IV/IM, 8 mg PO).

Sore throat Common after intubation; needs reassurance and simpl analgesia. Cold water ↓.

Muscle pain Often follows suxamethonium use in anaesthetic inductio Again, reassurance and simple analgesics.

Hypotension Usually caused by autonomic suppression by a GA. Treat b placing 'head-down'. If necessary, speed up IV infusion for a short while.

Chest infection CXR, culture sputum, and start on ampicillin or cefuroxim until culture results available.

Confusion A symptom, ∴ look for the cause, e.g. infection, electrolyt imbalance, alcohol withdrawal, hypoxia, or dehydration, and correct. Onl consider sedation, e.g. haloperidol 1–5 mg (care in the elderly), afte action has been taken to deal with the cause and the patient constitutes threat to themselves or others.

Rarer general complications

Urinary retention Comparatively rare, even after major maxillofacial surger Early mobilization and adequate analgesia helps; if not, use temporar catheterization (p. 592).

Superficial vein thrombosis Follows 'tissued' cannulae or irritant IV injec tions. Observe for infection, treat pain, and consider supportive strapping

DVT Signs are painful, shiny, red, swollen calf, usually unilaterally but ma be bilaterally. 'At risk' are immobile patients especially following pelvi surgery, patients with cancer, women on the pill, the elderly, and th obese. Confirm by doppler US or ascending venography. Prevent by usin a low molecular weight heparin (dalteparin, enoxaparin) pre-op and 5 day post-op &/or pressure stockings, and ensure early mobilization. Stop th pill prior to any major surgery. Rx: bed rest, leg strapping and elevation, ana gesia and heparinization (give 5000 units stat IV followed by 50 000 units i 50 ml normal saline by syringe driver infusion starting at 1000 units/ (1 ml/h) and adjust according to the KCT/APTT, keep between 1.5–2. times the control values). The major risk of DVT is the development c pulmonary embolus. This classically presents 10 days post-op when th patient has been straining at stool and may occur despite no apparen DVT. Symptoms are pleuritic chest pain, dyspnoea, cyanosis, haemoptysi and a ↑ jugular venous pressure. Signs of shock are often present, rangin from very little in the young who can compensate, to cardiac arrest! Usuall a clinical Δ, confirmed after heparinization, analgesia, and O_2 have bee instituted, by CXR, blood gases, spiral CT, or lung ventilation—perfusion scan &/or pulmonary angiography. ECG will sometimes show deep S waves in I, pathological Q waves in III, and inverted T waves in III (SI, QIII, TIII). Must be followed up by 3–6 months anticoagulation with warfarin, so involve a haematologist.

Less serious but more common are *post-phlebitic limb*, varicose veins, limb swelling, and skin discoloration. May lead to varicose eczema.

Local complications following oral surgery

Local pain, swelling, infection, and trismus are the commonest. Antral complications may follow maxillary surgery. These are considered in the relevant chapters.

Principal sources BMA/RPSGB September 2003 BNF. Walton's *Textbook of Dental Pharmacology and Therapeutics*, OUP. Consumers Association *Drugs and Therapeutics Bulletin*. HMSO *Prescribers Journal*. BDA/BMA/RPSGB/DPF/BNF 2000–02.

NB Although available on the Internet BNF.org is **NOT** recommended for use in clinically critical situations. BNF 48 now has an amalgamated BNF/DPF in preparation for extending dentists prescribing powers in 2005.

Relevant chapters and pages Chapter 11: Medicine relevant to dentistry; Chapter 13: Analgesia, anaesthesia, and sedation; asepsis and antiseptsis, p. 382; antiseptics and antibiotics in periodontal disease, p. 232; fluorides, p. 32; sugar-free medications, p. 126.

Generic: pharmaceutical name.
Proprietary: trade name.
Depending on patents, a generic drug may have more than one proprietary name.

Poisons information

UK National Poisons Information Service: 0870 600 6266
Drugs in sport: www.uksport.gov.uk/did 0800 5280004
drug-free@uksport.gov.uk

Medicines information services

Birmingham	0121 311 1974
Bristol	0117 928 2867
Ipswich	0147 370 4430/1
Leeds	0113 245 0530
Leicester	0116 255 5779
London	0207 955 5000 and 3594/5892
	0208 869 3973
Newcastle	0191 232 1925
Southampton	0238 079 6908/9
Cardiff	0292 074 2979
Aberdeen	0122 455 2316

Dundee	0138 263 2351
Edinburgh	0131 242 2920
Glasgow	0141 211 4407
Belfast	0289 063 2032
Dublin	00 3531 473 0589

UK medicines information pharmacists' group: www.ukmi.nhs.uk

Prescribing

The following pages are a brief guide to the clinical use of some of the more commonly used and useful drugs in hospital and general dental practice. Doses are for healthy adults.

Prescribing in general dental practice Extremely useful information is available in the DPF, which is updated every 2 yrs. Use this as the first line of enquiry when unsure about any topic concerning drugs. Drugs listed in the DPF can be prescribed in the UK within the NHS on form FP10 D (GP14 in Scotland, HS47 in Northern Ireland). Any other required drugs must be prescribed privately or via the patient's GMP. Many are available more cheaply OTC at pharmacies.

Prescribing in hospital The BNF is the definitive reference and should always be available for consultation. Use this to check dose alterations in children and the elderly, and for more detailed tables of drug interactions, C/I, and unwanted effects. Very detailed guidance for children is usually available on paediatric wards (e.g. Alder Hay booklet). Any drug in the hospital pharmacy may be prescribed by a hospital dentist for in-patients, patients being discharged, and out-patients. The only exception is controlled drugs for addicts, which must be prescribed by specially licensed doctors, usually a psychiatrist.

In hospitals, there are three methods of prescribing: **1** A hospital drug kardex recording both prescriptions and dispensing, kept on the ward for in-patients. **2** A take-home prescription form redeemable only at the hospital pharmacy for patients being discharged from the ward. **3** Hospital out-patient prescriptions, used in emergency departments and some out-patient clinics, redeemable at outside pharmacies.

Good prescribing Avoid abbreviations and write drug names legibly, using the generic whenever possible. Always describe the strength and quantity to be dispensed. When describing doses use the units micrograms, milligrams, or millilitres when possible. Do not abbreviate the term microgram or unit (when prescribing insulin) as these are easily misinterpreted.

Controlled drugs Each prescription must show, in the prescriber's own handwriting in ink: the name and address of the patient, the form, strength, dose, and total quantity of the drug to be dispensed, in both words and figures. When writing in general practice the prescription must also incorporate the phrase 'for dental treatment only'.

Prescribing in the elderly Doses should be substantially lower than for adults (often 50% lower).

Prescribing for children Children differ markedly from adults in their response to drugs, especially in the neonatal period when all doses should be calculated in relation to body weight. Older children can usually be prescribed for in age ranges, usually up to 1 yr, 1–6 yrs, and 6–12 yrs. All details of dosages should be checked in the BNF/DPF or paediatric booklet.

Prescribing in liver disease (p. 536) Try to avoid prescribing in patients with severe liver disease.

Prescribing in renal impairment (p. 538) Doses almost always need to be ↓ and some drugs are C/I completely.

Prescribing in pregnancy (p. 542) Avoid if possible.

Prescribing in terminal care, p. 596.

Dose and route abbreviations

Dose	*Route*
od once a day	**IM** intramuscular
mane in the morning	**INH** inhalation
nocte at night	**IV** intravenous
bd twice daily	**NEB** nebulization
tds three times daily	**PO** by mouth
qds four time daily	**PR** per rectum
prn as required	**PV** per vagina
	SC subcutaneous
	SUB sublingual
	TOP topical

Analgesics in general dental practice

▶ Consult BNF for dosages in children. See also p. 610. Most dental pain is inflammatory in origin and hence most responsive to drugs with an anti-inflammatory component, e.g. aspirin and the NSAIDs.

Of the peripherally acting analgesics in the DPF, aspirin, paracetamol, and ibuprofen are available cheaper direct to the public from pharmacies.

Aspirin Used in mild to moderate pain, it is also a potent antipyretic, which should **not** be used in children < 12 yrs (due to the rare but serious risk of Reye syndrome). Avoid in bleeding diathesis, gastrointestinal ulceration, and concurrent anticoagulant therapy. Ask about aspirin allergy, particularly in asthmatics. Often causes transient gut irritation (as do all NSAIDs). *Dose:* 600–900 mg 4 hourly PO.

Ibuprofen Popularly used for mild to moderate pain; has a moderate antipyretic action. Risks and side-effects are similar to that of aspirin but less irritant to the gut. *Dose:* 400–600 mg 6 hourly PO.

Paracetamol Similar in analgesic efficacy to aspirin but has no anti-inflammatory action and is a moderate antipyretic. Does not cause gastric irritation or interfere with bleeding times. Overdosage can lead to liver failure. *Dose:* 1000 mg 4 hourly PO.

Diflunisal A prescription-only drug available on the DPF, with similar properties and problems to aspirin. *Dose:* 250–500 mg bd with food PO.

The addition of **codeine** to the minor analgesics, while never being proven to be of advantage, may have marginal benefits in some cases. No combination analgesics are currently prescribable on the DPF.

There are very few indications for the use of opioid analgesics in general dental practice. Although **dihydrocodeine** remains in the DPF it has been demonstrated to be hyperalgesic in certain types of dental pain.[1]

Pethidine In tablet form (the only form in the DPF), is worse than dihydrocodeine in terms of side-effects.

Carbamezipine (p. 632) Prescribable in the DPF.

NB While all NSAIDs *may* exacerbate asthma and there is a higher incidence of NSAID allergy in asthmatics, the CSM recognizes that this *does not* constitute a C/I for the use of these valuable analgesics. Frank allergy to NSAIDs or proven exacerbation of asthma *is* a C/I.

1 R. A. Seymour 1982 *Lancet* **i** 1425–6.

Analgesics in hospital practice

In addition to those available in the DPF, some drugs available only within hospitals are of considerable value.

Diclofenac sodium is available in tablet, IM injection, suppository, and in once-daily, slow-release form. It is a mid-potency NSAID, and a useful alternative to high-dose lower potency NSAIDs or an opioid which has no anti-inflammatory effect. *Dose for tablets*: 50 mg tds after food; IM injection: 75 mg bd for no more than 2 days (it's a painful injection); suppositories: 100 mg PR od. Soluble tablets available.

Ketorolac trometamol 30 mg/ml injection, has advantage of small volume of injection. However, ↑ unwanted effects have been noted.

Opioid analgesics

The opioids act centrally to alter the perception of pain, but have no anti-inflammatory properties. They are of value for severe pain of visceral origin, post-op (acting partly by sedation), and in terminal care. However, they all depress respiratory function and interfere with the pupillary response, and are C/I in head injury. All opioids cause cough suppression, urinary retention, nausea, constipation by a ↓ in gut motility, and tolerance and dependence. The risk of addiction is, however, greatly overstated when these drugs are used for short-term post-op analgesia and in the terminal care context. Fear of creating addicts should **never** cause you to withhold adequate analgesia.

Codeine phosphate A moderate opioid analgesic useful for short-term analgesia and less likely to mask a head injury; 30–60 mg 4 hourly IM/PO. May be some advantage when used in combination (8/15/30 mg) with simple analgesics or NSAIDs.

Morphine In oral form (tablets, elixir, or slow-release tablets MST), the drug of choice in the management of terminal pain. Always prescribe a laxative (macrogols are currently in favour: see BNF). *Dose*: dependent on previous analgesia, but often starts at 10 mg morphine 4 hourly or 30 mg MST bd. When used IM or IV for acute or post-op pain: 10–20 mg 2–4 hourly; give an antiemetic.

Papaveretum A mixed opium alkaloid, frequently prescribed, but appearing to have no advantage over morphine. The presence of noscapine created a C/I in women of childbearing age. Noscapine-free equivalent (Omnopon 10 + 20) now available.

Buprenorphine A mixed agonist/antagonist with similar problems to pethidine and pentazocine. Unique in that it can be given sublingually. *Dose*: 200–400 µg 8 hourly.

Diamorphine (heroin) The most powerful opioid analgesic. Causes less nausea and hypotension than morphine and is very soluble. This is a great advantage, allowing it to be infused in tiny amounts SC or IV via infusion pump. Its ability to mobilize venous reserves makes it the drug of choice in MI and heart failure. Like morphine it is reversed by naloxone, dose 1–2 mg IV repeated up to 10 mg max (if that hasn't worked, you've got the diagnosis wrong).

Tramadol An opioid which acts by two central methods. Lower side-effect profile. 50–100 mg po 4 hourly. *Slow* IV 50–100 mg 4–6 hourly.

►Chronic and post-op pain require *regular*, not as-required, analgesia, given in adequate amounts and within the therapeutic half-life of the drug.

PCA (p. 596) A system for post-op pain control allowing patients to deliver small regular doses of IV/SC morphine/diamorphine. Gold standard post-op analgesia.

Anti-inflammatory drugs

These are among the groups of drugs that may be either analgesics or co-analgesics (drugs which are not analgesic in themselves but may aid pain relief either directly or indirectly). The two major groups are the NSAIDs (p. 612) and the corticosteroids.

Steroids are used in various forms, topical, oral, intralesional, and parenteral, and all have uses in dentistry.

Topical steroids

Hydrocortisone lozenges 2.5 mg lozenges dissolved in the mouth qds.

Triamcinolone in carboxymethylcellulose paste 0.1% paste applied in a thin layer qds. Sticks only to dry mucosa and is rapidly rubbed off the palate and tip of tongue. Both these preparations are available in the DPF and are of use in the management of recurrent apthous ulcers, lichen planus, etc. They are low-potency steroids and unlikely to have any of the systemic side-effects of steroids, such as ↑ of diabetes, osteoporosis, psychosis, euphoria, peptic ulceration, immunosuppression, Cushing syndrome (p. 540), or adrenocortical suppression.

Benzydamine A topically active NSAID. Used as spray or mouthwash to ↓ pain from inflammatory mucosal conditions.

Betamethasone phosphate tablets Prepared as a 0.5 mg soluble tablet (Betnesol) made into a 1 mg in 10 ml mouthwash rinsed qds, or a *betamethasone* inhaler designed for use in asthma, but can be used to spray on aphthae (1 spray = 100 μg). Repeatable to a maximum of 800 μg.

Hydrocortisone 1% and oxytetracycline 3% Ointment or spray (hydrocortisone 50 mg oxytetracycline 150 mg per aerosol unit) qds, are useful Rx for aphthae and related conditions seen in hospital. Hydrocortisone 1% cream is also available with miconazole 2% in DPF.

Intralesional steroids

Triamcinolone acetonide 1 ml (40 mg) injected into lesion. Needs LA. Used in granulomatous cheilitis, intractable lichen planus, and keloid scars.

Intra-articular steroids

These can be used to induce a chemical arthroplasty in arthrosis of the TMJ (p. 502).

Hydrocortisone acetate 5–10 mg single injection.

Triamincinolone Can be used intra-articularly.

Systemic steroids

Main indication is prophylaxis in those with actual or potential adrenocortical suppression. Occasionally used in erosive lichen planus, severe aphthae, e.g. Behçet syndrome (p. 440) or arteritis (p. 546).

Hydrocortisone sodium succinate Used for prophylaxis; dose 100 mg IM 30 min pre-op.

Prednisolone 30 mg PO as enteric-coated tablets given with food in ↓ dose. Regimen dependent on the condition treated.

Methylprednisolone 40 mg/ml. Various regimens described for control of oedema, post major surgery.

Dexamethasone 4 mg/ml. Various regimens described for control of oedema, post surgery.

Other immunosuppressants

Azathioprine and **thalidomide** are sometimes used in specialist centres. Topical tacrolimus used for erosive lichen planus.

Antidepressants

Another group of drugs which can be used as co-analgesics. In conditions such as atypical facial pain they may be used as the sole 'analgesic'. However, there are no antidepressants prescribable in the DPF.

In the past, there has been considerable debate about the potential interactions between the commonest antidepressants, the tricyclics, and the monoamine oxidase inhibitors (MAOIs), and adrenaline contained in LA (which constitutes the most commonly professionally administered drug anywhere). To date, there is *no clinical evidence* of dangerous interactions between the adrenaline in LA preparations commonly used in dentistry and the tricyclics or the MAOIs.[1] In hospital practice, the two most commonly used antidepressants are amitriptylne (a sedative tricyclic antidepressant) and dothiepin (a related compound).

Amitriptyline Use with caution in patients with cardiac disease (as arrhythmias may follow the use of tricyclics) and avoid in diabetics, epileptics, and pregnant or breast-feeding women. It can precipitate glaucoma, ↑ the effect of alcohol, and cause drowsiness (which can impair driving). In common with other tricyclics it can cause sedation, blurred vision, xerostomia, constipation, nausea, and difficulty with micturition, although tolerance to these side-effects tends to develop as Rx progresses. There is often an interval of 2–4 weeks before these drugs reach a level that exhibits a clinically evident antidepressant effect. *Dose:* 50–75 mg either as a single dose nocte or in divided doses, maximum 150–200 mg daily. Children and elderly half-dose.

Dothiepin has similar properties and unwanted effects to amitryptiline. It has, however, been demonstrated to be of value in the Rx of 'facial arthromyalgia' (a composite group of TMPDS and atypical facial-pain patients).[2] *Dose:* initially 75 mg nocte, increasing to 150 mg daily if needed. Half-dose in elderly.

Nortriptyline A less sedating tricyclic. *Dose:* 10–30 mg nocte; can be increased.

Tranylcypromine A MAOI that may be of value in treating facial pain unresponsive to tricyclics. *Dose:* 10 mg tds before 16.00 h.[3]

Motival A combination drug that may be of value in atypical facial pain (fluphenazine 0.1 mg, nortriptyline 10 mg) nocte.

MAOIs can precipitate a hypertensive crisis induced by dietary and drug interactions (sympathomimetics, opioids, especially pethidine, and foods containing tyramine, e.g. cheese, meat, or yeast extracts). LA is, however, safe.

Selective serotonin re-uptake inhibitors (SSRIs) Much less-sedative antidepressants, given as single dose a.m. Fluoxetine (Prozac) is best known (20 mg daily) and also abused (overprescribing and used to prolong effects of MDMA or Ecstasy). Paroxetine 20 mg mane and sertraline 50 mg mane are similar.

---

1 DPF 2000–02. In BNF **40** 2000.
2 C. Feinmann 1984 *BDJ* **156** 205.
3 M. Harris 1993 *BDJ* **174** 129.

Antiemetics

There are no antiemetics prescribable in the DPF; however, they form an essential part of in-patient hospital prescribing. The common indication is the control of post-op nausea and vomiting, which may be due to the procedure, anaesthetic, post-op analgesia, or blood in the stomach.

Prochlorperazine A phenothiazine antiemetic which acts as a dopamine antagonist and blocks the chemoreceptor trigger zone. Avoid in small children as the drug's major side-effect, the production of extrapyramidal symptoms, is especially common in this group. *Dose*: 12.5 mg IM 8 hourly, 20 mg initially followed by 10 mg tds PO. Buccal absorption 3–6 mg bd. Not licensed for IV use.

Metoclopramide has both peripheral and central modes of action. It ↑ gut motility, thus emptying the stomach. Acute dystonic reactions may occur, especially in young women and children; a bizarre acute trismus is sometimes seen as one of the manifestations. *Dose*: 10 mg tds PO, 10 mg IM 8 hourly. High-dose intermittent and continuous IV regimens are used for antiemesis in centres using cytotoxic chemotherapy.

Domperidone is less likely to cause central unwanted effects such as sedation and dystonia, as it does not cross the blood–brain barrier. Acts on the chemoreceptor trigger zone and is particularly useful for chemotherapy patients. *Dose*: 10 mg 4 hourly. May be used as part of a combination regimen, e.g. domperidone, prednisolone, and nabilone (a synthetic cannabinoid).

Ondansetron A selective 5-HT$_3$ receptor antagonist which is very effective in prevention and Rx of post-op nausea and vomiting. *Dose*: 4 mg single IV dose or 8 mg PO. Granisetron and tropisetron are similar 5-HT$_3$ receptor antagonists.

Hyoscine, antihistamines, and major tranquillizers all have antiemetic properties but are rarely indicated. If unable to control emesis with one agent use two, acting at separate sites *after* excluding intestinal obstruction, e.g. due to opioid constipation.

Cyclizine is often combined with opioid preparations as an anti-emetic—however, it can aggravate heart failure. Cheap. *Dose*: 50 mg tds IM or PO.

Do not forget the benefits of a nasogastric tube in preventing nausea and vomiting from a distended or irritated stomach. Constipation can also cause nausea—remember to exclude it as a cause.

Anxiolytics, sedatives, hypnotics, and tranquillizers

The short-term control of fear and anxiety associated with dental Rx is an entirely appropriate use of the benzodiazepines. It should not be confused with the long-term control of anxiety which is rife with problems of dependence and drug withdrawal. A benzodiazepine may also be a valuable adjunct in the management of TMPDS, where it acts as both a muscle relaxant and an anxiolytic (p. 482). IV and oral sedative techniques prior to surgery, p. 650.

Diazepam Has long half-life and is cumulative on repeated dosing. Like all benzodiazepines, can cause respiratory depression, ∴ patients should be warned not to drive or operate machinery while on this drug. *Dose for anxiety/TMPDS*: 2 mg tds, maximum 30 mg in divided daily doses. Paradoxical disinhibition may occur in children and its use in the < 16s is not advised. Diazepam in lipid emulsion (Diazemuls) is the IV Rx of choice in status epilepticus (p. 574). A rectal preparation is popular for paediatric sedation in some countries (p. 648).

Midazolam A water-soluble benzodiazepine of about double the potency of diazepam. Its main use is in IV sedation (p. 648). Also popular as a paediatric sedative for suture removal.

Nitrazepam A long-acting hypnotic which tends to cause a hangover effect. *Dose*: 5–10 mg nocte.

Temazepam Shorter-acting hypnotic. *Dose*: 10–30 mg nocte. Main indication is pre-op or as pre-medication. An OP sedation technique is described p. 650. Gelatine capsule preparations should no longer be used as they can be melted down for IV abuse.

In hospital practice

The following may also be prescribed:

Chlordiazepoxide Sometimes used instead of diazepam in TMPDS. It has the same side-effect profile. *Dose*: 10 mg tds, ↑ to maximum of 100 mg daily, in divided doses. It is drug of choice in the stabilization of alcohol dependent in-patients.

Lorazepam Sometimes used as a pre-med by anaesthetists. *Dose*: 2 mg nocte, 2 mg 1 h pre-op. Alternative to diazepam in epileptics.

Chlormethiazole A hypnotic sometimes used to ↓ severe insomnia in the elderly. *Dose*: 1–2 capsules nocte (each cap = 192 mg). Main indication is in management of alcohol withdrawal. Regimen: day 1: 3 caps qds; day 2: 2 caps qds; day 3: 1 cap qds. Acute withdrawal is sometimes managed by IV infusion; however, this is a dangerous technique, not to be undertaken lightly.

Zopiclone A non-benzodiazepine hypnotic. *Dose*: 7.5 mg nocte. Problems similar to benzodiazepines. May be of practical help when local policy controls use of temazepam.

Haloperidol Very useful in control of acute psychosis, in a dose of 10–30 mg IM. Less painful than, and does the same job as chlorpromazine but main problem is extrapyramidal side-effects.

Flumazenil A specific benzodiazepine reversal agent (p. 648). Dosages should be ↓ in elderly. Avoid in children.

Trimeprazine An antihistamine; a useful sedative for children. *Dose:* 2–3 mg/kg 1–2 h pre-op.

Chloral hydrate (Chloral Elixir, paediatric) 5 ml used as a sedative for removing facial sutures.

Antibiotics—1

Principles of antibiotic use

When prescribing, consider: **1** the patient; **2** the likely organisms; **3** the best drug. Patients influence choice, in that they may be allergic to various drugs, have hepatic or renal impairment, be immunocompromised, be unable to swallow, be pregnant or breast-feeding, or taking an oral contraceptive; consider also age and severity of the infection. The infecting organism should ideally be isolated, cultured, and its sensitivity to antibiotics determined, but this is only feasible in hospital practice. In reality, most infections are treated blind, ∴ it is essential to know the common infecting organisms in your field, and their sensitivities. You also need to know the drugs' modes of action, absorption, unwanted effects, development of resistance, interactions, and techniques available for delivery. The best drug is the one which is safe in that patient, specific to the infecting organism, and can be given in a reliable convenient form. Remember prophylaxis (p. 598) differs from Rx with antibiotics, and antibiotics do not replace the drainage of pus in abscesses.

Benzylpenicillin Inactive orally and only used IM or IV. *Dose:* 600–1200 mg IV/IM qds. Drug of choice in streptococcal infections. Like all penicillins is bactericidal: it interferes with cell-wall synthesis. Good tissue penetration except for CSF. Its most important unwanted effect is hypersensitivity, which is usually manifested as a rash, rarely as fatal anaphylaxis. Patients allergic to one penicillin will be allergic to all; 10% will be allergic to cephalosporins as well. A history of atopy (e.g. asthma) ↑ risk.

DPF prescribable antibiotics

Phenoxymethyl penicillin Oral equivalent of above. *Dose:* 250–500 mg qds PO Has a narrow spectrum, but is now largely superseded by

Amoxicillin Has a broad spectrum similar to **ampicillin**, but is better absorbed and achieves higher tissue concentrations. *Dose:* 250–500 mg tds PO. Both ampicillin and amoxicillin cause a maculopapular rash in patients with glandular fever, lymphatic leukaemia, or possibly HIV infection (this is **not** true penicillin allergy). Amoxicillin is drug of choice in prophylaxis against infective endocarditis (p. 598). May interfere with the action of oral contraceptives. All penicillins decrease excretion of methotrexate, ∴ ↑ risk of toxicity.

Tetracycline One of a group of broad-spectrum antibiotics with a problem of ↑ bacterial resistance. It is likely to promote opportunistic infection with *Candida albicans*, particularly when used topically, as has been recommended for the Rx of aphthae. Other problems are the deposition of tetracyclines in growing bone and teeth, causing staining and hypoplasia (∴ avoid in children <12 yrs and pregnancy) and erythema multiforme It is also particularly likely to render the oral contraceptive ineffective. *Dose:* 250–500 mg qds PO. Absorption inhibited by chelation with milk, etc., ∴ should be taken well before food. May be of value in periodontal disease (p. 232). Doxycycline 200 mg day 1, then 100 mg od PO and oxytetracycline 250–5000 mg qds PO are prescribable.

Erythromycin A similar spectrum to penicillin, but bacteriostatic. Active against penicillinase-producing organisms. Formerly an alternative to amoxicillin for endocarditis prophylaxis (superseded by clindamycin). Nausea is a major problem. *Dose:* 250–500 mg qds PO/IV.

Oral cephalosporins Of little value in dental practice, but cefalexin 250–500 mg bd or tds PO and cefradine 250–500 mg qds PO are prescribable. Clindamycin and metronidazole are also in DPF; see p. 626.

Antibiotics—2

Clindamycin Should be used cautiously in the management of dental infections, due to the risk of antibiotic-induced colitis. Useful in staphylococcal osteomyelitis in conjunction with metronidazole (which inhibits overgrowth with *Clostridium difficile*). Has replaced erythromycin for single-dose prophylaxis of infective endocarditis (p. 598).

Metronidazole An anaerobicidal drug, and as such effective in many acute dental and oral infections. Classical dose for NUG is 200 mg tds PO 3 days. For other anaerobic infections is more often used as 400 mg bd/tds (depending on severity) PO. Available in tablets, IV infusion, or suppository. Main problem is severe nausea and vomiting if taken in conjunction with alcohol (disulfiram reaction). Remember, it is NOT effective against aerobic bacteria.

Antibiotics of use in hospital practice

(in addition to the aforementioned)

Flucloxacillin A penicillin active against penicillinase-producing bacteria. Dose 250–500 mg qds PO/IV. Can be combined with ampicillin as co-fluampicil.

Co-amoxiclav Is amoxycillin plus clauvulanic acid. The latter destroys beta-lactamase (penicillinase) and hence widens the range of amoxicillin to include the commonest cause of resistance in infections of the head and neck. Dose 1–2 tabs tds PO or 600–1200 mg tds IV. Problems as for amoxicillin.

Cefuroxime A parenteral broad-spectrum cephalosporin often used in combination with metronidazole for surgical prophylaxis in contaminated head and neck procedures. *Dose*: 750–1500 mg tds IV (500 mg bd PO).

Gentamicin A bactericidal aminoglycoside antibiotic, active mainly against Gram −ve organisms. Complementary to the penicillins and available as a topical (ear use) or parenteral preparation. Major problem is dose-related ototoxicity and nephrotoxicity (monitor levels if used for > 24 h). *Dose*: up to 5 mg/kg monitored use local guidelines. Endocarditis prophylaxis, p. 602.

Co-trimoxazole Has few indications in the head and neck which have not been replaced by trimethoprim alone (200 mg bd). It is used, however, in ear, sinus, and urinary infections, but C/I in pregnancy and folate deficiency (as it is a folate antagonist).

Chloramphenicol Useful topically in bacterial conjunctivitis (0.5% eye drops, 1% eye ointment, apply 3 hourly). Systemic use is strictly limited due to toxicity. Ointment is an excellent wound dressing.

Vancomycin A unique bactericidal antibiotic. Two main uses are orally in the Rx of antibiotic-induced colitis (120 mg tds 10 days PO), and for prophylaxis of patients at high risk from infective endocarditis (p. 602). Ototoxic nephrotoxic, prone to cause phlebitis at infusion sites, and makes people feel generally unwell, ∴ not to be used lightly.

Teicoplanin Similar to vancomycin. Lasts longer. Can be given IV or IM. Fewer unwanted effects and kinder on patient, but more expensive.

Antifungal and antiviral drugs

Antifungals

The main fungal pathogen in the mouth is *Candida albicans* (p. 438).

Amphotericin Best used as lozenges 10 mg dissolved slowly in the mouth qds 10–15 days. Double dose if needed.

Nystatin Available as pastilles or mixture. *Dose:* 100 000 units qds either by sucking a pastille qds or using 1 ml of the mixture and holding it in the mouth before swallowing.

Miconazole Useful drug, particularly in management of angular cheilitis, as it is active against streptococci, staphylococci, and candida. Miconazole oral gel 25 mg/ml is of use in chronic mucocutaneous and chronic hyperplastic candidosis. *Dose:* place 5–10 ml in the mouth and hold near the lesions before swallowing, qds. Miconazole cream is used topically for angular cheilitis.

Fluconazole Available in both oral and IV formulations for severe mucosal candidosis in both normal and immunocompromised patients as a second line to topical preparations. Avoid in pregnancy. *Dose:* 50 mg od PO 7–14 days, 200–400 mg IV od. **Itraconazole** and **tioconazole** are other new antifungal drugs.

There are recognized potentially serious interactions between miconazole, fluconazole, and related drugs and: antibacterials, anticoagulants, antidiabetics, antiepileptics, antihistamines, anxiolytics, cisapride, cyclosporin, and theophylline. Check what your patient is currently taking. Candidal resistance to fluconazole is now recognized—get C&S if Rx not working.

Antivirals

Most viral infections are treated symptomatically. One drug is available for the Rx of orofacial viral diseases:

Aciclovir Active against herpes simplex and zoster; relatively non-toxic and can be given systemically or topically. *Dose:* herpes labialis: apply aciclovir cream to site of prodromal or early lesion 4 hourly for 5 days; herpetic stomatitis: 200 mg (400 mg in immunocompromised) PO 5 times daily for 5 days; herpes zoster: 800 mg PO 5 times daily for 7 days.

Idoxuridine Available as idoxuridine 5% in dimethyl sulfoxide. Regarded as being of little value nowadays. Other anti-herpes drugs include: **famciclovir** and **valaciclovir** (both pro-drugs). **Ganciclovir** Active against all herpesviruses, EBV, and CMV; however, it is very toxic and ∴ has no indications in dentistry. **Zidovudine (AZT)**, may prevent AIDS dementia complex. Other nucleoside reverse transcriptase inhibitors include abacavir, didanosine, lamivudine, stavodine and zalcitabine. Protease inhibitors and non-nucleoside reverse transcriptase inhibitors are also in use. There is no known cure but these drugs slow or halt disease progression. **Inosine pranobex** is licensed for use in treating mucocutaneous herpes simplex in conjunction with podophyllin. **Interferon** is an interesting drug, with no indications in dentistry.

Antihistamines and decongestants

Antihistamines

Rarely used in the usual range of dental practice. Sometimes indicated in the management of allergy, especially hayfever, for pre-medication and sedation in children, occasionally as antiemetics, possibly in the management of over active gag reflex, and as part of the emergency Rx of angio-oedema and anaphylaxis (p. 570). Main differences between the antihistamines are duration of action and degree of accompanying sedation and antimuscarinic effects.

Chlorpheniramine A sedative antihistamine. Dose: 4 mg qds PO.

Promethazine Also a sedative antihistamine. Dose: 10 mgs qds PO or 20–30 mg nocte when used as a hypnotic. On sale to the public as a hypnotic.
The sedative effects of these drugs potentiate alcohol and ability to drive or operate machinery safely. They should be used with caution in glaucoma, prostatic hypertrophy, and epilepsy.
Although these drugs are available in the DPF, probably the most useful antihistamines are not. These include:
A wide range of non-sedating antihistamines; e.g. cetirizine, loratadine are available as OTC generics to the public, largely replacing **terfenadine** due to its greater unwanted effects.

Trimeprazine A sedative antihistamine which may be of some value in the itching of uraemia, and frequently used by anaesthetists as a pre-med in children. Adult dose: 10 mg bd/tds; paediatric pre-med: 5–10 mg, dependent on age.

Decongestants

Valuable in the management of sinusitis and particularly in the closure of oro-antral fistulae.

Ephedrine nasal drops Produce vasoconstriction of mucosal blood vessels and ↓ the thickness of nasal mucosa, thus relieving obstruction. Avoid in patients taking MAOIs. Other problems: prolonged use leads to a rebound vasodilatation and a recurrence of nasal congestion, and long-term use results in tolerance and damage to nasal cilia. Dose: ephedrine nasal drops 0.5–1%, 1–2 drops into the relevant nostril qds for 7–10 days. For symptomatic nasal decongestion and as an adjunct to the management of oro-antral fistulae (p. 422) inhalation of **menthol** and **eucalyptus** is valuable. Dose: 1 teaspoonful of menthol and eucalyptus inhalation BP is added to a pint of hot water, and the warm, moist air is inhaled with a towel over the head.

Xylometazoline and oxymetazoline nasal drops and spray 0.1% are a more potent alternative to ephedrine, but more likely to cause a rebound effect. Systemic decongestants are of dubious value and contain sympathomimetics. They do not, however, cause rebound. For prescribed, short-term use, thereby avoiding risk of rebound, xylometazoline or oxymetazoline are drugs of choice; spray into relevant nostril tds.

Miscellaneous

A number of drugs not fitting into any specific category are important in managing oral and dental disease. These include:

Carbamazepine Primarily an antiepileptic drug which is of considerable value in the management of trigeminal and glosso-pharyngeal neuralgia. C/I in those sensitive to the drug, patients with atrioventricular conduction defects, porphyria, and should be used with extreme caution in patients on MAOIs who are pregnant, or who have liver failure. May interfere with the oral contraceptive. Common unwanted effects are gastrointestinal disturbances, dizziness, and visual disturbances. Rarely, rashes may occur, as can leukopenia. Do a FBC soon after starting carbamezipine: blood dyscrasia usually occur in the first 3 months. *Dose:* 100–200 mg bd; can be ↑ gradually to 200 mg tds/ qds. Maximum 1600 mg daily in divided doses. Important to be sure of your diagnosis before starting patients on long-term carbamezipine (p. 462). A slow-release preparation with fewer unwanted effects is available.

Vitamins There is no indication for first-line Rx with vitamins in dental practice. Deficiency due to inadequate dietary intake in the UK is exceedingly rare. Although it can occur in the elderly and alcoholics, these people should be fully investigated and not treated empirically. Severe gingival swelling, stomatitis, glossitis, or pain should be fully investigated before using vitamin supplements. The only preparations available in the DPF are

Vitamin B compound tablets, strong A combination of nicotinamide 20 mg, pyridoxine 2 mg, riboflavine 2 mg, thiamine 5 mg. Dose: 1–2 tablets tds.

Ascorbic acid tablets BP (vitamin C) ↑ iron absorption and prevents scurvy.

Artificial saliva Valuable adjunct in the management of xerostomia, especially after radiotherapy and in Sjögren syndrome. A slightly viscous, inert fluid which may have a number of additives, such as antimicrobial preservatives, fluoride, flavouring, etc. Useful preparations are Glandosane and Saliva Orthana, aerosol sprays sprayed sublingually 4–6 times per day. The latter contains fluoride. Regular sips of water may be of more practical long-term help. DPF has Artificial Saliva DPF 60 ml unit. Use: all should be sprayed into the floor of mouth area to act as a 'puddle' for redistribution. Do *not* spray all over mucosa. Use qds.

Topical anaesthetics Two main uses:
1 For preparation of a site prior to injection, e.g. of LA. Lignocaine 5% ointment or spray is the most useful. Flavoured benzocaine pastes are available in some countries (not UK).
2 EMLA and amethocaine (Ametop®) can be used on mucosa. Carmellose gelatine paste acting as a mechanical barrier is useful in areas where it will adhere. Many OTC agents are available; few are of great potency. To ↓ pain from minor oral lesions (e.g. for HSV 1 or aphthae). Benzydamine rinse is a mainstay.

Fluorides Fluoride supplementation is discussed on p. 34. It is important when using rinses, and particularly gels, that the fluid is not swallowed, since there is a risk of toxicity (p. 32).

Retinoids Used in some centres to manage erosive lichen planus and leukoplakia; have proved disappointing.

Alarm bells

When prescribing any drug for patients already compromised by concomitant disease or drug therapy, it is essential to exclude possible interactions. This can be achieved fairly quickly by consulting the comprehensive BNF.

Interactions with the most commonly given drug (LA) are covered on p. 640.

Common drugs with relative contraindications in liver disease
Aspirin
All benzodiazepines
All opioids
All sedatives
All antihistamines
All NSAIDs
Erythromycin
Metronidazole (decrease dose)
Paracetamol
Tetracyclines
Terfenadine

Common drugs with relative contraindications in renal failure
Aciclovir (↓ dose)
All penicillins (↓ dose)
All opioids
Amphotericin
Cephalosporins (↓ dose)
Co-trimoxazole (↓ dose)
Benzodiazepines (↓ dose)
NSAIDs
Tetracyclines

Common drugs with relative contraindications in pregnancy
Aspirin
Benzodiazepines
Carbamezipine
All opioids
Co-trimoxazole
NSAIDs
Metronidazole
Tetracyclines

Common drugs with relative contraindications in breast-feeding
Antihistamines
Aspirin
Benzodiazepines
Carbamezipine
Co-trimoxazole
Metronidazole
Tetracyclines

These lists are not comprehensive and some of the drugs mentioned can be used in suitably modified dose or under specific circumstances. These tables are designed to ring alarm bells, and encourage you to both think and consult the BNF.

Adverse reactions

Almost any drug can produce these, and many are missed. Try to avoid polypharmacy, and never prescribe without being aware of a patient's full medical history. Always enquire about drugs, including self-prescribed medication.

Report suspected adverse reactions to Medicines and Healthcare products Regulatory Agency (MHRA): email: info@mhra.gsi.gov.uk phone: 0800 731 6789, or in writing to:

CSM Freepost, London SW8 5BR
CSM West Midlands SW 2991, Freepost, Birmingham B18 7BR
CSM Mersey, Freepost, Liverpool L3 3AB

CSM Northern, Freepost 1085, Newcastle NE1 1BR
CSM Wales, Freepost, Cardiff CF4 1ZZ

Report • **all** serious adverse reactions;
• **any** reactions to 'black triangled' drugs in the BNF/DPF.

Emergency drugs

Oxygen	Cylinder size D (340 l) or E (680 l) plus reducing valve, flow-meter, tubing, and oxygen mask.
Adrenaline	1 mg in 1 ml (1:1000) solution (IM injection)
Hydrocortisone sodium succinate	100 mg powder, plus 2 ml water for injection (IM injection)
Chlorpheniramine maleate	10 mg in 1 ml solution (IM injection)
Glucagon	1 mg powder, plus 1 ml water for injection (IM injection)
Glucose or sugar	Drink, tablets, or gel (PO administration)
Salbutamol inhaler	0.1 mg per dose (INH administration)
Glyceryl trinitrate	0.5 tablets or 0.4 mg per dose spray (SUB administration)
Aspirin	300 mg tablets (PO administration)
Midazolam	10 mg in 2 ml solution (IV/IM injection)

Analgesia, anaesthesia, and sedation

NB Since the report of the GDC in 2001[1] the status of general anaesthesia in dental practice, and inevitably the medico-legal aspects of anaesthesia and sedation in the UK have altered considerably. This varies widely from country to country. General principles, however, remain the same.

Principal sources   J. Meechan 1998 *Pain and Anxiety Control for the Conscious Dental Patient*, OUP. *Department of Health Working Party on General Anaesthesia and Sedation in Dentistry* (Poswillo Report) 1990.

Relevant pages in other chapters   LA for children, p. 82; emergencies in dental practice, p. 560.

Definitions

General anaesthesia (GA)   A state of unrousable unconsciousness to which analgesia and muscle relaxation is added to produce 'balanced anaesthesia'.

Analgesia   The absence of pain.

Sedation   An altered level of consciousness in which the patient, although awake, has a ↓ level of fear and anxiety.

---

1 GDC *Maintaining Standards: General Anaesthesia and Resuscitation* (Amendment November 2001).

Indications, contraindications, and common sense

When dealing with LA, GA, and sedative techniques, indications, and contraindications are often relative, and the following should be thought of as guidelines rather than immutable laws.

LA The technique of choice for simple procedures or when a GA is C/I. LA is C/I in:

- uncooperative patients (of any description);
- infection around the injection site;
- patients with a major bleeding diathesis;
- most major surgery;

Adverse reaction to LA is a C/I, but in reality once allergy to preservatives in the solution is excluded, LA allergy probably does not exist.

Conscious sedation

This is an extension of LA technique using drugs and patient-management techniques. It is of benefit to anxious or mildly uncooperative patients and is a kind supplement to apicectomy or third-molar removal. C/I include:

- Cardiorespiratory, renal, liver, or psychiatric pathology.
- An unescorted patient or one unable or unwilling to conform to the requirements of conscious sedation (p. 650).
- A demonstrated adverse reaction to sedative agents.
- Pregnancy, during which benzodiazepines should be avoided.

GA Indicated when LA or LA and sedation is ineffective or inappropriate (as above). C/I include:

- All those for conscious sedation.
- Presence of food or fluid in the stomach (most anaesthetists require at least 4 h between last feed and GA).

The anaesthetist usually prefers hospital admission for patients with the following:

- Cardiovascular or respiratory disease (especially MI < 6 months ago).
- Uncorrected anaemia, sickle cell trait or disease.
- Severe liver or renal impairment.
- Uncontrolled thyrotoxicosis or hypothyroidism.
- Poorly controlled diabetes, adrenocortical suppression.
- Porphyria.
- Pregnancy.
- Neurological disorders, e.g. myopathy or multiple sclerosis.
- Cervical spine pathology such as rheumatoid arthritis or cervical spondylosis.
- Certain drugs, e.g. steroids, antihypertensives, MAOIs, anti-coagulants, narcotic analgesics, antiepileptics (need to avoid using methohexitone), lithium, alcohol. Malignant hyperpyrexia, scoline apnoea, and other unwanted reactions to anaesthetic agents.
- Causes of upper airway obstruction such as angio-oedema, submandibular cellulitis, Ludwig's angina, and bleeding diathesis affecting the neck. (In fact, these are indications to secure the upper airway.)
- Previous problems with anaesthesia.

Ask about previous GA and any problems. Note drugs used as repeated administration of halothane may induce hepatitis and should be avoided within a 3 month period (CSM). While all these conditions create problems with anaesthesia they may not preclude it absolutely within the hospital setting. They do, however, indicate the need for careful assessment and early prior consultation with the anaesthetist.

Local analgesia—tools of the trade

While any disposable needle and syringe system can be used to give LA, the vast number of LAs given in dental practice (>50 000/dentist/lifetime) has led to some very useful modifications.

LA cartridges Two sizes, 1.8 and 2.2 ml, come pre-sterilized. Commonest solution used is lignocaine 2% with adrenaline 1:80 000. A latex-free version is available for patients with latex allergy.[1]

Cartridge syringes Use with above, resterilizable. Used with ultra-fine disposable needles. Major advantage is the ability to perform controlled aspiration during LA injection (although the consistency with which this is achieved has been questioned).

Lignocaine/adrenaline Most commonly used preparation (2% lignocaine 1:80 000 adrenaline), gives effective pulpal analgesia for 1.5 h and altered soft-tissue sensation for up to 3 h. Extremely safe; maximum dose (adult) 500 mg (10×2.2 ml cartridges). Also available in ampoules 1%+2% lignocaine plain or 1:200 000 adrenaline. There are theoretical criticisms that the maximum dose is too high but these have not been borne out in practice.

Prilocaine/octapressin Similar but slightly less duration and effect compared to lignocaine/adrenaline. May cause methaemoglobinaemia in excess. Maximum safe dose (adult) 600 mg (8×2.2 ml cartridges). In reality, there are few hard indications for the use of prilocaine over lignocaine.

Mepivacaine Short-acting LA advocated for restorative work but has not really caught on. Maximum safe dose 400 mg.

Bupivacaine Long-acting LA (6 h plain, 8 h with adrenaline); useful as a post-op analgesic. Maximum safe dose 2 mg/kg. Only available in ampoules. **Levobupivicaine** is a similar drug.

Articaine At least as effective as lignocaine; said to diffuse through bone better. No hard evidence of superiority.

Topical analgesics Lignocaine is the only really useful topical analgesic among the above. It is available as a spray or a paste which is applied to mucosa several minutes prior to injecting. There is a high incidence of contact eczema in people frequently exposed to these preparations, so do not apply with bare fingers. Benzocaine in lozenge or paste form is used for mucosal analgesia. Amethocaine is a topical analgesic for use on mucous membranes. Cocaine 4% solution is used as a nasal mucosal analgesic and vasoconstrictor.

Emla cream, a eutectic mix of lignocaine and prilocaine, is an invaluable skin topical analgesic, used prior to venepuncture in children. Apply to puncture site and cover with 'Opsite' or equivalent dressing for at least 30 min. Amethocaine (Ametop) is similar.

Handling equipment One cartridge and needle per patient. Discard cartridge if a precipitant is seen in the solution or if air bubbles are present.

---

1 Astra Pharmaceuticals.

Store in a cool dark place and use before expiry date. Warm cartridge to ↓ discomfort and load into the syringe immediately prior to use. Aspirate before injecting. The ↑ risk associated with needlestick injuries has spawned a number of devices to aid resheathing the needle. It is simpler to hold the cover in a pair of artery forceps.

Local analgesia—techniques

The inferior dental block and local infiltrations are the mainstay of LA technique; however, numerous others are available as alternatives, supplements, and fallbacks.

IDB (inferior alveolar block) Technique of choice for mandibular molars; also effective for premolars, canines, and incisors (the latter if supplemented by infiltration). Aim is to deposit solution around the inferior alveolar nerve as it enters the mandibular foramen underneath the lingula. The patient's mouth must be widely open. Palpate the landmarks of external and internal oblique ridges and note the line of the ptyerygomandibular raphe. With the palpating thumb lying in the retromolar fossa, the needle should be inserted at the midpoint of the tip of the thumb slightly above the occlusal plane lateral to the ptyerygomandibular raphe. The needle is inserted ~0.5 cm and if a *lingual nerve block* is required 0.5 ml of LA is injected at this point. The syringe is then moved horizontally ~40° across the dorsum of the tongue and advanced to make contact with the lingula. Once bony contact is made the needle is withdrawn slightly and the remainder of the LA injected. It should never be necessary to insert the needle up to the hub. Note that the mandibular foramen varies in position with age (children, see p. 82). In the edentulous, the foramen, and hence the point of needle insertion, is relatively higher than in the dentate.

Gow–Gates technique Blocks sensation in Vc by depositing LA at head of condyle.[1] Akinosi approach: LA deposited above lingua.[2]

Long buccal block The long buccal nerve is anaesthetized by injecting 0.5–1 ml of LA posterior and buccal to the last molar tooth.

Mental nerve block The mental nerve emerges from the mental foramen lying apical to and between the first and second mandibular premolars. LA injected in this region will diffuse in through the mental foramen and provide limited analgesia of premolars and canine, and to a lesser degree incisors on that side. It will provide effective soft-tissue analgesia. Place the lip on tension and insert the needle parallel to the long axis of the premolars angling towards bone, and deposit the LA. **Do not** attempt to inject into the mental foramen as this may traumatize the nerve. LA can be encouraged in by massage.

Sublingual nerve block An anterior extension of the lingual nerve can be blocked by placing the needle just submucosally lingual to the premolars, use 0.5 ml of LA.

Posterior superior alveolar block A rarely indicated technique. Needle is inserted distal to the upper second molar and advanced inwards, backwards, and upwards close to bone for ~2 cm. LA is deposited high above the tuberosity after aspirating to avoid the ptyerygoid plexus.

Nasopalatine block Profound anaesthesia can be achieved by passing the needle through the incisive papilla and injecting a small amount of solution.

1 Gow–Gates 1973 OS, OM, OP **36** 321.
2 Akinosi 1977 *BJOS* **15** 83.

This is extremely painful (hints on how to overcome pain on palatal injections below).

Infra-orbital block   Rarely indicated. Palpate the inferior margin of the orbit as the infra-orbital foramen lies ~1 cm below the deepest point of the orbital margin. Hold the index finger at this point while the upper lip is lifted with the thumb. Inject in the depth of the buccal sulcus towards your finger, avoid your finger, and deposit LA around the infra-orbital nerve.

Infiltrations   The aim is to deposit LA supraperiosteally in as close proximity as possible to the apex of the tooth to be anaesthetized. The LA will diffuse through periosteum and bone to bathe the nerves entering the apex. Reflect the lip or cheek to place mucosa on tension and insert the needle along the long axis of the tooth aiming towards bone. At approximate apex of tooth, withdraw slightly and deposit LA slowly. For palatal infiltrations, achieve buccal analgesia first and infiltrate interdental papillae; then penetrate palatal mucosa and deposit small amount of LA under force.

Intraligamentary analgesia   Individual teeth can be rendered pain free by injecting small amounts of LA along the periodontal membrane via a specially designed system (high-pressure syringe and ultra-fine needles). Has the advantage of rapid onset and specific analgesia to isolated teeth; it is a useful adjunct to conventional LA and in some hands may replace it for minor procedures. Disadvantages include post-injection discomfort due to temporary extrusion and an apparent ↑ incidence in 'dry socket'.

Electronic dental anaesthesia (EDA)   An aggressively marketed technique based on the principles of TENS. Uses electrodes, buccally and lingually, which carry a minute electrical current to interfere with local nerve conduction and hence pain appreciation. May be of value in restorative procedures and others not requiring the profound analgesia or vasoconstrictive effects of LA.

Intraosseous analgesia   A recently reintroduced technique which produces profound single-tooth analgesia. Needs specialized equipment and technique.

▶ When developing LA technique there is no alternative to seeing, doing, and doing again.

Local analgesia—problems and hints

Failure of anaesthesia

There are enormous differences in individual response to a standard dose of LA, both in the speed of onset, duration of action, and the depth. Soft-tissue analgesia is more easily obtained, needing a lower degree of penetration of solution into nerve bundles, than does analgesia from pulpal stimulation. A numb lip does not ∴ indicate pulpal anaesthesia.

Causes of failure are:

- Poor technique and inadequate volume of LA.
- Injection into a muscle (will result in trismus which resolves spontaneously).
- Injection into an infected area (which should not be done anyway as this risks spreading the infection).
- Intravascular injection; clearly of no analgesic benefit. Small amounts of intravascular LA cause few problems. Toxicity, p. 570.
- Dense compact bone can prevent a properly given infiltration from working. Counter by using intraligamental or regional LA.
- Infrequently, anastomosis from either aberrant or normal nerve fibres not transmitted with a blocked nerve bundle.

Pain on injection

This is to a certain degree inevitable, but can be ↓ by patient relaxation; application of topical LA; stretching the mucosa; and slow, skilful, accurate injection of slightly warmed solution in reasonable quantities. Causes of pain include:

- Touching the nerve when giving blocks, resulting in 'electric shock' sensation and followed by rapid analgesia (it is extremely rare for any permanent damage to occur).
- Injection of contaminated solutions (particularly by copper ions from a pre-loaded cartridge). Avoid by loading the cartridge immediately prior to use.
- Subperiosteal injections are painful and unnecessary, ∴ avoid.

Other problems with administration

Lacerated artery May be followed by an area of ischaemia in the region supplied, or painful haematoma. Rare.

Lacerated vein Followed by a haematoma which resolves fairly quickly.

Facial palsy Can be caused by incorrect distal placement of the needle tip, allowing LA to permeate the parotid gland. The palsy lasts for the duration of the LA.

Post-injection problems

Lip and cheek trauma Tell patient to avoid smoking, drinking hot liquids, biting lip or cheek. Assure them the sensation will pass in a few hours and that their face is not swollen (whether adult or child). If the advice goes unheeded and they return with traumatized mucosa, Rx: antiseptics/antibiotics and simple analgesia.

Needle-tract infection Rare. Broad-spectrum antibiotic if needed.

General points

Thick nerve trunks require more time for penetration of solution and more volume of LA. In nerve trunks autonomic functions are blocked first, then sensitivity to temperature, followed by pain, touch, pressure, and motor function. Concentration of analgesic ↑ rapidly around the nerve at first and provides soft tissue analgesia; however, this is reached substantially before the levels needed for pulpal analgesia, which takes several minutes and will wear off first (usually within an hour of a standard lignocaine/adrenaline LA). Disinfection of mucosa prior to LA is not required in reality; however, sterile disposable needles are absolutely mandatory due to risks of cross-infection. LA for children, see p. 82. Faints, p. 562.

Sedation—relative analgesia

RA is the most commonly used and safest form of sedation in dentistry. It has two aspects: **1** the delivery of a mixture of nitrous oxide and O_2 **2** a semi-hypnotic patter from the sedationist. In dentistry, two different techniques of nitrous oxide sedation have been described: **1** inhalational sedation with a fixed concentration of nitrous oxide; **2** RA in which nitrous oxide is titrated to the patient. In the authors' view RA is the most useful.

Nitrous oxide

Has both sedative and analgesic properties; the former is the most useful. The analgesic effect requires high levels of nitrous oxide. It is an inert gas which does not enter any of the body's metabolic pathways and is distributed as a poorly soluble solution. This allows very rapid distribution; peak saturation is reached within 5 min and is similarly eliminated (90% in 10 min).

Indications It is of particular value in anxious patients undergoing relatively atraumatic procedures and in children, for whom the benzodiazepines are less suitable.

Contraindications Few, but upper airway obstruction, e.g. a cold. Pregnancy first trimester makes the procedure difficult and pre-existing vitamin B_{12} deficiency would C/I its use. Other C/I, e.g. complex medical history, are relative and may limit nitrous oxide use in practice but not in hospital.

Nitrous oxide pollution The major problem associated with RA. It is essential to have a scavenging system in place as nitrous oxide accumulation can lead to B_{12} deficiency and demyelination syndromes. There is a real potential hazard to pregnant staff working in confined conditions with this gas.

Aim

To produce a comfortable, relaxed, AWAKE, patient who is able to open their mouth on request with no loss of consciousness or the laryngeal reflex. During the procedure patients will experience general relaxation, a tingling sensation often in the fingers or toes, and describe feeling mildly drunk. There is often a sense of detachment and distortion of the sense of time. Rarely, patients may dream despite being awake, and these can be sexual fantasies, which is another reason for always having a second person in the surgery.

Technique

An RA machine will not deliver less than 30% O_2. Start by delivering 100% O_2 via a nasal mask and set flow control to match their tidal volume (flow rates 6–8 1/min for adult, 4 1/min for child). Then give 10% nitrous oxide for 1 min, ↑ (if needed) to 20% for 1 min, ↑ to 30% (if needed) for 1 min and so on. Most patients achieve adequate levels of sedation at 20–30%, some may require less, a few rather more. Remember that RA relies on the reassuring banter of the operator more than any of the other sedation techniques, and many view this as hypnosedation. Give LA and carry out Rx. To discontinue, turn flow to 100% O_2 and oxygenate patient for 2 min. Then remove mask and get the patient to sit in a recovery room for 10 min, by which time 90% of nitrous oxide will have been blown off and they will be safe to leave the surgery.

Sedation—benzodiazepines

General pointers, problems, and hints

Benzodiazepines are both sedative and hypnotic drugs which are usefu for sedation of patients. Two techniques are generally used: oral and IV.

Elderly patients tend to be very sensitive to benzodiazepines and dose are best halved in the >60 age group initially. Interestingly, children show not only resistance to these drugs but sometimes paradoxical stimulatior and benzodiazepine sedation is not recommended for the <16s.

Post-op drowsiness is perhaps the biggest problem, as patients may b influenced by, e.g., diazepam for up to 24 h after administration (this tim is ↓ with midazolam). There is also a re-sedation effect caused by enterc hepatic recirculation.

Poswillo Committee Its report redefined 'sedation' as the 'single injectio of a single drug'. In terms of IV sedation in an out-patient setting this is th surest way to avoid problems provided the 'single injection' is titrated an incremental.

IV sedation The most efficient and effective method of extending the us of LA in dental Rx; however, it requires substantial skill and confidence i venepuncture and administration of the drugs; ∴ an inexperienced operato or a patient with needle phobia, form relative C/I. As do inability t be accompanied, the need to be in a responsible position within 24 of sedation (e.g. looking after young children on own, driving, etc. patients with liver or renal impairment, glaucoma, psychoses, pregnancy or a demonstrated allergy to the benzodiazepines.

Certain drugs interact, including cimetidine, disulfiram, anti-parkinsonia drugs, other sedatives, narcotic analgesics, antiepileptic drugs, antihista mines, and antihypertensives. Patients on these may be best treated (an then cautiously) in a hospital environment. Patients addicted to alcohol c other drugs may require a substantial dose modification; usually a big ↑ Those being sedated need to give written informed consent. Always provid written post-op instructions because the patients will not remembe verbal ones. The role of operator sedationist is a perfectly sound and lega occupation, but note that a second appropriate person, i.e. one trained i CPR, must be present. At no time should the patient lose consciousnes during IV sedation. The addition of any drug, especially opioids, converts technique with a wide safety margin into one with a very narrow margi and confers *no* routine advantage.

Multiple drug techniques should only be carried out by trained anaes thetists. There is no need to starve patients prior to being sedated, althoug many local policies dictate this and oral medication should be continue Rectal sedation is popular in some countries using a prepackaged solutio of diazepam (Stesolid) given PR dose 2–10 mg.

Flumazenil A specific benzodiazepine reversal agent. *Dose:* 200 µg IV ove 15 sec followed by 100 µg at 60 sec intervals until reversal occurs. **NI** This drug has a shorter half-life than the drugs it will reverse, ∴ multipl doses may be required. Patients **should never** be reversed, then le unsupervised. This is an essential emergency drug for IV sedationists.

Benzodiazepines—techniques

Oral sedation
This is of use for managing moderately anxious patients. There are problems, however, with absorption time and the risk of sedation occurring too early or too late. There is again a risk of patients having sexual fantasies under the influence of these drugs. Two drugs are used:

Temazepam 30 mg, 1 h pre-Rx produces a degree of sedation similar to that seen with IV techniques.

Diazepam, either divided regimen, 5 mg night before, 5 mg morning of Rx, and 5 mg 1 h pre-Rx; *or* as 10–15 mg 1 h prior to Rx. Both drug and technique are highly variable in consistency and quality of sedation achieved. Both doses may have to be modified depending on the size and age of the patient.

IV techniques
A far greater control of the duration and depth of sedation can be consistently achieved with this approach. Gives excellent sedation with detachment for ~30 min with amnesia for the duration of Rx. The major disadvantage is a potential for respiratory depression, post-Rx drowsiness, and amnesia (a reversal agent is available but not suitable for routine reversal of conventional sedation, p. 648). Skill with venepuncture is a prerequisite of the technique. Diazepam has been entirely superseded by diazepam in lipid emulsion (diazemuls) as diazepam is not water-soluble and is very irritant.

Midazolam A water-soluble benzodiazepine of roughly double the strength of diazepam. Has a much shorter half-life, with no significant metabolites, creating a quicker and smoother recovery, and it is more amnesic than diazepam. It is supplied in both 2 ml and 5 ml ampoules, both containing 10 mg midazolam (5 ml ampoule is preferable, as it is easier to control the increments, given at 1 mg/increment). Drug of choice.

Diazepam in lipid emulsion Diazepam is metabolized to desmethyldiazepam which has a long half-life. It is presented in a 2 ml ampoule containing 10 mg diazepam, given in slow IV increments (usually 2.5 mg via a butterfly) until signs of sedation are observed. Suggested maximum dose 20 mg.

IV technique
Relax the patient and have them sitting in the chair. Place a tourniquet around the most convenient arm and ask them to dangle the arm at their side. Any useful veins on the dorsum of the hand will become quickly evident. While this is happening, get your equipment ready: sticky tape, spirit wipe, butterfly, and drug in syringe. Look at the hand; is there a reasonable straight segment of vein? (If not, cut your losses and look elsewhere.) If there is, secure the hand with your non-dominant hand, palmar surface to palmar surface, with your thumb in a position to tense the skin overlying the selected vein. Stroke the back of the hand and tap the vein to engorge it. Prepare the skin with spirit wipe; get your 'second appropriate person' to help remove the needle cover and inform the patient there will be a slight scratch. Introduce the butterfly tip at a shallow angle

through skin, then ↓ the angle further and move along the line of the vein until it has entered, as revealed by a flashback into the extension tubing. Then introduce the length of the needle along the vein carefully, so as to avoid cutting through, and secure with tape. Remove air by aspirating blood into the tubing and release tourniquet. Place the patient in the supine position and give a small bolus (2–3 mg diazepam, 1–2 mg midazolam). Wait for 1 min and then give further increments until adequate level of sedation is achieved. Leave the butterfly in to maintain venous access. Loss of laryngeal reflex constitutes oversedation and means you must stop and ensure the airway is patent, only proceeding if there is no respiratory depression and the airway can be protected.

Monitoring A 'second appropriate person' must be present. Pulse and BP should be monitored. Pulse oximetry is mandatory. An itchy nose is an early sign of 'complete' sedation. Hiccups constitute oversedation.

Post-sedation Allow time for recovery (30–60 min) in calm surroundings. The patient must be accompanied home and forbidden to drive or assume a responsible position for 24 h.

Anaesthesia—drugs and definitions

Anaesthesia is a triad of unconsciousness, muscle relaxation, and analgesia

IV anaesthetic agents

Thiopentone (dose 4 mg/kg) Although an ultra-short-acting barbiturate anaesthetic, its half-life is 6–12 h. It is a poor analgesic and relatively sparing to the laryngeal reflexes, requiring a greater depth of anaesthesia to prevent laryngospasm. Highly irritant on injection but cheap and very popular as an in-patient induction agent. It will abolish epileptic seizures in induction doses.

Propofol (dose 2.5 mg/kg) A true ultra-short-acting anaesthetic as it is completely metabolized within minutes. Less irritant than the others and the drug of choice for day-case anaesthesia.

Etomidate (dose 0.3 mg/kg) An IV induction agent often used for patients with compromised cardiovascular systems. Can be associated with involuntary movements, cough, and hiccup. Avoid in traumatized patients.

Ketamine (dose 1–2 mg/kg) Can be given IM at higher doses (unique among anaesthetic agents for this). Tends to maintain the airway and causes little respiratory depression. Its use is limited by a high incidence of severe nightmare hallucinations in adults, which are eased by midazolam.

Inhalational anaesthetics

Nitrous oxide Excellent analgesic but weak anaesthetic, mainly used to supplement other inhalational anaesthetics or in RA. Problem created by its rapid excretion if used for perianaesthetic analgesia; wears off rapidly so no post-op analgesic benefits.

Halothane Largely superseded by newer agents. Weak analgesic. Causes hypotension and dysrhythmias. The concomitant use of injected adrenaline should be avoided in non-ventilated patients breathing halothane as it ↑ risk of VF. Very rarely hepatotoxic after repeated anaesthetics in adults. Extremely rarely *de novo*.

Enflurane Weaker anaesthetic than halothane but less likely to produce dysrhythmias or hepatitis. Avoid in epileptics.

Isoflurane Close relation of enflurane but more potent. Causes less cardiac problems than halothane. Commonly used hospital agent may cause coughing with inhalational induction.

Sevoflurane Newer agent with rapid onset and recovery. Good for inhalation induction and becoming increasingly inhalational agent of choice.

All inhalational agents cause muscle relaxation.

Muscle relaxants

Used to create laryngeal relaxation for intubation; this stops patients breathing, and they must then be ventilated until the agent wears off or is reversed.

Suxamethonium Used for emergency cases for rapidly securing airway. Short-acting depolarizing muscle relaxant; quick, good recovery but cannot be reversed. Main problems for the patient are muscle pains, which arise 24–48 h after administration. These can be very severe and are more likely in the ambulant. It can also cause severe bradycardia, especially on repeat dose in children. Metabolized by plasma cholinestese, absence of which can lead to suxamethonium sensitivity, p. 542. Causes an ↑ in K^+, ∴ know U&Es in all but very routine cases.

Pancuronium, atracurium, vecuronium, and rocuronium   All non-depolarizing muscle relaxants; slower acting and longer lasting, but can be reversed using neostigmine.

Mivacurium   A short-acting non-depolarizing agent which, it was hoped, would fill the role of suxamethonium. Disappointing in practice.

Analgesics   Opioids are mainstay, and include:
- Morphine; long acting, mainly used for post-op analgesia.
- Fentanyl; first of the short-acting opioids.
- Alfentanyl; purely used as anaesthetic opioid due to short duration.
- Remifentanyl; continuous infusion needed because of ultra-short duration; ideal for anaesthesia but not post-op pain relief.

Anaesthesia and the patient on medication

Certain drugs should ring alarm bells when patients require a GA. These include:

Monoamine oxidase inhibitors Should be stopped 2 weeks prior to GA.

Antiepileptic drugs Must be continued up to, during, and after GA however, methohexitone should be avoided.

Antihypertensives Should be continued, but ensure the anaesthetist is aware they are being taken.

Bronchodilators Should be continued. Give inhaler with pre-medication and ensure nebulizer is available post-op.

Cardioactive drugs Should all be continued. Warn the anaesthetist, as these patients often benefit from a pre-op anaesthetic assessment.

Cytotoxics Patients on these rarely need GA, but if they do they need FBC, U&Es, LFTs. Suxamethonium should be avoided.

Diabetic drugs For management, see p. 600.

Lithium Measure levels. Omit prior to major surgery.

Oral contraceptives Think about DVT prophylaxis, although experience suggests the risk is remote. BNF recommends discontinuing 4 weeks prior to major elective surgery; this is generally unnecessary for maxillofacial/oral surgery. Be guided by local policy. HRT does *not* need to be stopped.

Sedatives and tranquillizers If the patient takes a regular dose these can be maintained, but warn the anaesthetist.

Corticosteroids Patients on long-term steroids require supplementation p. 542, 572, 602.

Oral anticoagulants Stop and heparinize for all major surgery. Monitor clotting. INR for warfarin. KCT for heparin.

Anaesthesia—hospital setting

With the exception of the out-patient GA service provided by dental hospitals, GA in a hospital setting is similar to that for any other surgical service. The provision for, and the care of the patient immediately prior to, during, and after the anaesthetic is the domain of the trained anaesthetist. The input from the hospital junior is the same, whether in a dental or surgical specialty, and is mainly covered on p. 584. The fundamental problem for any dental, oral, or maxillofacial anaesthetic is that the surgeon and anaesthetist both need to have access to the same anatomical site: the shared airway. The means by which this is overcome in hospital practice is by endotracheal, particularly nasendotracheal intubation, muscle relaxation, and ventilation.

Endotracheal intubation secures the airway by placing a tube into the trachea via the nose, mouth, or a tracheostomy. This tube has an inflatable cuff which prevents aspiration of debris and is connected to an anaesthetic machine to allow delivery of O_2, nitrous oxide, and an inhalational anaesthetic. Most anaesthetists also use a throat pack to supplement the cuff, **which must be removed at the end of the operation**. Intubation is a specialist skill and must be learned by practice; skilled practitioners can perform blind nasendotracheal intubation, which is of enormous value in cases with trismus; most cases are, however, performed by direct vision of the vocal cords using a laryngoscope with the patient's neck fully extended. The major risk of intubation is intubating the oesophagus **and not recognizing it**. Other complications include: traumatizing teeth; vocal cord granulomata; minor trauma to the adenoids; rarely, pressure necrosis of tracheal mucosa and laryngeal stenosis.

The laryngeal mask airway The LMA has become an acceptable method of maintaining the airway. Structurally, it is a curved tube with a large cuff at its end. It is a device which is inserted orally without direct vision following the normal curve of the pharynx. Its onward progression is stopped by the upper end of the oesophagus and at this point the cuff is inflated, forming a seal around the entrance to the larynx. Patients must be starved as it does not protect against aspiration. It occupies a substantial volume in the mouth. The necessity of movement of the LMA to allow surgical access may displace the cuff, possibly causing laryngeal obstruction. Expensive, but autoclavable up to 40 times. It requires quite deep anaesthesia both to pass and maintain the LMA, which may prolong anaesthesia inappropriately.

The LMA should only be used by those trained in intubation.

Muscle relaxation Essential for successful intubation in elective patients. These drugs are covered on p. 652. For most oral surgery, once intubated ventilation is aided by small doses of non-depolarizing muscle relaxant. An alternative is a continuous infusion of a very short-acting opioid (e.g. remifentanil).

Ventilation May be hand or mechanical. The latter is more precise and convenient for the anaesthetist. It involves a machine providing intermittent +ve pressure ventilation.

Monitoring There are increasingly sophisticated non-invasive techniques available: pulse oximetry to measure the percutaneous saturation of haemoglobin with O_2 (a normal person breathing air will have a saturation >95%); capnograph to measure end-tidal $PetCO_2$ (normal: 5.2 kPa or 40 mmHg); ECG and automatic BP machines. It must be stressed, however, that these machines do not replace, only ↑, the ability of the anaesthetist to use clinical observation of pulse, colour, skin changes, and ventilatory pattern. Minimum standard of monitoring set by Royal College of Anaesthestists is: BP, ECG, SaO_2, end-tidal CO_2.

Malignant hyperpyrexia,   p. 542.

Anaesthesia—practice setting

Since the GDC's 2001 amendment to *Maintaining Standards: General Anaesthesia and Resuscitation*, the administration of GAs in dental practice setting has been effectively abolished. This has seen a huge pressure to ↑ the number of specialist (particularly) paediatric day units concentrating on paediatric exodontia and minor oral surgical work. This is often integrated with the community service for special-needs dentistry patients out-patient (ambulatory) setting.

The ideal team to provide exodontia under GA is a small skilled group, e.g. anaesthetist, dentist, and nurse, who have received appropriate postgraduate training and have suitable facilities.

Out-patient anaesthesia is given to healthy patients; the majority of anaesthetics, from induction to recovery, are a few minutes. The LMA is frequently used as an airway adjunct for day-case extraction, avoiding the need for muscle relaxation and intubation.

Controversial points

Pollution with anaesthetic gases In the hospital environment it is possible to scavenge the majority of gases as patients are either intubated, or have an LMA or a relatively leak-proof face mask. This is not the case in a dental surgery, as the patients are breathing through a nasal mask and, invariably, through their mouths.

Hazards of inhaling anaesthetic gases These are not well established. It is true that patients continuously breathing nitrous oxide for 24 h or so begin to have suppression of the bone marrow and that chronic recreational abuse can cause subacute combined degeneration of the spinal cord. The short-term and intermittent long-term effects of exposure to nitrous oxide, halothane, enflurane, and isoflurane are, however, simply not known. It remains common sense that no one should work in a polluted atmosphere. The current guidelines are HC (76) 38.

Selected principal recommendations of the Poswillo Committee

Sedation

1 Sedation be used in preference to GA whenever possible.
2 For sedation by inhalation, the minimum concentration of O_2 be fixed at 30%.
3 Flumazenil be reserved for emergency use.
4 Intravenous sedation be limited to the use of one drug with a single titrated dose to an endpoint remote from anaesthesia.
5 The use of IV sedation in children be approached with caution.
6 Dentists must be aware of the significance of pulse oximetry readings.
7 All patients treated with the aid of sedative techniques be accompanied by a responsible person.
8 Undergraduates should have experience of managing at least 5 cases of IV sedation and 10 cases of inhalation sedation, and be proficient in venepuncture.
9 Interested dentists should complete a recognized course in IV sedation within 2 years of qualification.

2001 GDC recommendations on GA and dentistry

These reinforce and extend the Poswillo recommendations. A *referring* or treating practitioner who breaches these recommendations will now be liable to a charge of serious professional misconduct.

Points to note

Referring

- A full PMH must be taken.
- A full explanation of risks and alternatives must occur before referral.
- Justification for the use of GA must be made in the referral letter.
- A copy of the letter must be retained.

Facilities to treat

- Access to critical care.
- Written protocol and training in ALS.
- Anaesthetist must be on GMC Specialist Register or working under supervision of same.
- Is supported by an Operating Department Practitioner.

Treatment

- Rx must only be provided if the treating dentist believes it is appropriate.
- The dentist should be supported by a dental nurse or equivalent.

The likely outcome should be a ↓ in numbers of GAs for dental procedures, and safer GAs but with a vast ↑ in cost and a major ↑ in hospital workload.

Dental materials

Relevant pages in other chapters   Materials used in endodontics, p. 322.

Principal sources   J. F. McCabe 1998 *Applied Dental Materials*, Blackwell. E. C. Combe 1999 *Dental Biomaterials*, Kluwer.

    Many materials texts list the requirements for an ideal cement, filling material, impression material, etc., and then conclude that it doesn't exist. We will try to resist this temptation.

Properties of dental materials

Definitions

Stress Internal force per unit cross-sectional area acting on the material. Can be classified according to the direction of the force: tensile (stretching), compressive, or shear.

Strain Change in size of a material that occurs in response to a force. It is the change in length divided by the original length.

Yield strength (or elastic limit) The stress beyond which a material is permanently deformed when a force is applied.

Elastic modulus A measure of the rigidity of a material, defined by the ratio of stress to strain (below elastic limit).

Stiffness An indication of how easy it is to bend a piece of material without causing permanent deformation or #. It is dependent upon the elastic modulus, size, and shape of the specimen.

Toughness The amount of energy absorbed up to the point of #. A function of the resilience of the material and its ability to undergo plastic deformation rather than #.

Resilience The energy absorbed by a material undergoing elastic deformation up to its elastic limit.

Hardness Resistance to penetration. A number of hardness scales are in use (e.g. Vickers, Rockwell). Between these scales hardness values are not interchangeable.

Creep The slow plastic deformation that occurs with the application of a static or dynamic force over time.

Wear The abrasion (±chemical) of a substance.

Fatigue When cyclic forces are applied a crack may nucleate and ↑ by small increments each time the force is applied. In time the crack will ↑ to a length at which the force results in # through the remaining material.

Thermal conductivity Ability of a material to transmit heat.

Thermal diffusivity Rate at which temperature changes spread through a material.

Coefficient of thermal expansion The fractional ↑ in length for each degree of temperature ↑.

Wettability Ability of one material to flow across the surface of another, determined by the contact angle between the two materials and influenced by surface roughness and contamination. The contact angle is the angle between solid/liquid and liquid/air interfaces measured through the liquid.

Evaluation of a new material

Before it reaches the dental supply companies a new material should have undergone the following tests:

- *Standard specifications* (i.e. physical properties), e.g. compressive strength, hardness, etc. The actual values obtained are mainly of value in comparing the new material with those already in use and which are performing satisfactorily. Compliance with an international (ISO) standard indicates fitness for dental use.

- *Laboratory evaluation*   Should be relevant to the clinical situation, but this is easier said than done!
- *Clinical trials*   Usually conducted under optimal conditions. Many materials have been less successful under the conditions imposed by clinical practice, particularly those with demanding placement techniques.

Clinically, the important questions to ask the rep include:
- Shelf-life.
- Details of the chemical constituents.
- Handling characteristics, e.g. presentation, mixing, working time, setting time, and dimensional changes on setting.
- Performance in service.
- Cost.
- Does the material meet the relevant ISO standard?

Then decide whether this new material has any significant advantages over the material you are familiar with. Being new doesn't always mean it's better!

Amalgam

An amalgam is a mixture of Hg and another metal. Dental amalgam i
made by mixing together Hg with a powdered silver–tin alloy to produce
plastic mass that can be packed into a preparation before setting. Despite
toxicity scares and the introduction of universal resin composites
amalgam is still widely used, mainly because the use of resin composites in
posterior teeth is not allowed under NHS regulations.

Types of amalgam

There are two ways of classifying amalgam:

Particle shape Can be lathe-cut (irregular), spheroidal, or a mixture of
the two. Spheroidal particles give a more fluid mix which is easy to con
dense, can be carved immediately, and take 3 h to reach occlusal strength
(compared to >6 h for lathe-cut amalgams). Spheroidal amalgams are
preferable for large Class V and pinned restorations.

Particle composition The first (conventional) alloys introduced had a low
copper content (5%). Research showed that the weakest (tin–Hg or
gamma-2) phase of the set amalgam could be eliminated by ↑ the propor
tion of copper, so a variety of high copper (6–25%) amalgams have been
introduced. These are more expensive, but superior in terms of corrosion
resistance, creep, strength, and durability of marginal integrity. There
are two types of high-copper alloy: (1) a single composition alloy of
silver–tin–copper; (2) a blended (dispersion) mix of silver–tin and
copper–silver alloys. Of these, (1) is the most resistant to tarnishing.

Handling characteristics

Mixing or trituration This is carried out mechanically, in one of two ways
1 Pre-encapsulated by manufacturer, with automatic vibrator. The
  preferred method.
2 Using an amalgamator which dispenses Hg and alloy in correct
  proportions and mixes them. However, the amalgamator requires
  re-filling by hand which ↑ likelihood of Hg spillage occurring. The
  duration of trituration varies from 5 to 20 sec.

Condensation Carry out incrementally, either by hand instrument
(lathe-cut or spheroidal) or mechanically (lathe-cut only). Both are equally
effective but the latter is quicker. Preparations should be overfilled so that
the Hg-rich surface layer is removed by carving.

Carving With spherical alloys this can be commenced immediately, but
with lathe-cut a delay of a few minutes is advisable. Burnishing is now back
in vogue.

Polishing Polished amalgams look good, but whether polishing is necessary
is still the subject of debate. **NB** Maximum strength takes 24 h to develop.

Marginal leakage

Whilst amalgam corrosion products will form a marginal seal in time
microleakage can be ↓ by the use of either a conventional cavity varnish

(e.g. Copalite) or a bonding agent (e.g. Amalgam-bond or Panavia-21). The latter (an anaerobic resin adhesive) also bonds to set amalgam.[1] Alternatively, sealing over the completed restoration with a fissure sealant has been suggested, and this is a possible solution to the 'ditched', but caries-free amalgam.

Toxicity

'There is insufficient evidence to justify the claim that Hg from dental amalgam has an adverse effect on the vast majority of patients'.[2] However, recent advice has included avoiding the placement of amalgam fillings during pregnancy.[3]

The greatest risk appears to be related to the inhalation of Hg vapour, ∴ attention should be paid to the following:

- Avoid spilling Hg (p. 728).
- Waste amalgam should be stored in a screw-top bottle under old radiograph (X-ray) fixing solution.
- When removing old amalgams, safety glasses, masks, and high-volume aspiration are a wise precaution.

Types of amalgam

Average composition (%)	Silver	Tin	Copper	Zinc
Conventional	68	28	4	0–2
High copper	60	27	13	0

Types of amalgam currently available

Conventional   Lathe-cut.

Conventional   Spherical.

High-copper dispersion   Lathe + spherical.

High-copper single   Spheroidal.

High-copper single   Lathe-cut.

D. C. Watts 1992 *J. Dent* **20** 245.
B. M. Eley 1993 *BDJ* **175** 161.
Department of Health 1998 Letter no. PL/CDO(98).

Resin composites—constituents and properties

The modern resin composite is a mixture of resin and particulate filler, the handling characteristics of which are determined largely by the size of the particles and method of cure.

Constituents

Resin Most resin composites are based on either Bis-GMA or urethane dimethacrylate plus a diluent monomer, TEGDMA.

Filler Confers the following benefits on the resin composite:
- ↑ compressive length, abrasion resistance, modulus of elasticity, and # toughness.
- ↓ thermal expansion and setting contraction.
- ↑ aesthetic qualities.

Resin composites can be subdivided according to particle size:

Macrofilled (or conventional) Contains particles of radio-opaque barium or strontium glass 2.5–5 μm in size, to give 75–80% by weight of filler. Good mechanical properties, but hard to polish and soon roughens.

Microfilled Contains colloidal silica particles 0.04 μm in size and 30–60% by weight. Retains a good surface polish, but is unsuitable for load-bearing situations, has poor wear resistance, and ↑ contraction shrinkage.

Hybrid Contains a mixture of conventional and microfine particles designed to optimize both mechanical and surface properties. Contains 75–85% by weight of filler.

Most composites are of the hybrid type; however, materials with smaller particles (nanofillers) have recently been introduced.

Initiator/activator
1 Chemically cured: benzoyl peroxide (or sulfinic acid) initiator + tertiary amine activator. **2** Light-cured: amine + ketone activated by blue light (460–70 nm).

Other constituents include pigments, stabilizers, and silane coupler to produce bond between particles and filler.

Important properties of composites
1 Polymerization shrinkage of 1–4%.
2 Thermal expansion is significantly greater than enamel or dentine, and without acid-etch bond can result in marginal leakage.
3 Elastic modulus should be high to resist occlusal forces. Modulus of hybrid type is greater than other resin composites, amalgam, or dentine. However, resin composites are still brittle and # if used in thin section.
4 Wear resistance is greatest in hybrids.
5 Radio-opacity is particularly useful, especially for posterior resin composites.

Resin composites—practical points

Method of polymerization

Chemical (self-cure) No additional equipment required, but mixing of two components introduces porosity and the working time is limited.

Light activation Provides long working time, command set, and better colour stability, but requires a light source, has a limited depth of cure, and the temperature ↑ during setting can be as high as 40°C. Three types of light source are currently available: quartz tungsten halogen (QTH), plasma arc light (PAC), and light-emitting diode (LED). Current evidence suggests that a QTH is the preferred option and that PAC and LED lights confer no advantage at present.

Dual-cure Curing is initiated by a conventional light source, but continues chemically to help ensure polymerization throughout the restoration.

Practical tips
- Replace bulbs every 6–12 months. Some lights correct for the effects of bulb ageing.
- Air attentuates light beam, ∴ position as close to tooth as possible.
- Preparations >2 mm depth should be cured incrementally.
- Precautions are necessary to protect eyes from glare, ∴ use safety specs, get the patient to close their eyes, and the DN to look away. Alternatively, use a hand-held shield or one attached to the light tip.
- Efficiency of light source can be tested by curing a block of composite. Practical depth of cure is half thickness of set material.
- The greater the intensity of the light source the greater the depth of cure.

Finishing Ideally, a mylar strip to produce the contour of the restoration. Then refine with microfine diamond or multi-blades tungsten carbide finishing burs (under water spray), finishing strips, and then polish with aluminium oxide coated discs (Shofu, Soflex). Shofu points or finishing pastes are useful for inaccessible concave surfaces.

Problems with resin composites

1 Difficult to obtain satisfactory contact points and occlusal stops. Modern placement techniques have largely overcome this.
2 Polymerization shrinkage.
3 Depth of cure of light-cured materials is limited. This is a particular problem in posterior teeth.

Indirect composite inlays may circumvent the last two problems (p. 272)

Fissure sealants Composite resins containing little or no filler, which are either self- or light-cured. Clear or opaque types are available, the former having better flow characteristics (whether this is an advantage depends upon the position of the tooth). Success depends upon being able to achieve good moisture control for the acid-etch bond.

Flowable resin composites are now available. They are predominately resin with a reduced % of filler particles, and consequently shrink considerably on curing. Some advocate using them as liners or in the bottom of proximal preparations, but the high shrinkage precludes this. RMGIC is preferable in proximal preparations, which are below the CEJ (bonded-base approach), however, they have a place in the marginal repair of restorations.

Acid-etch technique

Recent research would suggest that:
- Success depends upon adequate moisture control, as contact with saliva for as little as 0.5 sec will contaminate etch pattern.
- A prophylaxis prior to etching is not required unless abundant plaque deposits are present.
- 30–50% buffered phosphoric acid provides the best etch pattern.
- An etching time of 15–20 sec is adequate for both primary and permanent enamel, and 15 sec for dentine is recommended.
- The etch pattern is easily damaged, $\therefore$ using a probe to aid etchant penetration of pits and fissures, or applying etchant by rubbing vigorously with a pledget of cotton wool, is C/I.
- There is no difference in bond strength whether an etchant solution or gel is used. Gels take twice as long to rinse away but have the advantage of greater viscosity and colour contrast.
- Rinse for at least 15 sec.
- Remineralization of etched enamel occurs from the saliva, and after 24 h it is indistinguishable from untreated enamel.
- Etched enamel is porous and has a high surface energy. The etch pattern consists of three zones (from surface inwards):

Etched zone (enamel removed)	10 μm
Qualitative porous zone	20 μm
Quantitative porous zone	20 μm

$\therefore$ composite resin tags may penetrate up to 50 μm into enamel to give micromechanical retention.

NB Many of the newer dentine adhesive systems do not have a separate acid-etch stage. These systems use a combination of acidic primers and bonding resins, either as a single stage or applied separately (Prompt L Pop, ibond, xeno bond).

Dentine-adhesive systems (dentine bonding agents)

The advantages of bonding to dentine (e.g. preservation of tooth tissue) have fuelled considerable research effort. The problems that have had to be overcome include the high water and organic content of dentine; the presence of a 'smear layer' after dentine is cut; and the need for adequate strength immediately following placement, to withstand the polymerization contraction of resin composite. These difficulties have been approached in a number of ways, making the topic of dentine bonding confusing, a situation which has been exacerbated by the pace of new developments and by the claims of the manufacturers.

Indications

- Marginal seal where preparation margin in dentine or cementum, e.g. cervical (Class V), proximal (Class II) box.
- Retention and seal of direct resin-composite restorations.
- Retention and seal of indirect porcelain and composite inlays.
- Dentine adhesives have also been used for repairing # teeth, cementing ceramic crowns and veneers, and as an endodontic sealer.

The smear layer consists of an amorphous layer of organic and inorganic debris, produced by cutting dentine. It ↓ sensitivity by occluding the dentine tubules and prevents loss of dentinal fluid. It purportedly has an ↑ inorganic content compared to dentine. The smear layer is partially or completely removed &/or modified during dentine bonding.

Mechanism of dentine bonding

Most dentine adhesive systems aim to modify and partially remove the smear layer, by the application of an acidic primer. This demineralizes the underlying surface, exposing the collagen and opening up the dentinal tubules. It is important to keep this surface moist to prevent the collagen becoming flattened (for foodie readers: the collagen should resemble *al-dente* spaghetti). This layer is then infiltrated using a resin with bi-functional ends: one hydrophilic end, which is able to bond to wet dentine and one hydrophobic end capable of bonding to the composite resin. In this infiltrated hybrid layer molecular entanglement of the collagen and resin occurs, providing the basis for the bonding system.

Practical points

- Follow manufacturer's instructions.
- For better results use a matched resin-composite and adhesive system.
- When a dentine adhesive is used polymerization shrinkage of resin composite is more likely to result in cuspal deformation and ∴ post-op pain. An incremental filling and curing technique will help to ↓ this problem.

- Pre-curing the adhesive bonding agent before placing the composite ↑ bond strength.[1]
- No technique produces zero microleakage.

For a concise review of adhesive systems, the article by Watson and Bartlett is recommended.[2]

1 J. F. McCabe 1994 *BDJ* **176** 333.
2 T. F. Watson and D. Bartlett 1994 *BDJ* **176** 227.

Glass ionomers—properties and types

Glass ionomer has been officially renamed glass polyalkenoate. However, we have continued with glass inonomer (GI) as abbreviating glass polyalkenoate could lead to confusion with gutta-percha (GP).

Setting reaction
Alumino-silicate glass + polyalkenoic acid → calcium + aluminium poly alkenoates (base + polyacid → polysalt + water).

The set material consists of unreacted spheres of glass surrounded by silicaeous gel, embedded in metal polyalkenoates. Fluoride is released from the cement to give cariostatic properties.

Presentation
1 Powder + liquid.
2 Powder (with anhydrous acid) + water.
3 Encapsulated.

Itaconic acid is added to ↑ rate of set, and tartaric acid to sharpen set. In some products polymaleic acid replaces polyacrylic and one new material is based on polyvinyl phosphoric acid.

Properties
Adhesion To enamel and dentine by: **1** ionic displacement of calcium and phosphate with polyacrylate ions; **2** possible absorption of polyalkenoic acid onto collagen. Some authors recommend pre- conditioning the dentine, e.g. with 10% polyalkenoic acid (GC Dentin Conditioner) for 30 sec. Whether this ↑ adhesion is controversial. GI cement also bonds to the oxide layer on SS and tin.

Cariostatic Due to fluoride release throughout the lifetime of the restoration. GI are also able to take up fluoride when the IO concentration is raised, the 'reservoir effect'. However, the therapeutic benefit of fluoride release has yet to be shown to be effective.

Thermal expansion Similar to enamel and dentine.

Strength Brittle material. Tensile strength is only 40% of resin composite.

Radiolucent Except for the cermets, which are rarely used.

Abrasion resistance Poor, but ↑ all the time, especially with the high viscosity versions.

Biocompatibility This is being questioned following reports of pulpal inflammation when used as a luting cement, but this is not a problem clinically.[1]

Applications
GI are unable to match the aesthetics and abrasion resistance of the resin composites, and brittleness limits their use to non-load-bearing situations. However, their adhesive and fluoride-releasing properties have resulted in a range of applications and matching formulations.

1 R. van Noort (ed.) 1994 *J Dent* **22** 8.

Type I   Luting cements for crowns, bridges, and orthodontic bands.

Type II   Restorative cements. There are two subtypes: (a) aesthetic; (b) reinforced. Can also be used as a fissure sealant, for the restoration of deciduous teeth (p. 84) and for repairing defective restorations.

Type III   Fast-setting lining materials. Defer placement of amalgam for at least 15 min and composite for 4 min. In load-bearing situations or where lining is exposed to the oral environment (e.g. in sandwich technique), use of a type II reinforced cement or RMGIC is preferable.

Type IV   Includes the light-cure and dual-cure GI (use of a light source optimizes the properties of the dual-cure materials, although they will self-polymerize without). It has been suggested that the light-cured GI have higher bond strengths than self-cure GI.[1]

1 C. G. Plant 1988 *BDJ* **165** 54.

Glass ionomers—practical points

Practical tips

- A dry field is essential.
- Encapsulated systems ensure optimal mixing and allow placement via syringe tip, e.g. Ketac-fil.
- Cement should be inserted before its sheen is lost.
- GI sticks to SS, ∴ use powder as a separator.
- Cellulose or soft metal strips provide the best finish.
- Water balance during setting is critical. Absorption of water results in dissolution, and dehydration leads to crazing, ∴ cement must be protected with waterproof varnish (**NB** Copalite is not waterproof). Alternatively, use light-cured bonding resin, which acts as a lubricant for finishing and can then be cured.
- Although most manufacturers claim that trimming can be started 10–15 min after placement, it is better to defer for > 24 h.

Cermets

These are similar to GI, except that the ion-leachable glass is fused with fine silver powder. Mixing with a polymeric acid gives a cement consisting of unreacted glass particles to which silver is fused, held together by a metal–salt matrix.

Properties
- Adhesion to enamel and dentine.
- Radio-opaque.
- ↑ wear resistance compared to GI, but equivalent strength.
- Cariostatic.

Applications   Core build-ups; low-stress-bearing restorations; restoration of deciduous teeth.

Cermets, however, are rarely used and have been largely superseded by the RMGICs.

Resin-modified glass ionomers

These allow 'command' setting and help overcome the moisture sensitivit and low early mechanical strength associated with conventional GI. Th acid–base reaction of GI is supplemented by the addition of ~5% resi (HEMA Bis-GMA). The initial set of the material is due to the formation c a polymerization matrix, which is strengthened by the acid–base reactior They are easier to handle than conventional GI and may be polishe immediately after light-curing. Aesthetics approach those of resin-base materials, plus the advantage of fluoride release.[1] These materials can b used in conjunction with resin composite for placement in deep proxima preparation where the deepest parts of the preparation are below th CEJ. This type of open sandwich restoration fell into disrepute whe restorations were placed with traditional GI cement. The development c RMGICs has improved the technique, with good results reported at 7 yrs.

Compomer

Another recently introduced hybrid material. It combines the adhesive an fluoride-releasing properties of GI with the abrasion resistance of resi composite, with a touch of originality, 'compomer'. Compose of a single hydrophobic resin filled with acid-leachable glass particle Bonded with a bi-functional primer and light-cured. It is claimed that th chemical reaction takes place through uptake of water from saliva leadin to fluoride ions leaching out. It is difficult to think of a situation wher compomer could be used but a resin composite material could not. It hard, therefore, to give specific indications for this group of material except possibly for the restoration of deciduous teeth.

Giomers

This group of materials are more correctly described as resin composite with active filler particles. The filler particles are based on pre-reacte surface or fully reacted GI filler particles, which have been shown to b capable of sustained fluoride release. Possibly useful for high-caries ris individuals.

1 S. K. Sidhu 1995 *Dental Update* **10** 429.
2 J. W. van Diijken 1999 **78** 1319.

Cements

Used for a variety of purposes, including temporary dressings, preparatio liners, and as luting agents. With the exception of calcium hydroxide, th materials available are based on combinations of:

Powder Zinc oxide or fluorine-containing aluminosilicate glass (th releases fluoride and is stronger than zinc oxide).

Liquid Phosphoric acid (irritant) or eugenol (↑ solubility, obtunden or polyalkenoic acid (adhesive).

Setting occurs by an acid–base reaction. The set cement comprise cores of unreacted powder in a matrix of reaction products.

Now thought that the ability of a cement to prevent microleakage more important than its setting pH.

Based on zinc oxide eugenol (ZOE)

ZOE Powder of pure zinc oxide is mixed (in a ratio of 3:1) with eugen liquid to give zinc eugenolate and unreacted powder. Setting time is 24 l This is the weakest cement, but the eugenol acts as an obtundent an analgesic, ∴ it is useful as a temporary dressing, but not for RCT as no sea

Accelerated ZOE, e.g. Sedanol. Addition of zinc acetate to the powde ↓ setting time to 5 min.

Resin-bonded ZOE, e.g. Kalzinol. Addition of 10% hydrogenated resi to the powder ↑ strength.

EBA, e.g. Staline, Opotow. Addition of ortho-ethoxybenzoic aci (62%) to the liquid ↑ strength.

Zinc phosphate, e.g. De Treys Zinc. The powder consists of zinc an magnesium oxides, and the liquid 50% aqueous phosphoric acid. Th working time is ↑ by adding the powder in small increments. Popul because of its strength. Although its low setting pH theoretically C/I its us for vital teeth, in practice this does not seem to be a problem.

Zinc polycarboxylate, e.g. Poly-F, Durelon. The powder is a mixture c zinc and magnesium oxides and the liquid is 40% aqueous polyacrylic aci Recently, anhydrous acid formulations have been introduced, which ar mixed with water. The powder should be added quickly to the liquid. Th temptation to remove excess cement should be resisted until it has reache a rubbery stage. Adheres to dentine, enamel, tin, and SS.

Calcium hydroxide Chemically curing types comprise two pastes whic are mixed together in equal quantities. One paste contains the calciu hydroxide plus fillers in a non-reacting carrier, and the other polysalicyla fluid. The set material consists of an amorphous calcium disalicyla complex plus calcium hydroxide and has a pH of 11. In addition to bei bacteriostatic, calcium hydroxide can induce mineralization of adjace pulp. Light-cured formulations which are resin-based are available. Have bactericidal properties, but ↑ strength.

Gl (p. 674) This and RMGIC are the preferred luting cements for ca indirect restorations.

Strength Phosphate > EBA or polycarboxylate > resin-bonded ZOE accelerated ZOE > calcium hydroxide.

Practical points
- Generally, the thicker the mix, the greater the strength.
- Heat ↓ setting time, ∴ a cooled slab is advisable.
- To stop cement sticking to the instruments during placement, dip in cement powder (except calcium hydroxide) or use non-stick instruments.
- When luting, apply cement to crown or inlay before tooth.

Choice of cement

Temporary restorations Choice depends upon how long the dressing needs to last and whether any therapeutic qualities are required. Pure ZOE is useful for a tooth with a reversibly inflamed pulp, but resin-bonded ZOE is stronger. GI is preferable for semi-permanent dressings and because it seals the preparation margins.

Luting cement Zinc phosphate, GI, and polycarboxylate are all popular as luting cements. EBA cement is C/I because of ↑ solubility. Composite-based luting systems are available, which are often used in conjunction with dentine adhesive systems. Mandatory for cementing ceramic or porcelain inlays/onlays and ceramic veneers.

Lining cement Choice of lining depends upon the depth of the preparation and the material being used to restore it.

    Amalgam Minimal: preparation sealer (Gluma Desensitiser); moderate: RMGIC (vitrebond); deep: use a sub-lining of calcium hydroxide (direct or indirect pulp capping) and any of the cements listed above. Typically RMGIC is recommended as it seals as well as lines the preparation.

    Resin Composite Dentine adhesive system with direct or indirect pulp capping as indicated.

Pulp capping Hard-setting calcium hydroxide.

Sedative dressing ZOE &/or calcium hydroxide.

Bacteriostatic dressing Calcium hydroxide plus GI (stepwise excavation).

Impression materials

Classification

Non-elastic	Elastic	
Plaster	*Elastomers*	*Hydrocolloid*
Compound	Silicone	Reversible
ZOE paste	Polysulfide	Irreversible
Wax	Polyether	

Elastomers

Indicated when accuracy is paramount, e.g. crown and bridge work, an implants.

Condensation-cured silicone, e.g. Xantopren, Optosil. This material is relatively cheap compared with other elastomers, but prone to some shrinkag and should be cast immediately. Addition-cured silicones are preferred.

Addition-cured silicone, e.g. Aquasil, President, Dimension. This type c silicone is very stable, which means that impressions can be posted c stored prior to casting. A perforated tray is advisable as the adhesive supplied are not very effective. Up to five viscosities are manufactured allowing a range of impression techniques. **NB** Powdered latex glove (now rarely used) can retard setting of putty materials.[1]

Polysulfide, e.g. Permalastic. Messy to handle, but useful when a lon working time is required. Use with a special tray and, although stable, cas within 24 h. Not recommended.

Polyether, e.g. Impregum. Popular because it uses a single mix and a stoc tray (and smells of gin and tonic). The set material is stiff, and remova can be stressful in cases with deep undercuts or advanced periodontiti Absorbs water, ∴ do not store with alginate impressions. Can cause allergi reactions. Routinely used for implant cases and crown and bridgeworl especially when there are multiple preps.

Hydrocolloids

Reversible hydrocolloid is accurate, but liable to tear. Requires the purchas of a water bath.

Irreversible hydrocolloid (alginate) Setting is a double decompositio reaction between sodium alginate and calcium sulphate. Popular becaus it is cheap and can be used with a stock tray. However, it is not sufficient accurate for crown and bridge work. Impressions must be kept damp an cast within 24 h. Alginate can retard the setting of gypsum and affect th surface of the model.

Impression compound

Available in either sheet form for recording preliminary impressions, or i stick form for modifying trays. The sheet material is softened in a wate with warm water (55–60°C) and used in a stock tray to record edentulou ridges. The viscosity of compound results in a well-extended impressior but limited detail. Admix impression material (mix of greenstick and impression compound) is useful for denture cases with severe resorption.

Impression waxes

(E.g. Korecta) Produced in four grades. The very soft (orange) type is useful for the correction of small imperfections in ZOE impressions, or for recording -/P free-end saddles.

Zinc oxide pastes

Dispensed 1:1 and mixed to give an even colour. Used for recording edentulous ridges in a special tray or the patient's existing dentures, but C/I for undercuts. Setting time is ↓ by warmth and humidity.

Impression techniques

(For crown and bridge work)

► Time spent recording a good impression is an investment, as repeating lab work is costly.

Special trays Help the adaptation of impression material and ↓ the amount required, i.e. ↑ accuracy and ↓ cost. Can be made in cold-cure acrylic, or light-activated tray resin. Special trays are rarely used for crown and bridgework impressions, with stock trays used routinely.

For crown and bridge work an accurate impression of the prepared teeth is required. Usually the palate does not need to be included, so design the special tray accordingly or use a lower stock tray. For the opposing arch alginate in a stock tray will suffice.

Monophase technique (e.g. polyether) The same mix of medium-viscosity material is used for both a stock tray and syringe. Although less accurate than other methods, it is adequate for most tasks.

Double-mix technique (e.g. polysulfide, addition-cured silicone) A single-stage technique necessitating the mixing of heavy- and light-bodied materials at the same time, and use of a special or stock tray.
- Apply adhesive to tray.
- Mix light- and heavy-bodied viscosities simultaneously for 45–60 sec.
- Remove retraction cord or preferably leave in place and dry preparation, while DN loads syringe with light-bodied material.
- Syringe light-bodied mix around prep. A gentle stream of air helps to direct material into crevice.
- Position tray containing heavy-bodied material.
- Support tray with light pressure until 2 min after apparent set.

Putty and wash technique (e.g. silicone) The putty and light-bodied viscosities can be used with a stock tray, either:
1 *Single-stage* Similar to the double-mix technique above, or
2 *Two-stage* This involves taking an impression of the prep with the putty, using a polythene sheet as a spacer. This is then relined with the light-bodied material, which is also syringed around the prep. The trend is, however, away from putty wash towards monophase or a double-mix technique.

Cost In decreasing order:
- addition-cured silicone using putty/reline;
- polyether with special tray;
- addition-cured silicone using double mix and special tray;
- polysulfide with special tray;
- condensation-cured silicone using putty/reline;
- hydrocolloid.

Automixing dispensers This double-cartridge presentation is exceptionally popular. The two pastes are extruded and mixed in the nozzle when the trigger is pressed. Appears expensive, but ↓ waste and the mixture is void free. Many manufacturers are now producing their materials in this format.

Disinfection of impressions

Impressions should be rinsed to remove debris and then immersed in a solution of sodium hypochlorite (1000 ppm available chlorine) for 10 min.

Casting alloys

An alloy is a mixture of two or more metallic elements. The chemistry of alloys is too complicated for this book (and its authors), so for a fuller understanding the reader is referred to one of the source texts.

The properties of an alloy depend upon:
- The thermal treatments applied to the alloy (including cooling).
- The mechanical manipulation of the alloy.
- The composition of the alloy.

NB The properties of an alloy may differ significantly from that of its constituents.

The main examples of alloys in dentistry include amalgam (p. 664), steel burs and instruments, metallic denture bases, inlays, crowns and bridges, and orthodontic wires.

Casting alloys

A warm moist mouth provides the ideal environment for corrosion. To overcome this problem, dental casting alloys comprise an essentially corrosion-resistant metal (usually gold), with the addition of other constituents to enhance its properties. However, with the exception of titanium all have the potential to affect hypersensitive individuals.

Additions to gold alloys Copper ↓ density, ↓ melting point, ↑ strength and hardness, but ↓ corrosion resistance.

  Silver ↑ hardness and strength, but ↑ tarnishing and ↑ porosity.

  Platinum ↑ melting point, ↑ corrosion, and ↑ tarnish resistance.

  Palladium Similar properties to platinum, but less expensive.

  Zinc or indium Scavenger, preventing oxidation of other metals during melting and casting.

Dental casting gold alloys Noble metal (gold, platinum, palladium, iridium) content must >75%; 65% must be gold. Four types are defined by proof stress and elongation values from type I (low strength for castings subject to low stress) to type IV (extra-high strength).

Dental casting semi-precious alloys Have 25–74% noble metal content. Four types are defined by proof stress and elongation properties.

  Silver palladium Palladium (>25%), silver, gold, indium, and zinc. Cheaper than gold alloys and of equivalent hardness, but less ductile, more difficult to cast, and prone to porosity.

  Nickel chromium 75% nickel, 20% chromium. Used in crowns and bridge work. In latter ↑ rigidity compared to gold alloys is an advantage. However castings are less accurate than gold, and nickel sensitivity can C/I its use.

  Cobalt chromium 35–65% cobalt, 20–35% chromium. Modulus of elasticity twice that of type IV gold alloys. A good polish is difficult to achieve, but durable. Used mainly for P/-.

  Titanium Good biocompatibility; used exclusively for implants. Pure titanium casting is still being perfected.

Alloys for porcelain bonding

Requirements:
- Higher melting point than porcelain.
- Similar coefficient of thermal expansion to porcelain.
- Won't discolour the porcelain.
- High modulus of elasticity to avoid flexure and # of porcelain.

Indium is usually added to facilitate bonding to porcelain. Copper is C/I as it discolours the porcelain. A matched alloy and porcelain should be used.

High gold ↑ palladium or platinum content (to ↑ melting point) compared to non-porcelain alloys.

Medium gold 50% gold, 30% palladium. Widely used.

Silver palladium Cheap, but care required to avoid casting defects.

Nickel chromium Very high melting point and modulus of elasticity, but casting more difficult. **NB** Some patients are sensitive to nickel.

Casting

For gold (melting point <950°C)
- Wax pattern and sprue are invested in gypsum bonded material.
- Wax burnt out by slowly heating investment mould to 450°C.
- Alloy melted either by gas/air torch or electric induction heating and cast with centrifugal force.
- Casting allowed to cool to below red-heat.
- Quenched. Some alloys are used as cast and others heat-hardened.
- Cleaned with ultrasonics and acid immersion.

For nickel chromium and cobalt chromium alloys (melting points 1200–1500°C), need silica or phosphate bonded investment and either oxyacetylene torch or electric induction heating.

Casting faults A casting may be:
- dimensionally inaccurate;
- have a rough surface;
- be porous, contaminated, or incomplete.

Wrought alloys

Wrought alloys are hammered, rolled, drawn, or bent into the desired shape when they are solid.

Stainless steel Steel is an alloy of iron and carbon. The addition of chromium (> 12%) produces a passive surface oxide layer which gives SS its name. The SS used in dentistry is also known as austenitic steel (because the crystals are arranged in a face-centred cubic structure) or 18:8 steel (due to the chromium and nickel content). Available as:

1 Pre-formed sheets for denture bases. The SS is swaged onto the model by explosive or hydraulic pressure. This produces a thin (0.1 mm), light denture base resistant to #. Rarely used today.

2 Wires are produced by drawing the SS through dies of ↓ diameter until the desired size is achieved. This work-hardens the wire, but heat treatments are carried out to give soft, hard, or extra-hard forms. Manipulation of SS wire also work-hardens the wire in the plane of bending, ∴ trying to correct a bend is more likely to result in #. Main applications are orthodontics and partial denture clasps. SS can be welded and soldered.

Soldering SS Requires use of a flux (e.g. Easy-flo flux) to remove the passive oxide layer (this reforms after soldering). The ↓ part of the flame should be used, but do not overheat as this can anneal and soften the components.

- Melt a small bead of low fusing silver solder (e.g. Easy-flo solder) onto the wire.
- Mix up the flux with water to a thick paste and apply to the item to be added.
- Heat up the solder so that wire underneath is a cherry red.
- Bring the fluxed wire into the molten solder and remove the flame at the same time.

This is not easy and requires practice, which explains the popularity of electrical soldering.

Cobalt chromium Has a similar composition to the cast form (p. 688).

Cobalt chromium nickel Used in orthodontics as an archwire material (Elgiloy). It has the advantage that it can be hardened by heat treatment after being formed. Also used for post fabrication in post and core crowns (Wiptam wire).

Titanium Pure titanium is used in implant systems.

Titanium alloys Nickel and titanium alloy (nitinol) is useful in orthodontics as it is flexible, has good springback, and is capable of applying small forces over a long period of time. However, it is not easy to bend without #. Titanium molybdenum alloy (TMA) is also used for archwires and has properties midway between SS and nitinol.

Gold Expense limits the application of wrought gold alloys to partial denture clasp fabrication.

lloys for dentures

st cobalt chromium is the material of choice for partial denture connect-
s because of its high proof stress and modulus of elasticity: thin castings
e strong, rigid, and lightweight. Although wrought gold alloys are more
table for clasps, the advantage of being able to cast connector and clasps
one means that cobalt chromium is more commonly used (p. 340). Be
are of nickel allergy.

Ceramics—dental porcelain

Ceramics are simple compounds of both metallic and non-metallic oxide Although many of the materials used in dentistry are ceramics, the term commonly used to refer to porcelain and its derivatives. Dental porcel actually more closely resembles a glass, and comprises feldspar, qua (for strength and translucency), and kaolin (for strength and colour), p pigments. Most dental porcelain is reinforced with alumina partic (40–50% by mass) to provide greater strength. Unfortunately, this ↑ t opacity, ∴ the proportion of alumina in enamel porcelains is ↓. Duri construction of a PJC a platinum matrix is laid down on the die produc from the impression of the prepared tooth to act as a base. The porcela powder is mixed with water to form a slurry, which is built-up in laye onto the foil until the desired shape is achieved. The porcelain is co pacted by removing water from the preparation by blotting with absorbe paper or by flicking with a brush. This ↓ firing shrinkage. The crown is th fired to ↓ porosity, which ↑ strength and ↑ translucency. Glazing produc a glossy outer skin which resists cracking and plaque accumulation. It c be added as a separate layer or by firing at a higher temperature after t addition of surface glazes. The platinum foil lining is removed prior cementation to give space for the cement lute.

Other ceramic crowns are built-up on a refractory die (dentine-bond crowns), heat-processed core (Empress), or computer-generated sinter core (Procera).

Properties
- Firing shrinkage 30–40%, ∴ crown must be overbuilt.
- Chemically inert provided the surface layer is intact.
- Low thermal conductivity.
- Good aesthetic properties.
- Brittle. The main cause of failure is crack propagation which almost invariably emanates from the unglazed inner surface. This can be ↓ by (1) fusion of the inner surface to metal, as in the platinum foil and metal-bonded techniques; or (2) by the use of an aluminous porcelain core
- High resistance to wear.
- Glazed surface resists plaque accumulation.

Ceramics—practical applications

Porcelain jacket crown Now considered somewhat old-fashioned. A co of aluminous porcelain is laid down first, onto which 'dentine' and the 'enamel' porcelains are built up. For strength a minimum porcelain thic ness of 0.8 mm is required and a 90° butt joint at the margin.

Porcelain fused to metal crown The porcelains used for bonding to a met substrate have additional alkali oxides added to ↑ the coefficient thermal expansion to almost match the alloys used. Also, a porcela which fuses below the melting point of the alloy is required. Bonding the metal occurs by a combination of:
- mechanical retention;
- chemical bonding to the metal oxide layer on the surface of the alloy.

The ↑ strength of porcelain bonded to metal crowns is due to:
- the metal substructure supporting the porcelain;
- ↓ crack propagation by bonding the inner surface of the porcelain to metal;
- the outer surface of porcelain being under tension, thus ↓ crack propagation.

Glass ceramic or castable ceramics Semi-crystalline glasses, e.g. tetrasilic fluormica glass (Dicor), produced by adding a nucleating agent onto whic the glass crystals precipitate during cooling. This structure resists crac propagation, having a similar strength to core aluminous porcelain. A additional advantage is that the lost wax process can be used, so compe sation for firing shrinkage is not required. A wax pattern is built-up by th technician and invested and cast. Following cooling, the casting is reheate to allow crystal growth to occur. The castable ceramics have ↑ transl cency compared to porcelain, but dentine colour has to be created wit surface glazes, which requires time and skill. Glass ceramic crowns ar more expensive than PJC, but useful for young translucent teeth. Ho pressed (IPS-Empress I and II) and glass infiltrated (Inceram) ceramics d not match the strength of porcelain fused to metal.

All ceramic systems now also include flame-sprayed (Techceram) CAD-CAM (Procera) alumina cores onto which conventional porcelai are fired.

Porcelain veneers A thin shell of porcelain or castable ceramic ~0.5–0.8 m thick (p. 292). Their thin section limits their ability to hide underlying toot discoloration.

Porcelain inlays Promising alternative to conventional treatment pro cedures. Only limited long-term studies available.

Porcelain repairs Can be carried out using composite and a silane couplir agent. A number of proprietary kits (Cojet) are available.

Denture materials—1

Acrylic resin

Acrylic is the most commonly used polymer for denture bases. Not or can it be re-lined, repaired, and added to comparatively easily, but it is al aesthetic and lightweight. Acrylic is composed of a chain of methacryla molecules linked together to give PMMA.

Presentation Usually comprises a liquid and a powder mixed togeth The liquid is stored in a dark bottle to ↑ shelf-life.

Powder	Liquid
PMMA beads (< 100 mm)	Methylmethacrylate monomer
Initiator, e.g. benzoyl peroxide	Cross-linking agent
Pigments &/or fibres	Inhibitor, e.g. hydroquinone
	activator (self-cure only)

Manipulation The powder and liquid should be mixed in a ratio of ~2.! by weight. The mix passes through several distinct stages: sandy-strin dough-rubbery-hard (set).

The dough stage is the best for handling and packing.

In denture fabrication the wax pattern and teeth are invested in plaste The wax is then boiled out and the plaster coated with sodium alginate a separator. The resultant space is then filled to excess (to allow for co traction shrinkage of 7%) with acrylic dough under pressure. The acrylic then polymerized.

Mode of activation

Self-cure acrylics show less setting contraction, but more water absor tion than heat-cure. This may result in the final item being slightly over-size thus ↓ retention. Self-cure acrylics are more porous, only 80% as stror less resistant to abrasion, and contain a greater level of unreacted monom compared to heat-cure. The main applications of self-cure acrylics are f denture repairs and re-lines, and orthodontic appliances, although for th latter the greater strength of heat-cure is preferable.

Heat-cure Conventionally polymerization requires heating in a ho water bath for 7 h at 70°C, then 3 h at 100°C. The flask should be coole slowly to minimize stresses within the acrylic. However, resins with d ferent curing cycles (fast heat-cure) are now available. Microwave ener can be used to cure acrylic resin, but (apart from lunchtime) has no adva tage over a water bath.

Light-cure resins are supplied as mouldable sheets. Used for dentu bases or special trays.

Properties

- The glass transition (or softening) temperature of self-cure acrylic is 90°C, and for heat-cure 105°C.
- Poor impact strength and low resistance to fatigue #.
- Abrasion resistance not very good, but usually adequate.
- Good thermal insulator—undesirable as it can lead to the patient swallowing foods which are too hot.
- Low specific gravity (i.e. not too heavy).

Radiolucent. Attempts to ↑ radio-opacity have not been very successful.

Absorbs water, resulting in expansion. Drying out of acrylic should be avoided.

Residual monomer (due to inadequate curing) weakens acrylic and can cause sensitivity reaction.

Good aesthetics.

e strength of a denture depends upon:

Design, e.g. adequate thickness, avoidance of notches.

Strength of the acrylic, i.e. low monomer content, ↓ porosity, adequate curing. Can be ↑ by using high-impact resin.

searchers are still evaluating methods of ↑ strength of denture resins. The dition of high-performance fibres (e.g. glass fibres) appears promising ick Tech).

Denture materials—2

Rebasing

Rebasing a denture base involves replacement of the fitting surfac. Rebases can be either:

1 Hard: heat or self-cure.
2 Soft: permanent: heat, self-cure, or light-cure.
       temporary (a) tissue conditioner: self-cure.
                      (b) functional impression material: self-cure.

The properties of self-cure materials are generally inferior, ∴ should on be used as a temporary measure.

Hard rebases   Heat-cure PMMA is preferred, but requires the patient do without the denture while it is being added. A self-cure material h obvious advantages: heat, but even the higher acrylics, e.g. butylmethacryla (Peripheral seal) should only be used as a temporary measure as they a weaker than PMMA and discolour.

Soft liners   require a material with a glass transition temperature belo or at that of the mouth so that it is soft and resilient. The majority of so liners are either based on silicone or acrylic (polyethylmethacrylate PMMA powder plus alkyl methacrylate monomer and a plasticizer), b the recently introduced polyphosphazene fluoroelastomer liners lo promising.[1]

Plasticized acrylic	Silicone polymers
Good bond to denture	Bond with denture base not reliable
Harden over time	Maintain resilience
More readily distorted	Absorb water: candida colonization
	More elastic

Heat, light, or self-cure types are available. The self-cure materials ha inferior properties, but all require replacement during the lifetime of th denture.[2] Cleaning, p. 362.

Tissue conditioners   usually comprise powdered polyethylmethacrylate which a plasticizing mix of esters and alcohol is added. No chemical rea tion takes place, the liquids merely soften the powder to form a gel a leach out over time, resulting in hardening. To ensure maximum tiss recovery the lining should be a minimum thickness of 2 mm and replac every few days. E.g. Coe-soft, Coe-comfort, Viscogel. Cleaning, p. 362.

Functional impression materials   The tissue-conditioning materials a usually used for this purpose, an impression being cast of the fitting surfac after a few days of wear.

1 F. Kawano 1992 *J Prosthet Dent* **68** 368.
2 E. R. Dootz 1993 *J Prosthet Dent* **69** 114.

Biocompatibility of dental materials

Before a new material can be marketed it must successfully pass both laboratory and clinical trials to evaluate its biocompatibility. Yet, some adverse effects only become apparent after the material has been in clinical use. Unless used with care many materials may prove a hazard to the patient or the dentist and his staff.

Hazards to the patient

Systemic Effects

Allergic reactions
- *Amalgam* Although genuine cases of amalgam allergy exist, these are rarer than the tabloid press would suggest. For proven cases resin composite or cast restorations should be used.
- *Nickel* Constituent of some alloys can cause contact eczema. Sensitive patients often have a history of allergy to jewellery or watch casings. Alternative alloys are available.
- *Acrylic monomer* Can cause an allergic reaction and should be considered in a patient complaining of a 'burning mouth'. The concentration of monomer is ↑ in poorly cured acrylic and greater in self- than heat-cure. Extended curing, e.g. 24 h, may ↓ concentration of monomer to an acceptable level; if not a cobalt chrome or SS denture base will be required.
- *Epimine* In polyether impression material.

If an allergy is suspected, refer to a dermatologist.

Directly toxic
- Beryllium, present in some nickel alloys, is known to be a carcinogen. Provided the alloy is not ground any risks are confined to the production laboratory. Beryllium-free alloys are becoming ↑ available.
- Fluoride in excess can be toxic (p. 32).

Ingestion or inhalation of air-borne dust must be avoided.

Local Effects
Eye damage Curing lamps can cause eye damage due to the glare. The simplest solution is to ask the patient to close their eyes and use a shield.

Thermal injury Can result: **1** to the pulp, e.g. caused by exothermic setting reactions; **2** to the mucosa, e.g. caused by dentures which are thermal insulators, as the patient may swallow drink/food that is too hot, or by the setting reaction of self-cure denture re-line materials; **3** to the soft tissues, e.g. by hot instruments.

Chemical injury Can be caused by noxious chemicals (e.g. etchant, hydrogen peroxide) being allowed to come into direct contact with the tissues.

Hypersensitivity reactions Can occur in response to the materials that cause systemic allergy.

Hazards to staff
In the surgery
- Allergic reactions, e.g. topical anaesthetics, latex gloves, methyl methacrylate monomer, dentine adhesive systems.

- Eye damage from light sources. Use eye protection or shielding.
- Alginate dust.
- Mercury vapour.
- Nitrous oxide.

In the laboratory

- Cyanide solution for electroplating.
- Vapours from low-fusing metal dies.
- Silicaeous particles in investment materials.
- Fluxes containing fluoride.
- Hydrofluoric acid used for etching porcelain veneers.
- Beryllium in some alloys.
- PMMA powders.
- Methyl methacrylate monomer.
- Casting machines.

Law and ethics

Relevant pages in other chapters   Hiring and firing staff, p. 726.

Principal sources   J. Seear 1991 *Law and Ethics in Dentistry*, Wright. GDC 2001 *Maintaining Standards*. BDA 2000 *Ethics in Dentistry*.

Definitions

Claimant   (or in Scotland, **pursuer**) The claimant in a civil action.

Defendant   (or **defender**) The person against whom a claim is made.

Legislation   The law laid down in Acts of Parliament.

Secondary legislation   The precise implementation of the general rules laid down in the Act (often published as Statutory Instruments).

Litigation   An action brought in a court of law.

Claim form   A document setting out the details of a proposed action, which is served to the defendant.

Affidavit   A written statement on oath.

Serious professional misconduct   Action or omission by a professional person which would be regarded as disgraceful or dishonourable by reputable colleagues. Examples of professional misconduct include fraud, indecent assault, and breaches of the Terms of Service.

▶ *On qualification*: (1) Register with the GDC (p. 718); (2) Join a defence organization (p. 714). Consider taking out sickness and accident insurance.

Legal processes

In England

Civil law in general, governs the rights and obligations between individual and corporations, e.g. debt recovery, breaches of contract, negligence. It i also concerned with the function of the State and of public authorities. I civil cases, the verdict is given on the balance of probabilities, i.e. each side argues their case and the decision is given to the version that is most likel to be true. The losing party is liable for the costs of both sides.

Depending upon financial value, cases are allocated to :
1 Small claims track: <£5000 (personal injury <£1000).
2 Fast track: <£15 000 (personal injury £1000–15 000).
3 Multi track: >£15 000.
4 County Court: <£15 000.
5 High Court: >£15 000.

Appeals are referred to the Court of Appeal (civil division) and, occasionally to the House of Lords.

Criminal law   Criminal prosecutions are undertaken when the 'law' ha been broken, e.g. speeding, fraud, assault. In criminal law, the case mus be proved beyond reasonable doubt. Depending upon the severity of the misdemeanour cases are heard in:
1 Magistrates' court. Appeals to Crown Court.
2 Crown Court (with a judge and jury). Appeals go to the Court of Appeal (criminal division).

Coroner's Court   This straddles the two systems and meets to conside unnatural and unexpected deaths, e.g. a death in the dental chair. The process is investigative (as opposed to the claimant versus defendan stance taken in the other courts).

In Scotland

In parallel with many European countries, criminal prosecutions are brought by the Procurator Fiscal, who, in addition to prosecuting ir the Sheriff and District courts, also fulfils a role similar to that of Coroner The nomenclature of the courts in Scotland is quite different from that o England.[1] Another disparity between the two systems is that in crimina cases in Scotland, an additional verdict of 'not proven' is possible. Ir Scotland there is no Coroner's Court, but in the event of an unnatura death in the dental surgery, a Fatal Accident Inquiry may be heard before a sheriff.

▶ Any unexpected death should be reported to the Coroner in England Wales, and N. Ireland, or to the Procurator Fiscal in Scotland, eithe directly or through the police (the Registrar of Deaths will notify the authorities if this has not already been done).

Dentists are no longer automatically exempt from jury service. It is possible to apply for exemption (using the form sent with the summons).

---

1 BDA Advice Sheet 2000 *Giving Evidence*.

Complaints[1]

The present NHS complaints procedure (currently under review) was introduced in April 1996 with the aim of ↓ bureaucracy and resolving complaints in their early stages (at a practice/hospital level).[2] The system also separates complaints from disciplinary procedures, and is the same for both clinical and non-clinical complaints. A complaints procedure for private treatment is under consideration by the GDC.

Every practice/hospital is required to have a:
- nominated complaints administrator;
- complaints procedure available on request (e.g. notices; leaflets);
- method of recording all complaints.

Time limits

Complaints must be made <6 months after the event or <6 months after the complainant realizes there was a problem, provided this is <12 months after the incident. Where a good case can be made, this latter time bar may be extended.

Stages

Local resolution   Once a complaint (oral or written) is received:
- At least an initial acknowledgement of receipt (if not a full explanation) is given. In practice sphere this must be in <2 working days.
- Where applicable an investigation is carried out.
- A written reply is sent to complainant: dental/medical practice in <10 (hospital <20) working days.

Independent review panel   can be sought by the patient if they are still dissatisfied, provided 'local' procedure has been exhausted. The Primary Care Trust/Board/Hospital Trust will appoint a Convenor who will decide (in <20 working days) whether a panel should be convened, or if further local resolution is appropriate. Review panel comprises Convenor and two independent members. For clinical complaints the panel will sit with two independent clinical assessors. Written report is sent to parties involved and the PCT/Board who will decide if any service improvements are to be recommended.

Healthcare Commission (HC)   In England, under new regulations introduced in July 2004, the independent review panel is replaced by the right to appeal to the HC. The HC staff will undertake the investigation, with expert advisors if necessary. Complainant has right to appeal to independent panel of 3 lay people from list held by HC.

NHS Ombudsman   If the complainant is still not satisfied, he can go to the Ombudsman.

Disciplinary procedures

If, following the instigation of a complaint and the report of an Independent Review Panel, the PCT/Board decides a dentist is in breach of their Terms of Service they can decide to remove him from their list or,

---

1 BDA Advice Sheet (B10) 1998 *Handling complaints*.
2 NHS (Complaints) Regulations 2004, Dept. of Health.

fer the matter to another PCT/Board for further investigation or, if
plicable, to a professional body or the police.

Where the breach of Terms of Service does not concern a patient's
mplaint the matter may be referred to another PCT/Board who will
t up a Disciplinary Committee with a legally qualified chairperson, two
y, and two dentally qualified members. A written report is sent to the
ferring PCT/Board, who will decide if any action is required. A dentist
n appeal against the report of a Disciplinary Committee.

mplaint by a GDP to recover unpaid fees There are two approaches to
s: (1) issue a County Court Summons (the Citizen's Advice Bureau have
 explanatory leaflet), or (2) employ a debt-collection agency. The latter
considerably easier.

mplaint by GDP against GDP The Local Dental Committee may be asked
 arbitrate. Advice can also be sought from the defence organizations.

Further advice is available in the BDA's Advice Sheet on Dental
sciplinary Committees.

Consent

► Treatment without any consent = assault.
► Treatment with general consent, but without explanation of what involved may = negligence.

It is a general legal and ethical principle that valid consent must b obtained before starting treatment, a physical investigation, or providin personal care, for a patient. To be valid, consent should be 'informed', i. the patient should understand the treatment to be carried out (and an aftercare or precautions necessary) and be made aware of any alternativ forms of treatment. An explanation of commonly occuring risks or sid effects should be given, but these should be put in context.[1, 2]

Consent can be given in writing, verbally, or be implied.

Consent should always be obtained by a clinician who can explain th risks and benefits of treatment—not by auxiliary staff.

Written consent Preferable, especially when extensive treatment planned and essential before a GA is given. However, a signature on consent form does not itself prove the consent is valid: the form simp records the patient's decision and that the consenting process has take place.

Verbal consent Should be the minimum obtained for treatment. Th benefits of having a third party present at all times are obvious.

Implied consent By attending an appointment and sitting in the dental cha a patient gives implied consent to a dental examination (but not treatment).

Consent for children

Those aged 16 and 17 are presumed to have the competence to giv consent for themselves. Younger children who understand fully what involved in the proposed procedure can also give consent (although the parents will ideally be involved). In other cases, someone with parent responsibility must give consent on the child's behalf, unless they cann be reached in an emergency. If a competent child consents to treatment, parent cannot override that consent (the 'Gillick competence' principle Legally, a parent can consent if a competent child refuses, but it is like that taking such a serious step will be rare. For children in care consult a authorized representative of the local authority.

Consent for adults who are not competent to give consent

No-one can give consent on behalf of an incompetent adult. Howeve you may still treat such a patient if the treatment would be in their be interests. People close to the patient may be able to give you informatic on some of these factors. Where the patient has never been competen relatives, carers, and friends may be best placed to advise on the patient needs and preferences. If an incompetent patient has clearly indicate in the past, while competent, that they would refuse treatment in certa

---

1 Department of Health, 2001, *12 key points on consent: The law in England*.
2 Department of Health, 2001, *Reference guide to consent for examination or treatment*.

circumstances (an 'advance refusal'), and those circumstances arise, you must abide by that refusal.

Some specific problems
- Treatment of an unconscious patient is valid under the legal doctrine of 'necessity', but is limited to emergency care.
- If a patient's photographs are to be used for a lecture or presentation, written consent should be obtained.

Contracts

A contract is defined as an agreement between parties and can be either verbal or written. In law, both are equally binding, but as the parties may have differing recollections of what was said, the advantages of a written agreement are apparent.

Between dentist and patient Although in the past the majority of contracts were made verbally (as with consent), a written treatment plan and charge estimate which is signed by the patient puts the NHS contract between dentist and patient on a firmer legal footing. Once the time limits for Service Committee complaints are past an NHS form can be thrown away unless it covers private treatment when it would be advisable to retain it for longer. For purely private patients it is wise to draw up a simple type written contract setting out the treatment to be done and the fee agreed.

Legally, the dentist is expected to exercise a reasonable degree of care while the patient also has a duty to keep appointments and pay the agreed fee.

Between dentist and PCT or Health Board A dentist working within the GDS is in contract with this body for every patient accepted for treatment under the NHS Terms and Conditions of Service. Breaches of this contract are investigated by a Disciplinary Committee and, if applicable, the clinical freedom of the dentist may be restricted or a fine levied.

Between principals and associates, or between partners Because of the importance these should be written with the help of a solicitor. The BDA (address p. 780) has sample agreements for partnerships, assistantships, associateships, and for expense-sharing arrangements, and in cases of dispute can arrange arbitration. A barring-out clause is a common inclusion designed to prevent unfair competition by a rival practice being set up in the near vicinity. However, these need to be fair (e.g. 1 mile radius in a busy suburban area for 1 yr) to be enforceable. Consideration should be given to emergency arrangements; what is to happen to a dentist's continuing care and capitation patients when he/she leaves; and the NHS payments (maternity pay, sick pay, and course allowances). Arrangements for payment of fees for any remedial or replacement work also need to be agreed and included. Fee assignments where the money earned by an associate is paid directly by the DPB to the practice principal, who then pays the associate after taking off their percentage and laboratory fees, are another potential minefield. Careful consideration should be given to include safeguards in case the practice runs into financial difficulties.

Between dentist and staff This should include a job description, pay, holiday entitlements and arrangements, bonuses for additional qualifications and loyalty, sickness allowances, pensions, disciplinary rules, and termination procedures with details of notice required by each party. Advice sheets are available from the BDA.

Negligence

Professional negligence is defined as a failure to exercise reasonable care in one's professional capacity.

Often these cases hinge on what 'reasonable care' constitutes; however, if a dentist can show that his actions were in line with those of a large number of his colleagues, he is unlikely to be held negligent (Bolam test).

For a negligence case to win, the onus is on the claimant's or pursuer's lawyer to prove the following:

- The dentist owed a duty of care to the patient.
- There was a breach of that duty.
- Damage occurred to the patient as a result (no damage, no case).

Where no demonstrable loss has occurred a patient has no recourse in the law and can only voice his complaint to the PCT or Health Board. The ploy of attempting to shift the onus of proof onto the defendant by pleading *res ipsa loquitur* (the facts speak for themselves) is rarely successful.

If the case is proved, financial compensation will be awarded by the court, taking into account the damage that occurred and the steps necessary to put it right.

Criminal negligence   For criminal proceedings to be started the negligent action must be very serious and have some accentuating factor, e.g. the dentist was drunk or drugged, or disregarded well-known safety principles.

Contributory negligence   When the actions of a patient have been partially (or completely) to blame for the damage that occurred, then contributory negligence can be pleaded; e.g. failure to follow post-op instructions.

Vicarious liability   An employer can be held responsible for any negligence by an employee which occurs during his employ. This means that a dentist is responsible for the actions or omissions of his staff; e.g. DN, receptionist, technician. However, as every individual is responsible for his own acts, a charge of negligence could be brought against both employee and employer. Vicarious liability and Crown Indemnity are discussed on p. 714. A GDP is also responsible for the safety of the practice premises (p. 728).

Time bar   Usually 3 yrs; however, this does not begin to run until the patient knows, or ought to have known, of the damage that is said to have been done. For children the time bar does not start until 18 yrs of age; there is no time bar in the case of mental disability. A patient may petition the Court to set aside the time bar if they can show reasonable grounds for this to be done.

The steps involved in a civil action for damages

- Usually the first intimation of trouble is a solicitor's letter (known as a letter before action). This should be dealt with only after consultation with a defence society. Notification of a Legal Aid application should also be passed on.
- If the patient's solicitor proceeds, a letter of claim or summons will be served. As there is a time bar (usually 14–21 days) within which notification of a defence to the claim must be given to the court, it is important to respond quickly via a defence organization.

- The defence society will then make their own investigation into the claim, if necessary seeking the advice of an 'expert'. Should the case appear not to be defensible, then the society will try to settle the matter out of court. Where they judge that no negligence has occurred the case will be allowed to proceed to a full hearing.
- Prior to the trial, counsel for the defence will need to establish the full facts of the case. This can be time-consuming.
- At the end of the trial the verdict will be given on the balance of probability, and the level of compensation set as appropriate.

There but for the grace of God go I? It must be remembered that doctors and dentists are human beings and not infallible. The law does realize that unforeseen accidents can happen. The defence organizations advise: 'In circumstances where complications and errors arise it is proper that objective, factual information, with appropriate clinical reassurance is provided. Adequate explanations assist in reducing fear and uncertainty which may give rise to complaints and claims.'[1]

The importance of clear, concise, and contemporaneous notes cannot be over-emphasized. Record cards, X-rays, and study models (where appropriate) are invaluable.

---

1 Medical Protection Society, *Annual Report 1986* and *1987*.

The protection and defence organizations

These non-profit-making organizations serve to provide the medical and dental professions with advice, indemnity, and defence in legal proceedings involving professional matters (they also contribute significantly to the social life of medical and dental students). In the UK there are three:

Medical and Dental Defence Union of Scotland.
Medical Defence Union.
Dental Protection (part of Medical Protection Society).

Their addresses are given on p. 780.

All dentists in the GDS should join one of these organizations upon qualifying. Because of the rising cost of medical litigation, in 1989 the Health Authorities took over liability for the acts or omissions of doctors and dentists working in their hospitals and Salaried Primary Care (Crown Indemnity), and this has subsequently passed directly to those hospitals which are Trusts. However, dentists in Hospital and Salaried Primary Care are advised to maintain some personal cover as Crown Indemnity does not cover 'good Samaritan' deeds, representation at Coroner's inquests, Fatal Accident Inquiries, and private practice (including medico-legal reports). In addition, PCT or Trust lawyers may try to settle without going to court, thus preventing defendants from proving their innocence of the charge. The defence societies have therefore introduced several levels of cover.

Professional ethics and etiquette[1]

▶ Do as you would be done by.

Although not imposed by legislation, ethical behaviour is necessary, t maintain the standing of the profession in the eyes of the public. Th above precept should apply in all aspects of life, but the following ar more specific examples of how it pertains to dentistry:

- The needs of the patient should be of overriding concern.
- Professional confidentiality should be observed, except where to withhold information which could be construed as acting against the public interest.
- Do not criticize colleagues.
- Do not solicit patients from other dentists.
- When consulted for emergency treatment by a colleague's patient: treat as necessary to alleviate pain and refer the patient back with an explanation of what was done.
- Refer to suitably qualified colleagues, cases which are beyond your competence and require specialist advice and/or treatment.
- Avoid false certification and misleading statements.
- Although the restrictions on advertising have now been lifted, all adverts must still be legal, decent, truthful, and have regard for professional propriety.
- It is the duty of a dentist leaving a practice to make the necessary arrangements for the continuing care of his patients.

NB Clinicians who behave unethically may have to account for their action to the GDC.

1 BDA Advice Sheet 2000 *Ethics in Dentistry.*

The General Dental Council and the Dentists' Register

▶ The practice of dentistry is limited by law to registered dental and medical practitioners and enrolled ancillary workers.

▶ A dentist shall be liable to have his name erased from the Dentists' Register if, either before or after he is registered, he has been convicted of a criminal offence or has been guilty of serious professional misconduct (Dentists Act 1984).

The GDC is a statutory body set up by the Dentists Act to regulate the practice of dentistry. Its size has recently been reduced from 44 to 29 members, which include 15 elected dentists, 4 elected professionals complementary to dentistry (PCDs), and 10 lay members. There are 13 specialist lists.

Functions of the GDC

To maintain the Dentists' Register   This is a list of those who have attained the appropriate qualification and paid their annual retention fee. A name may be erased if a person is found guilty of certain offences or if the retention fee is not paid.

To supervise the standards of dental education   This involves regular visits to the UK dental schools, with the power to withdraw recognition standards are not met.

Discipline   Currently the GDC can act in cases where a dentist may have committed 'serious professional misconduct', or in health issues which affect his fitness to practice. (There is a proposal that in future it be able to deal with poor performance as well.)

There are four stages when a complaint is made to the GDC (it may not progress to all stages):

1 Professional Standards Officer decides if case suitable for GDC or not.
2 Preliminary Screener (experienced dentist).
3 Preliminary Proceedings Committee considers evidence from complainant and dentist
4 Professional Conduct Committee decides if allegations have been proved beyond reasonable doubt. Sanctions include suspension or erasure from the register. The dentist can appeal to the Privy Council.

▶ It is unwise for a dentist to enter a plea of guilty in criminal matters, for charge for which he has a defence, as this will be taken as an admission of guilt by the GDC.

Changes to the GDC

The Health Act 1999 allows the Dentists Act to be amended through a section 60 order. Already a Fitness to Practice Panel has been appointed which is independent of the GDC. It is composed of 35 members (15 dentists, 15 lay people, and 5 PCDs).

Wise precautions, or how to avoid litigation

▶ When in doubt contact your defence organization.

- Good records are invaluable. They should be concise, factual, and objective, and contain details of any treatment and advice given (especially that which the patient is unwilling to accept). All appointments made and failed should be noted. Keep your opinions about difficult patients to yourself; committing them to writing on their dent records is unwise. The Data Protection Act 1998 allows patients acce to manual and electronic records. Patients can apply for a copy of the records (a fee of < £10 and the cost of copying can be charged) and to have incorrect data removed.
- Take adequate radiographs whenever clinically necessary.
- Clinical records, to include X-rays and models, should be kept for at least 11 yrs; for children, they should be retained until age 25, or for 11 yrs, whichever is the longer.
- Protect the patient's eyes and airway.
- Check the medical history at every recall.
- Keep up to date. Continuing with outmoded techniques could render dentist liable to a charge of professional misconduct. Similarly, be war of using controversial or unproven procedures or materials.
- When treating a patient it is essential to have a third person present a all times to act as a chaperon. This is particularly important if using sedation, as reports of patients having erotic fantasies under the influence of nitrous oxide, diazepam, or midazolam can no longer be regarded as amusing anecdotes.[1]
- For any expensive or complicated procedures, obtain written consent
- Refer a patient when it is their best interests.
- Take adequate precautions against cross-infection for patients, staff, a yourself (p. 748).
- Where a GA is being administered this must be by a medically qualifie anaesthetist, with a written protocol for referral and management of the patient. This must include appropriate arrangements for immediat transfer of the patient to a critical care facility.
- Read current guidance issued by the GDC (www.gdc-uk.org).
- Comply with the Ionizing Radiation Guidelines (p. 750).

   ▶ If you are sued, make copies of all relevant documents and recor. The originals should then be kept in a safe place. One copy should forwarded to your defence society. It is also wise to compile a dia of any relevant events, noting down all that you remember. Nev alter records under the threat of litigation. Significant alteration made at any time, should be dated and initialled.

Advice lines
Dental Protection: 0207 7399 1400.
Dental Defence Union: 0207 202 1500.
Medical and Dental Defence Union of Scotland: 0141 221 5858.

1 M. Fields 1990 *BDJ* **169** 4.

Forensic dentistry

Theoretically, forensic dentistry encompasses all aspects of dentistry an the law, but here we will confine ourselves to the application of dent science to criminal investigations.[1]

Identification As the dental tissues survive the effects of fire, water, an time well, dental identification is helpful where other means of distin guishing a person have been lost, e.g. following incineration or burial. No only can the teeth be used to indicate the approximate age of a victim, b also the condition of the dentition, including any filled or missing teet can be compared with dental records to aid identification. Occasional the dental chart of an unknown person is publicized in the dental pre with an appeal from the police for help in identification. In this situation must be remembered that dental treatment may have been carried o subsequently and that additional restorations or missing teeth, as com pared with the GDP's records of a suspected victim, do not necessar exclude identification. Information can also be obtained from studying th skull and jaw bones, e.g. age, sex, racial origin, and the time elapsed sin death. Comparative radiographs may be as individual as fingerprints.

From a forensic point of view the value of accurate up-to-date record and identification marks in dentures, are self-evident.

Occasionally, a practitioner may be requested by the police to reve the dental records of a live, but missing person. The advice of a defen society should be sought, as legally a patient's confidential records shou not be revealed without a Court Order.

Bite marks in inanimate objects left at the site of a crime have on occasio contributed to the conviction of the perpetrator. If the 'evidence' a perishable foodstuff, then a permanent record can be made either casting in stone or rubber base material, following photography.

Bite marks in human skin can occur in assault or non-accidental inju cases. Considerable aggression is required to penetrate the skin. It important to first establish any identifying features of the teeth that caus the bite and then compare them with the dentition of any suspects. Goo photographs, including a linear scale, are essential, and if the victim is aliv need to be repeated 24 hrly as the clarity of the bite may improve wi time. In addition, any saliva associated with the mark can be analysed see if it indicates the blood group of the assailant.

1 K. Whittaker 1989 *A Colour Atlas of Forensic Dentistry*, Wolfe.

Practice management

Relevant pages in other chapters   Contracts, p. 710; biocompatibility of dental materials, p. 700.

Principal sources   K. J. Lewis 1989 *Practice Management for Dentists*, Wright. R. Rattan 1996 *Making Sense of Dental Practice Management*, Radcliffe Medical Press. J. O. Forrest 1984 *A Guide to Successful Dental Practice*, Wright. The BDA have an excellent range of leaflets covering many of the topics in this chapter.

Management skills

Management technique courses are now big business. Although it wou be easy to dismiss them as a way of making a quick profit (for the perso giving the course), in fact underneath the jargon there is a good deal sound business sense.

What are the benefits of good management? ↑ efficiency, ↓ stress, and job satisfaction—for the whole dental team. A happy practice environment not only more pleasant to work in, but the *bonhomie* will also be transmitte to patients.

Keys to successful management

Good communication While the benefit of good communication with patien is acknowledged, the importance of discussion with other members of t dental team receives less emphasis. A few jokes about the receptionis latest boyfriend (strange though he may be) is not communication. F teamwork to be successful the opportunity for all staff to discuss problem and ideas for improvements needs to be created. This usually means settin aside some time within the working week for regular staff meetings. It helpful if these meetings have some sort of structure—which does not me that the dentist dominates proceedings, rather that all staff are encourag to submit ideas for an agenda. On occasion, some guidance may be nece sary to prevent these meetings developing into factional warfare, but wi care the opportunity to discuss problems will ensure the smooth running the practice. One approach is to prepare a handbook of procedures with the practice, for the benefit of new staff.

Delegate those tasks that do not require your training and expertise. addition to ↓ stress and freeing you for the more demanding tasks, this al ↑ job satisfaction for ancillary staff, provided they are given the training a time to cope with their new responsibilities; e.g. getting the hygienist to the fieldwork involved in deciding which new ultrasonic scaler to buy.

Teamwork The importance of building a mutually supportive team c readily be appreciated by trying to work in an environment where everyo has been forced to protect their corner. Successful leadership involv encouraging staff to develop their potential both as an individual and as valued member of the team, and encouraging discussion as to what the go are to be and how to achieve them. Motivation to work as a team can be fo tered by monetary incentives linked to the performance of the practice (s below), but it is wise to find out what motivates individual members of t practice as money may not be the most important factor for all employees.

Staff training This should not only involve the newly appointed; training existing staff to extend their skills more tasks can be delegate Patient management and communication skills of both reception a nursing staff can also be developed. A manual of procedures and routin applicable to the practice can be useful and staff should be encouraged contribute and help update this. In-house training days with speake either from within the practice, or invited, are appreciated.

Adequate training is mandatory for staff involved in taking radiograp (p. 750).

y   Motivation can often be enhanced by financial incentives.[1] Therefore structuring payment to comprise: **1** a fixed hourly rate; **2** an individual nus, which is related to attendance, sickness record, and productivity id as a percentage of the hourly rate; and **3** a group bonus which is a ed proportion of the profits of the practice; all staff have an inducement reduce overheads and improve efficiency in the practice.

. M. Scola 1990 *BDJ* **169** 334.

Hiring and firing staff

Hiring

1 Define what tasks the practice team would like the new member of staff to perform (but do not limit possible applications only to Superman). Decide on the criteria for an ideal candidate, as this will selection later.

2 Draw up a job description. Consider including details of practice, th role of the new member of staff in the team, required skills, in-job training to be provided, hours of work, pay, and other benefits.

3 Advertise post in local press and hospitals. Remember to include a realistic closing date for applications.

4 Short-list candidates.

5 Interview, preferably with two or three people on the panel. This should be structured so that candidates are asked the same questio to aid comparison. Notes should be made, because after several interviews the candidates may begin to merge! Hopefully a suitable person will be found and they should be offered the job in writing, subject to references, ASAP. If no one is acceptable, go back to **1** ar reassess requirements.

6 Draw up a provisional contract, including how assessment is to be carried out at the end of the trial period (usually 6–8 weeks is long enough). Both employee and employer should retain a signed copy.

7 Orientate and train the new member of staff, giving plenty of time fc feedback in both directions.

8 Before end of trial period, reassess, and if progress satisfactory drav a formal contract (p. 710).

9 When recruiting staff, do not discriminate on grounds of disability, s gender reassignment, race, religion, marital situation, or whether the have children or not.

Always put all matters regarding employment in writing.
The BDA have an excellent advice sheet on recruitment.

Firing

The BDA have advice sheets on dismissal and redundancy and the Advis Conciliation and Arbitration Service (ACAS) will also give guidance. from a practical and emotional point of view, dismissal of staff is not and if taken to tribunal, can be expensive. The Trade Union and Lal Relations Acts allow dismissal only for unsatisfactory conduct, ineptit and contravention of the law.

If problems arise with an employee, to prevent a claim of unfair disr use the following procedure:

- Tell employee formally that their conduct is unsatisfactory, giving a timetable for improvement, advice, and help.
- Give written warning that if there is no improvement, dismissal will fol
- Give written notice as per contract.

The minimum statutory notice required depends upon length of ser <1 month = no notice; 1 month to 2 yrs = 1 week, 2–12 yrs = 1 weel each complete year worked. >12 yrs = 12 weeks. For gross misconc instant dismissal is acceptable.

Redundancy is dismissal for reasons other than the personal behaviour of the employee. Statutory redundancy payments are required for staff who have been employed continuously for >2 yrs (full or part-time). The amount paid depends upon pay, length of service, and age. Staff in this category are also entitled to paid time-off to look for a new job or undergo training.

Health and safety[1]

Health and Safety At Work Act 1974

This Act states 'It shall be the duty of every employer to ensure, so far as is reasonably practicable, the health, safety, and welfare at work of all employees.'

In addition to requiring that all equipment and systems of work are s and that information, training, and supervision are provided, the A demands a written statement of policy with regard to health and safe for premises employing >5 members of staff. In addition, to the work environment, the Act requires practice premises to be maintained in a s condition (see RIDDOR below).

Practice inspections are usually carried out by appointment, althou this is not legally required. Employees are also expected to take reaso able care for their own and other people's safety—refusal to comply grounds for dismissal.

Hazard Anything with the potential to cause harm.

Risk The likelihood that someone will be harmed by a hazard.

Risk assessment A systematic evaluation of what could cause ha (e.g. equipment, chemicals, work activities) in the workplace and ensur precautions are in place to minimize these risks.

COSHH

The Control of Substances Hazardous to Health regulations were introduc in 1989. Employers are required to assess all substances (e.g. vapou microorganisms) in the workplace which are potentially hazardous, and ta steps to prevent or ↓ any risks to the health of employees. The follow procedure is recommended:

1 Identify hazardous substances.
2 Record frequency and quantity of use.
3 Assess the risk.
4 Monitor the medical condition of staff, where necessary.
5 Prevent or control risk.
6 Provide staff training.
7 Record the assessment.

Hg spillage Hg use should be confined to impervious surfaces where a spillage will be limited, ideally a lipped tray lined with foil. Staff should w gloves when handling Hg-containing substances. Lead from radiograp packets can be used for absorbing small spillages along with a paste of eq parts calcium hydroxide and flowers of sulfur and water, or a propriet spillage kit can be purchased. Any waste Hg or amalgam should be sto in a sealed, labelled container, for the disposal of which the practice ha written contract.

X-rays, see p. 750.

Cross-infection control, see p. 748.

---

1 BDA Advice Sheet, *Health and Safety Law for Dental Practice.*

Hepatitis B/C:- employer's responsibilities Dentists are responsible for ensuring that any of their staff who carry out procedures that could bring them into contact with blood (e.g. assistants, hygienists, dental nurses) should be immunized against hepatitis B. Any health-care worker who becomes e-antigen +ve is obliged to cease practising.

Latex allergy Affects ~1% of the population and 10% of health-care workers. The range of latex-free products is ↑.[1]

Blood/body fluid spillage The management of this requires written protocols (see p. 740).

RIDDOR

In accordance with the Reporting of Injuries, Diseases and Dangerous Occurrences Regulations, any serious accidents or injuries to staff or patients should be immediately reported to the Health and Safety Executive and, if made verbally, followed up in writing on form F2508 (from HMSO bookshops). Less serious incidents which result in absence from work of <3 days, should also be notified within 7 days. A written record should be kept of all accidents in the practice.

Disposal of waste

Under the Environmental Protection Act, dentists are responsible for segregating waste, storing it safely, and arranging for its disposal. The Health and Safety Executive recommends that clinical waste for incineration should be stored in yellow containers and disposed of by a registered collector. Non-clinical waste should be stored in black containers.

Employers' liability

A certificate of insurance must be displayed on the premises. PCTs/Health Boards are now empowered to carry out practice inspections—the above issues are likely to be high on the agenda of any such inspection.

Medical Devices Directive

A dental prosthesis or orthodontic appliance is now viewed as a custom-made device requiring a written prescription from the dentist. All dental labs need to register with Medical Devices Agency.

E. A. Field 1998 *BDJ* **185** 65.

Financial management

Find a good accountant and a friendly bank manager, preferably on the recommendation of another practitioner.

It is advisable to develop a structured system for dealing with fees and estimates, tailored to the individual practice, which is understood and adhered to by all staff.

Delegating many aspects of calculating and collecting fees from patients, to trained and motivated staff should make the practice more cost-effective. However, failure to monitor the situation adequately can, at best, result in a false sense of security.

Book-keeping is time-consuming but necessary. Many book-keeping tasks can be performed by computer, either with an integrated practice management system or stand-alone software. Suggested minimum:

- Fees due and fees received.
- Bank deposits.
- Patient lists.
- List of all FP17s sent to the DPB and their individual values. This can then be checked against schedules when they are returned. As it is a major headache if these forms are lost in the post, the DPB recommend sending a few at a time, by registered or recorded delivery or via computer line.
- Income/expenditure. This should include all monies received and all bills paid (e.g. lab fees, wages) and be compiled monthly by the principal, in order to develop a feel for the financial situation. Suitable ledgers (e.g. Admor) can be purchased from stationers. It is wise to seek the advice of your accountant as to the methodology, since accurate accounts will make his job easier (and ∴ cheaper).
- Petty cash transactions should be recorded, together with relevant receipts. The money (£50) is best stored in a separate locked box. For larger sums a practice cheque can be cashed.
- Wages.
- Staff absences and sickness records.

Banking It is helpful to bank all monies at the end of each day, as the bank statement then indicates the daily takings. To encourage settlement of fees, it is wise to accept payment in any form, i.e. cash, cheque, or credit card. Although credit cards incur a commission, patients with cash-flow problems may be happy to accept this form of payment as a face-saver, then their lack of funds becomes the credit company's problem. It is good policy to negotiate overdraft facilities in advance to cover those occasions where cash-flow problems arise.

Budgeting An annual forecast and budget should be prepared jointly with the accountant.

Bad debts These can often be prevented by having a definite House Policy which is widely advertised to patients and adhered to; e.g. payment in part at the beginning of Rx and the balance on completion; or payment in full, up front. At the examination appointment patients should be given a written estimate and reminded when payment is due. If a patient forgets at the last visit they should be asked to sign a form con?rming that the R has been satisfactorily completed and that they agree to pay (£x) within 7 days. If payment is still not forthcoming, reminders (with an ↑ chill factor) should be sent out at 7, 14, and 28 days. If there is still no joy, send in the debt collectors, but beware of a counter claim of negligence.

Tax This is really where a good accountant comes in. By providing him with information on income and expenditure on a monthly basis, he will be able to provide advice on what to do before the end of the financial year to minimize the taxman's percentage.

Insurance Essential for property, contents, equipment, indemnity, staff, loss of income, and personal insurance.

Consumer Credit Act 1974 requires those extending credit to the public by allowing them to pay for goods or a service in instalments to obtain a licence. Provided payment is in <4 instalments it is possible to gain exemption. For further details, contact the Office of Fair Trading.

Running late

Running late happens occasionally to everyone, usually when you were hoping to finish early to rush off to do something else. A common reaction is to cut corners, a strategy which can misfire and as a result waste even more time. Another response to being overstressed is to try too hard to hurry, not pausing to plan time effectively. There are no immediate simple solutions, but if another member of staff is free, e.g. hygienist or dental nurse, you may be able to delegate some simple tasks.

If running late is becoming a habit, it is imperative to stop and re-assess your working practices, either before your patients get fed up waiting or your BP rises too far. The first step is to re-evaluate the times booked for each common procedure; are you being realistic? If the answer is yes, then the problem lies with the receptionist's perceptions of your superhuman abilities, and some gentle re-education is necessary. After erring on the generous side for the length of time required for each Rx, go through the appointment book and block out some buffer zones in each session for emergencies, catching-up with paperwork or, if for no other reason, a breather. The frequency and length of these will depend upon the severity of the original problem.

Some additional hints to ↓ everyday stress:
- Have an appointment book, divided into 5 min blocks to provide flexibility.
- A working day comprising a longer morning and a shorter afternoon is more productive.
- If you are so busy that longer procedures have to be booked well in advance, designate some specific sessions for them each month (thus ↓ the temptation to squeeze them in).
- For busy sessions, try and utilize two surgeries.
- Schedule more complex work for the morning and less stressful work (e.g. check-ups) for the end of sessions.
- For last-minute cancellations, have a list of patients who are willing to come in at short notice.
- Define the working day and try not to extend beyond this.
- Coffee-breaks and lunchtime should not always be used to catch up on other work; be kind to yourself and have a rest occasionally.
- It is very common to run late after holidays. It is helpful if you ask the receptionist to pretend that you are having at least an extra couple of days off and book these last of all. Then you will be able to cope with fitting in urgent patients on your return and not feel stressed.

Emergencies can be defined as the patients who are willing to attend at any time. The patient who tries to stipulate when they are seen is not an emergency. If buffer zones are built into your timetable, fitting in the true emergencies should not be a problem. For emergencies out-of-hours there should be a number to contact for advice and, if appropriate, Rx.

Marketing

With the introduction of the recent NHS reforms, the concept that the general public are consumers of health care has resulted in the busy practitioner having to add marketing to his skills. Whether NHS, private or independent, the success or otherwise of a practice is going to depend on its ability to attract and keep patients.

Advertising Relaxation of the GDC restrictions on advertising has opened up a range of opportunities. Advertising does not need to be brash; after all, it is merely a means of letting the public know about the existence of a practice and the services that are available. Apart from the 'yellow pages' this information can be disseminated via:

1 Leaflets (p. 736) These can be distributed to existing patients and possible sources of new recruits, e.g. nurseries, doctors' waiting rooms.
2 Open days. These allow apprehensive patients to find out more about painless dentistry without the need to have an examination or Rx.
3 Practice website. With ↑ popularity of the internet this can be an efficient and dynamic medium for practice promotion.
4 Adverts in local publications: but follow the GDC guidelines.
5 The best advert is a satisfied patient who will recommend you by word of mouth.

First appearances count This starts before the patient arrives at the surgery as most patients will make their initial enquiry by phone. So the phone should always be answered promptly, in person (not by an answer machine), with a friendly and welcoming greeting. When the prospective patient arrives at the surgery the external and internal decor, together with the welcome they receive, will play a role in determining a patient's impression of the professionalism of the practice. It is relatively cost-effective to decorate non-dental areas, ∴ ensure that the exterior of the premises looks well cared-for, with a professional-looking plate. The reception and waiting areas should appear cosy and inviting. Choose light, warm colours and comfortable seating to give a relaxing ambience. Plants, provided someone remembers to water them, also help. A small area for children to play in with toys and some books, or if possible a crèche, are good practice builders. A range of interesting magazines (look at the range available at your optician's, rather than the doctors' waiting room) and practice leaflets on different aspects of dental care/health should be available.

Staff The receptionist must be friendly and helpful (even on Monday mornings). It is worth spending some time with the receptionist, deciding on stock responses to some of the more common problems that arise (e.g. dealing with the angry patient) and to ↑ their knowledge of dental techniques available so that patients' queries can be answered correctly. It is also helpful if the receptionist can ask new patients how they heard about the practice, so as to better target future marketing strategies.

The presentation and attitude of all the staff is of vital importance. An attractive and functional uniform in the practice colour or bearing the practice logo is bound to impress.

Emergencies Although it is tempting to exclude non-registered patients from receiving out-of-hours emergency Rx, it is a good practice-builder to see any patient in pain, as some of them will become regular attenders.

Market Research   It is vital to know your patient base. Is there a significant group which may need special attention (e.g. elderly or young families)? What extra sevices would your patients like to see (e.g. implants; a creche)? What do they feel about your opening times—is there another group of patients who might attend if the opening times were extended/changed?

Remember, the most important marketing aid is without doubt the personal touch.

Practice leaflets

What information to include?

Compulsory information (in NHS practice):

- Practice name, address, and telephone number.
- For all dentists at the practice:name, sex, qualifications, and date of firs registration.
- Hours, and appointment system.
- Whether any dentist provides only orthodontic Rx.
- Whether suitable for patients who cannot climb stairs and has wheelchair access.
- Any foreign languages spoken by the dentist (holiday Spanish probably doesn't count!).

Further *optional* information can be included in the leaflet:

- Practice philosophy.
- Map showing location of practice.
- e-mail and website address.
- Emergency arrangements and contact phone number.
- Further information on the special interests of the dentists, both denta and non-dental.
- Illustrations of the practice, and photos of staff and facilities.
- Details of charges: for broken appointments also, if applicable.
- Methods of payment accepted.
- Whether both NHS and private Rx available.
- Special facilities and Rx available, e.g. sedation, crèche.

How to set about producing a leaflet Broadly speaking there are tw approaches: either get professional help (e.g. designer, photographe printer) or DIY, using a desk-top printing package on the practice compute However, the two are not mutually exclusive and all practices should, least, consider taking advice from a designer. Before seeking help it important to have some idea of what you want. For example:

- Only one leaflet, or the first of a series?
- What is your potential market (young families with small children, olde professionals and their families)?
- Black and white, or two or more colours?
- Glossy booklet or a folded A4 sheet?
- How much money do you want to spend?
- How many copies do you need (to avoid being lead astray by the bulk discounts)?
- How is the leaflet to be distributed?

It is wise to shop around and examine the work of several professiona before choosing.

Design and layout The leaflet aims to create the impression of a cari practice, and to inform. The key to success is simplicity. One helpful tip to have a practice logo &/or house style (or colours), replicated in oth items of practice stationery. This idea of a corporate image is not new, b has worked well in the business world. A designer will be able to sugge styles and layouts best suited to your projected market, as well as he with the text wording. Photos and illustrations will ↑ the cost, but also the impact, as will using more than one colour.

Sponsorship   Worth considering, to give full flight to your creative aspirations. Try approaching toothbrush manufacturers, dental supply companies, or local firms that you deal regularly with.

Points to watch
- Don't say that a dentist has specialist expertise unless registered on a specialist list with the GDC.
- Don't advertise other services or goods.
- Don't include names of practice staff other than dentists.
- Be legal, decent, honest, and truthful.

Computers and dental practice

These wonders of modern technology can, with the right software an
some skill, function as a secretary, accountant, appointment book, filir
cabinet, calculator, publisher, etc., etc., BUT when they go wrong th
repercussions can be quite spectacular. It is not possible in a book
this size to cover the subject adequately; the intention is rather to poir
the reader in the right direction.

▶ Befriend a computer buff, particularly one who is readily available
  by phone.
▶ Garbage in: garbage out.
▶ Back up your data regularly
▶ Register with Data Protection.

Definitions

Hardware Computer equipment, i.e. display screen, central pre
cessing unit (CPU), keyboard, and printer.

Software Computer programs.

Hard disk Computer's memory, usually located within CPU.

Floppy disk Additional, removable source of memory and data.

CD Compact disc, used to store/supply data, e.g. for programs or fc
backup.

DVD Digital versatile disc; can store large amounts of data for image
video, and backup.

Mouse Hand-held device used move to a cursor on the screen
open/close programs, manipulate text and graphics, etc.

Disk drive Slot in CPU into which floppy discs are entered and read.

Byte One letter or space in text. Gauges size of memory.

RAM Random access memory; the part of the computer which stor
programs. A program will not run if its requirements exceed available RAP

User-friendly Means that a program is easy to run (often a misnomer

Back-up Additional copies of important information.

Computers and dental practice

e-mail Electronic mail system between computers.

Modem Converts digital into audio signals to allow transmission
a telephone line.

Internet Global network of computers linked electronically
telephone line.

Surfing the net Spending time (that should be spent working) explorir
the Internet.

CAL Computer-assisted learning.

Functions of a computer are determined by the software that is use
A word-processing package makes letters and information leaflets ea

produce. A database package will compile and manage lists of patients, thereby facilitating recalls. A spreadsheet package can be used to produce accounts. An integrated program allows several functions to operate simultaneously without having to change from one package to another. Specific dental software can run dentally related functions, providing a full clinical and administrative system. Digital X-ray detectors and IO digital cameras can be linked to a computer. The images they produce can be invaluable for patient communication, and saved in the patient's record.

Where to go for advice
Dental computer specialist: generally worth the extra expense.
Business computer specialist.
Local retailer.
Teach yourself; but be warned: computers can be addictive.

Choosing a system It is important to decide what you want the computer to do and how much you are prepared to spend. If an (expensive) multi-function practice management system is being considered, then the choice of hardware is less important and is often dictated by the software package. However, if a more cautious approach is planned (e.g. starting with word-processing only) then the choice of computer and operating system is more important. In this case, a computer with the largest memory you can afford and a good quality inkjet or laser printer is advisable. An agreement providing on-site maintenance in case of breakdown is a necessity, and training and back-up are essential. It is worth asking other practices which computers/which system they wish they'd bought instead!

Patient records can be stored on computer without duplicate manual records. If this is the case an audit trail must ensure that the data is not tampered with. It should not be possible to change or erase a record without this being recorded.

Data Protection Act 1998[1]
The act covers manual as well as computerized records. A dentist storing personal data on a computer system must register with the Data Protection Commissioner. And the practice should have a data protection policy.

Under the terms of the Act, data must be:
- obtained fairly and for a specific and lawful purpose;
- only used for specific and lawful purposes;
- should not be excessive but adequate and relevant;
- only disclosed to certain recipients;
- protected and held securely;
- accessible to patients on request.

Plans are in hand in the UK for all NHS dental practices to be linked to the National Programme for Information Technology.

The BDA produce a useful fact sheet, entitled data protection.

Independent and private practice

'Independent' is the term preferred by many for private practice, as it soun[ds] less avaricious. An ↑ proportion of dentists are turning to other methods [of] remuneration than the NHS; indeed the pace of change is so fast that it [is] difficult to provide information that will necessarily be relevant in th[e] future. ∴ these pages are limited to discussing general principles.

Researching the market

To develop the potential of a practice it is necessary first to fully evalua[te] its present position. An appreciation of the existing patient base can b[e] gained simply by going through the manual or computer records an[d] looking at the geographical spread and socio-economic groups. If mo[st] patients are part of a family group, then future developments need [to] provide advantages for parents and children; e.g. if changing to independe[nt] practice, then a family-based capitation scheme might be more applicable[.]

Also, the potential for attracting new patients to the practice, and th[e] competition from other practices in the area for those and existing patien[ts] should be assessed.

It is also important to research and take into consideration the sta[ff] views about any changes to be made to the practice, and to inform the[m] of the advantages these changes will bring.

Business planning

If the financial basis of a practice is to be changed a business plan will ne[ed] to be drawn up and discussed with the practice's accountants and banke[rs.] Two fashionable business planning tools are:

1 The planning cycle:

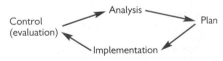

2 A SWOT analysis is a consideration of the Strengths, Weaknesses, Opportunities, and Threats, to and of a business.

Fee setting

This difficult exercise should be carried out in conjunction with the advi[ce] of the practice accountant. The following will need to be calculated:
1 Practice overheads.
2 Profit desired (realistically!).
3 Inflation.
4 Number of sessions worked per week.

From this the target hourly rate can be calculated. However, local mark[et] conditions need to be considered, which may necessitate a little round[ing] down of the profits desired, or a ↓ in overheads if that is possible. Once [a] realistic hourly rate has been calculated, *either* fees can then be dete[r]mined for each procedure by the average amount of time taken, to gi[ve] set price list, *or* patients charged according to the time taken. Laboratory charges and hygienist fees, as indicated, should be additional.

Types of independent practice

There are basically four different approaches:
A combination of independent and NHS practice. For example, exempt patients are seen on the NHS, whereas other adults are seen privately. In practice, this two-tier system can cause difficulties and friction.
Low-cost independent practice.
Traditional 'private' practice.
Insurance-based schemes.

Private dental schemes

This is one of the real growth areas in modern dentistry. At present there are five types:
Capitation-based (e.g. Denplan) Patients pay a monthly fee to the company (which is passed on to the GDP minus an administration fee), usually determined by their dental status and the practice's overheads. The dentist then provides Rx as indicated, but certain items, e.g. orthodontics and laboratory fees, may be excluded.
Insurance schemes Rx costs are reimbursed.
Corporate dental schemes
Savings schemes At present these are restricted to orthodontics.
Maintenance schemes Prevention and diagnosis covered by a monthly payment. Fees paid for item of service Rx. Insurance for trauma, out-of-hours emergency Rx, etc.

Prescribing for private and independent patients

When a private patient requires medicines as part of their Rx, a private prescription should be provided. Dentists can also supply or sell medicines to any patient, but are bound by pricing and other dispensing rules. Alternatively, common drugs can be given as required and their cost included in the overall fee.

Complaints

Patients are paying more for their Rx they will naturally have ↑ expectations of the service provided. In a large proportion of cases, a potential problem can be dealt with by better communication. So if patients are provided with the means to voice any complaints within the practice setting, an opportunity is given to resolve the situation early. It is now mandatory to have a written practice complaints procedure.

Vocational training

Vocational training (VT) is designed to give a supervised and mentored introduction into general dental practice.

Trainees work as salaried assistants and are ∴ not under any pressure to achieve a high-volume turnover. Each region organizes a day-release scheme (30 days or more per year), which covers the clinical and administrative aspects of NHS practice, as well as patient and financial management. But each trainee will also receive on-the-job training and supervision from their trainer, as well as tutorials on a weekly basis. Trainees do not have their own NHS number, so all patient fees go to the trainer. Salary is set at half of notional Target Annual Net Income (TANI), and the contract includes 4 weeks of holiday a year. On completion of VT a certificate is awarded.

Trainers To be accepted, a practice needs to satisfy the criteria set by the VT Committee and the trainer needs to be present not less than 3 days a week. Trainers are themselves trained for their roles in teaching and assessment. A grant of 15% of notional TANI is paid and the trainee's salary is reimbursed in full. Trainees are members of the NHS superannuation scheme and their contribution is deducted at source. Trainers are vicariously liable for the actions of their trainees.

Procedure GDPs with >4 yrs experience are eligible to become trainers. They are selected after a visit to the practice to check its suitability as a training environment, and its compliance with Clinical Governance requirements and wider legislation. They are also required to attend an interview. Details of each regional scheme are advertised to final-year students or are available from the Regional VT Adviser. Potential trainees are responsible for contacting practices on the approved list and arranging visits and interviews.

Contract A standard contract, which both parties are required to sign, is available from the BDA and course organizers. The contract runs for 12 months, at the end of which each party is free to make their own arrangements. It includes a binding-out clause which prevents the trainee subsequently accepting as a patient someone he has treated at the practice, should they move to another practice.

Community vocational training This is also compulsory, and extends over 2 yrs. Each region has a nominated trainer. There is often some tie-in with the GDS VT course.

General professional training A 2 yr period of post-basic training in two or more disciplines. There are several modes of GPT available. The least structured is to complete VT and then apply for CDS or SHO posts. At the other extreme is a scheme that integrates general dental practice VT and house officer posts in the hospital service into a seamless 2 yr period of training.

Clinical governance, continuing professional development, clinical audit, and peer review[1]

These are the current buzzwords in terms of quality assurance and good clinical practice.

Clinical governance

Part of the NHS drive to ↑ the quality of health care and to make providers accountable for delivering a consistent standard of care.
- Practice-based quality assurance system.
- Mandatory for all GDS dentists.

To fulfil the GDS terms of service, ensure that:
- All dental care is of a consistent quality.
- Cross-infection control measures are effective.
- Legal requirements relating to health and safety are satisfied.
- Legal requirements relating to radiological protection are satisfied.
- Requirements of the GDC in respect of continuing professional development are satisfied.

It is also necessary to provide an annual report for the primary care trust, appoint a person responsible for operating the system, and display a written practice quality policy.

Continuing professional development (CPD)

Now a mandatory requirement for registration with the GDC.
- Recertification every 5 yrs.
- 250 hours of CPD in every 5 yr cycle (average 50 h/yr).
  — 75 h verifiable, e.g. appropriate courses;
  — 175 h non-verifiable/general CPD; e.g. reading professional journals.
- All dentists must maintain their own records, keep certificates, etc.
- Failure to comply may result in erasure from the Register.
- Funding is available within the GDS via the CPD allowance (currently 15 h/yr, minimum NHS gross stipulated).

The BDA produces a useful CPD Planner: *Continuing Professional Development: A Guide for the Dental Team.*

Clinical audit

What it is The systematic critical analysis of the quality of clinical care, covering procedures used for Δ and Rx, use of resources, and the outcome for the patient. The aim of clinical audit in dentistry aims to encourage dentists to self-assess different aspects of their practice, implement changes, and monitor them with a view to improving service and patient care.

What it is not Clinical audit is not the same as its commercial equivalent, which is the assessment of an institution's financial status against best practice. It is not a management tool for dictating clinical policy to clinicians. It is not judgemental, and should not be used for disciplinary measures.

1 BDA Advice Sheet, *CPD Clinical Governance, Audit and Peer Review.*

Aims and objectives Primarily, improvement of the quality of care provided. This is achieved by identifying less-than-adequate care and raising it to the standard of the agreed best.

General principles The basis is frank and open discussion without fear of criticism. It is essential to identify agreed standards against which the quality of care provided can be compared. These standards should not be fixed and immutable, so as to allow evolutionary change. It is imperative that the results of such discussion should lead to changes in practice when indicated. Confidentiality is an absolute prerequisite. Other crucial elements are genuine motivation and interest amongst the participating staff, honesty, and adequate data. Appropriate information technology, while of undoubted benefit, is not essential. An 'audit cycle' is illustrated below. Possible topics include cross-infection control, appointment systems, and clinical methodology.[2]

Peer review The object of peer review is to improve the quality of care provided in dental practice by encouraging communication between dentists and to identify areas in which change can be made.

Since May 2001 clinical audit and peer review have been mandatory in the GDS; 15 h required over 3 yrs. Funding is available through the DH.

British Standards 5750 BS5750 can be gained by any manufacturer or service sector organization that can demonstrate quality management systems. A number of dental practices have successfully achieved this standard.

Audit cycle

Meeting to agree a 'gold standard' of care for a
specific condition.
↓
Prospective analysis of care for that condition.
↓
Meeting to compare actual standard with 'gold standard'.
Identify areas where deficiencies exist and make
recommendations.
Agree to implement recommendations for improvement.
↓
Prospective analysis of care following implementation of
new recommendations.
↓
Meeting to compare actual standard with 'gold standard'.
'Gold standard' not met—re-enter cycle.
'Gold standard' met—is 'gold standard' good enough?
If yes—recognize, and periodic review only.
If no—agree new standard and re-enter cycle.

Evidence-based medicine/dentistry[1]

EBM/D is the latest 'hot topic' and involves making clinical decisions based on the best available evidence, which should include sound research, epidemiology, basic science, and clinical experience. EBM is essentially the same as:

Clinical effectiveness This involves using those clinical interventions which have been shown to be effective both by research and audit.

The 'gold standard' for research is a well-planned RCCT, but in many areas of clinical practice evidence from such trials is yet not available. In the meantime clinicians should continue to evaluate carefully the techniques they use and the results of studies reported in the literature, although the sheer volume of scientific literature makes keeping up to date a difficult task. Review articles are helpful, but in the past have tended to be rather subjective.

Systematic review A method of collating and assessing the results of research on a particular topic. This implies that a thorough search for suitable articles and indeed unpublished work has been made, and explicit criteria used to decide whether an article should be included or rejected.

Meta-analysis A systemic review which uses special statistical methods to combine the results of several studies. Only RCCTs should be included. By considering a number of studies the effects (and side-effects) of a Rx are magnified as the sum total of subjects is effectively ↑. Whether the findings are consistent for different population groups or Rx variations can also be evaluated. For example, if this technique had been used to evaluate the results of research into the use of streptokinase in the treatment of myocardial infarction a positive benefit would have been demonstrated almost 20 yrs before it became apparent from the individual studies.

The Cochrane collaboration This aims to collate the results of systematic reviews in all areas of health care and ensure that the findings are kept up to date. The results can be accessed electronically via the Cochrane library, which is available quarterly on computer disc, CD-ROM, and the Internet (p. 778). An Oral Health Group is currently investigating several topics of interest to the dental specialities.

Clinical guidelines Another fashionable topic. They are defined as 'systematically developed statements which assist clinicians and patients in making decisions about appropriate treatment for specific conditions'. They may be developed nationally or locally, but should always be seen as guidance and are ∴ aids to, but not a substitute for, clinical judgement. To be effective, clinical guidelines should be brief, practical, and based on the results of sound research. They should be reviewed regularly in the light of new research and their effectiveness audited.

---

1 D. L. Sackett 1997 *Evidence-Based Medicine*, Churchill Livingstone.
2 T. Mann 1996 *Clinical Guidelines*, NHS Executive.

Clinical guidelines can be drawn up by any group of clinicians; in dentistry this approach is mainly being co-ordinated nationally by the Royal Colleges &/or specialist societies. The National Institute for Clinical Excellence (NICE) is a government based body that also investigates the effectiveness of different Rx modalaties. See their guidelines relating to the removal of wisdom teeth (May 2000).

Prevention of cross-infection[1]

Cross-infection is the transmission of infectious agents between patients and staff within the clinical environment. Potential risks include not only hepatitis and HIV, but also other viruses (e.g. herpes) and bacteria (e.g. *Streptococcus pyogenes*). Transmission can occur by inoculation or inhalation. The BDA recommends:

1 Universal precautions: a standard cross-infection control policy for all patients. This is advisable because it may not be possible to distinguish the healthy carrier. Also, an effective policy will ↓ the risks to the dentist and his staff, as well as being a practice-builder.
2 Carriers of blood-borne viruses (hepatitis, HIV) can be treated in general dental practice, provided routine procedures are implemented rigorously.
3 Patients with manifestations of immunosuppression should be referred for specialist hospital care.
4 All staff should be trained in cross-infection control and every practice must have a written infection control policy.
5 It is unethical to refuse dental care on the grounds that it could expose the dentist to personal risk.

Immunization All clinical staff must be immunized against hepatitis B with a single booster 5 yrs after the primary course. Protection is indicated by HbsAb > 100 mIU/ml. Antibody levels < 10 mIU/ml indicate a non-responder. Poor responders have antibody levels of 10–100 mIU; it is not clear what protection is afforded by this level of response so an annual booster is recommended. You must keep documentary evidence of immunization and response for all staff. Staff should also be immunized against common illnesses.

Medical and social history Tact and discretion are required if truthful answers are to be obtained to sensitive questions.

Gloves[2] Should be worn routinely by dentist and DN. The BDA recommends a new pair of gloves for each patient. Wash hands in a disinfectant solution before gloving and cover any cuts with a waterproof dressing. Use handcream at the end of a session to prevent skin drying and cracking. Those with an allergy to latex can try vinyl, or wear undergloves of silk or nylon. Non-powdered gloves are advisable.

Surgery design and equipment[3] New and existing surgeries should include separate areas for dentist and DN, within which are designated 'clean' zones. Layout and equipment must be planned to allow easy cleaning, and to minimize the number of surfaces touched; e.g. taps or lights that can be turned on with infrared light switches or foot controls.

Cleaning and sterilizing instruments Disposable instruments and cleaning materials should be used wherever possible. Manufacturers are exhibiting considerable ingenuity in this area (e.g. single-use diamond burs, disposable handpieces). Reusable items (including handpieces) must be cleaned

1 BDA Advice Sheet, *Infection Control in Dentistry*.
2 M. A. Baumann 1992 *Int Dent J* **42** 170.
3 L. S. Worthington 1988 *BDJ* **165** 226.

sterilized after use (p. 382). Chemical solutions only disinfect and ould be restricted to those articles which cannot be sterilized by conntional methods. The BDA recommends plastic sheeting to cover handces and 3-in-1 tubing and equipment handles.

atment of work surfaces During use, instruments should only be placed a sterilizable tray or impervious disposable covering. Care is required to bid contamination of areas which are difficult to disinfect. A system of ing ↑ efficiency as only those areas which are likely to be contaminated ed to be cleaned and disinfected with a suitable viricidal disinfectant.

rosols Minimize these by high-volume suction. Wear gloves, eye otection, and masks. Flush aspirators and tubing through daily with a recmended disinfecting agent. Use of rubber dam ↓ splatter and aerosols.

od spillages Immediately cover with disposable towels, treat with 000 ppm sodium hypochlorite solution. After 5 mins dispose of in ical waste. Use protective clothing and household gloves.

posal of sharps Care is required to prevent needlestick injuries, and ferably a re-sheathing device should be used. Sharps must be placed in gid sharps container. Disposal can be arranged via PCT/Health Board.

edlestick injuries (p. 383) Allow wound to bleed, and wash. If a risk of ection, do serological tests of staff and patient. Get advice from consult microbiologist or consultant in communicable disease control.

oratory items Rinse and disinfect all impressions and appliances ording to the maunfacturer's recommendations prior to dispatch to the Proprietary products are available for impression disinfection.

nsmissible spongiform encephalopathies These include Creutzfeldt–Jakob ase (CJD) and variant CJD (VCJD/BSE). Patients with a known history of e of these conditions or those at risk (growth hormone Rx before 1985; ipients of dura mater grafts; or family history of this disease) are t treated in a specialist environment as routine autoclaving does : destroy the causative agent: prions. Current advice is available at w.dh.gov.uk

X-rays—the statutory regulations[1]

The Ionizing Radiation Regulations 1999 (IRR99)
The Ionizing Radiation (Medical Exposure) Regulations 2000 (IRMER)

Terminology

The **legal person** is responsible for implementing the regulations a
good working practice. Usually the practice owner.

The **radiation protection supervisor (RPS)** is appointed by the le
person and is responsible for implementing the local rules. Can be
appropriately trained dentist or PCD.

An **IRMER practitioner** is the dentist responsible for justifying
exposure, and ensuring the benefits outweigh the risks.

A **referrer** is a dentist who refers a patient to an IRMER practitioner
radiological examination.

An **operator** is any person who carries out all or part of the practi
aspects associated with a radiological examination, including taking
X-ray, developing films, identifying the patient, etc.

A **radiation protection adviser (RPA)** must be appointed in writing
provide advice on complying with legal obligations, e.g. testing of equipme
staff training, risk assessment, quality assurance program, etc.

With the introduction of these regulations to the statute books,
dentist (legal person) must:

1 Complete an inventory of X-ray equipment (including age,
manufacturer, model, and serial number) and notify Health and
Safety Executive.
2 Complete a risk assessment in consultation with the RPA to ↓
exposure of staff and patients. It should be documented and reviewe
at least every 5 yrs.
3 Ensure every IRMER practitioner and operator has appropriate traini
and undertakes continuing education. Update every 5 yrs and keep
records of training for inspection.
4 Appoint a RPS. Can be either the dentist or a suitably trained auxiliar
5 Complete a radiation protection file. This should include the local ru
and other documentation relating to radiation protection within the
practice, e.g. written procedures for patient protection, guidelines fo
referral for radiological examination, quality assurance programs,
records of training, etc.
6 Have a set of local rules, which must include name and contact detail
for RPA, details of controlled areas, and a contingency plan in the eve
of an equipment malfunction, working instructions.
7 Identify designated controlled areas. This is usually within a radius of
1.5 m, except in the direction of the beam, where it extends until the
beam is attenuated.
8 Ensure that all equipment is regularly serviced and a radiation safety
assessment carried out at least every 3 yrs (this can be done by post
the National Radiological Protection Board).

---

1 BDA Advice Sheet, *Radiation in Dentistry*.

9 Keep radiation dose As Low As Reasonably Practicable (ALARP). This has several aspects:
   - Be able to justify taking every radiograph.
   - There must be written guidance for exposure settings for all types of radiograph.
   - A clinical evaluation and report in patient's records for all films.
   - Avoiding repetition by recording all X-rays taken in the patient's records; send X-rays with patient for referrals.
   - Rectangular collimation, with minimum skin-to-focus distances as follows: <60 kV = 10 cm; >60 kV = 20 cm.
   - A quality assurance program to ↑ diagnostic yield and ↓ need for repeat X-rays.
   - Use of fastest film consistent with good diagnostic quality (ISO speed E or faster).
   - Routine use of film holders.

X-rays—practical tips and helpful hints

Practical tips

- When an exposure is made the raised dot on the packet should face the direction of the X-rays. When the processed film is viewed from the side with the raised dot, the patient's right is shown on the left of the film.
- In order of radio-opacity: air, soft tissues, cartilage, immature bone, tooth-coloured fillings, mature bone, dentine and cementum, enamel, metallic restorations.
- View films in subdued lighting against an illuminated background.
- The oblique lateral mandible is a useful view for the angle of the mandible and the molar region that can be carried out with a dental X-ray set. Two views (left and right) can be taken on a single film if a lead sheet is placed over half the cassette. *Technique*: get patient to extend neck and protrude mandible (to ↓ superimposition of cervical spine), position cassette parallel to lower border of mandible and 2 cm below it, and centre tube 2 cm below and behind the contralateral angle of the mandible.
- For soft-tissue views (e.g. after trauma) a very short exposure (often below the lowest setting on the X-ray set) is required. A slower occlusal film may be more practical.
- The incisive foramen will have a parallax shift in relation to an incisor apex.
- Routine use of a lead apron is no longer considered necessary. (p. 21)
- Dental radiographs are not C/I during pregnancy. (p. 21)

Processing

Manual   Do this either in a darkroom or a daylight processing tank. It important to always keep the developer and fixer baths in the same orde

Automatic   There are several dental types available which can process I and some EO films. It is faster as the first wash is eliminated and rolle squeeze off the solutions.

Method

Manual regimen:

- Remove packaging and put film carefully in holder.
- Place in developer. Length of time varies according to the manufacturer and the temperature, but is usually 3–4 min.
- Rinse.
- Place in fix for twice as long as it takes for film to clear.
- Wash. The recommended time is 10 min.

If a film is urgently required the films can be viewed 'wet' after 2–4 min the fixer, but they should be returned for complete fixing.

NB Avoid contamination of the developer with fix and change th chemicals at least once a fortnight.

Self-developing film   So called because the developer and fix are con tained within a sachet, which also contains the film. Following exposur tabs are pulled which release first developer and then fixer onto the film

e film is then removed and rinsed. Although this method obviates the
ed for processing equipment, the results are inferior so do not use it
utinely.

gital detectors allow an image to be viewed and stored on a computer
stem. Processing time is ↓ and the image can be manipulated to ↑ diag-
ostic yield. Exposure settings should be ↓ to the minimum compatible
th the diagnostic quality required of the image.

lm faults

n dark	• Fogged film: out-of-date or poorly stored film.
	• Overexposure.
	• Overdevelopment.
	• Temperature too high.
n pale	• Underexposed.
	• Underdeveloped: impatience, exhausted chemicals.
	• Temperature too low.
or contrast	• Overdevelopment.
	• Developer contaminated with fix.
	• Inadequate fixation &/or washing.
or definition	• Patient movement.
otches	• Dark blotches are due to developer splashes, and white blotches to fixer splashes.

e most common faults are overexposure and underdevelopment.
The article by Chadwick discusses the factors affecting b/w, and is
commended.[1]

. L. Chadwick 1998 *BDJ* **184** 80.

Syndromes of the head and neck

Principal sources R. J. Gorlin 1990 *Syndromes of the Head and Neck*, OUP.

Syndromes of the head and neck

Introduction

The aim of this section is neither to bemuse the reader nor to demonstrate esoteric knowledge, although both may appear to occur. The real importance behind the learning of names associated with conditions which may be of relevance to, or be picked up by, clinical examination of the head and neck, is that, once learned, some difficult diagnostic problems can be quickly solved and appropriate Rx instituted. We have retained eponyms where relevant (although this is not in keeping with current fashion) as they are, we feel, easier to learn and certainly more fun. Examiners have a tendency to remember their favourite eponymous syndrome and it helps to at least agree on the name. We have, however, avoided the use of the possessive when using eponyms because invariably others were involved in describing or elucidating the condition and the syndrome does not belong to the individual(s) associated with it. The following list is in no way comprehensive but takes you through conditions met by the authors either in their clinical practice or in examinations, and which could ∴ be considered worth knowing about.

Definitions

Malformation   A primary structural defect resulting from a localized error of morphogenesis.

Anomalad   A malformation *and* its subsequently derived structural changes.

Syndrome   A recognized pattern of malformation, presumed to have the same aetiology but not interpreted as the result of a single localized error in morphogenesis.

Association   A recognized pattern of malformation not considered to be a syndrome or an anomalad, *at the present time*.

Syndromes

Albright syndrome (McCune–Albright syndrome)   Consists of polyostotic fibrous dysplasia (multiple bones affected), patchy skin pigmentation (referred to as *café-au-lait* spots), and an endocrine abnormality (usually precocious puberty in girls). Facial asymmetry affects up to 25% of cases.

Apert syndrome   is a rare developmental deformity consisting of a cranial synostosis (premature fusion of cranial sutures) and syndactyly (fusion of fingers or toes). Severe mid-face retrusion leads to exophthalmos of varying severity. Early surgical intervention may be indicated for raised intracranial pressure or to prevent blindness from subluxation of the globe of the eye.

Behçet syndrome   (pronounced behh-chet, after Turkish doctor Hulusi Behçet) is, classically, oral ulceration, genital ulceration, and uveitis. Clinical can be made on finding any two of these. It is, in fact, a multisystem disease of immunological origin, although no hard diagnostic tests are yet available. It tends to affect young adults, especially males, and there is an association with HLA-B5. It undergoes spontaneous remission, although a variety of drugs including thalidomide are in use to treat it. See also p. 440.

...ler syndrome Maxillonasal dysplasia, severe mid-facial retrusion, and ...ent or hypoplastic frontal sinuses are the main features. There is no ...ociated intellectual defect.

...diak–Higashi syndrome is a combination of defective neutrophil func-..., abnormal skin pigmentation, and ↑ susceptibility to infection (leading ...severe gingivitis, periodontitis, and aphthae in young children). It is a ...etic disease.

...docranial dysostosis (cleidocranial dysplasia) is an autosomal dominant ...erited condition consisting of hypoplasia or aplasia of the clavicles, delayed ...fication of the cranial fontanelles, and a large, short skull. Associated ...ures are shortness of stature, frontal and parietal bossing, failure to pneu-...ize the air sinuses, a high arched palate &/or clefting, mid-face hypopla-..., failure of tooth eruption with multiple supernumerary teeth. Many of the ...h present have inherent abnormalities such as dilaceration of roots or ...wn gemination. Hypoplasia of 2° cementum may occur. The condition ...ly, though NOT exclusively, affects membraneous bone.

...du chat' syndrome is a chromosomal abnormality caused by deletion ...art of the short arm of chromosome No. 5, resulting in microcephaly, ...ertelorism, and a round face with a broad nasal bridge and malformed ...s. Associated laryngeal hypoplasia causes a characteristic shrill cry. ...re is associated severe mental retardation.

...uzon syndrome is the commonest of the craniosynostoses. It is an ...osomal dominant condition consisting of premature fusion of cranial ...ures, mid-face hypoplasia, and, due to this, shallow orbits with proptosis ...he globe of the eye. Radiographically the appearance of a 'beaten ...per skull' is characteristic. The enlarging brain is entrapped by the ...maturely fused sutures, and ↑ intracranial pressure can lead to cerebral ...aage and resulting intellectual deficiency. This and the risk of blindness ...fy early craniofacial surgery to correct the deformity.

...n syndrome (trisomy 21) is the commonest of all malformation ...dromes, affecting up to 1:600 births. Risk ↑ with maternal age. Down's ...dren account for 1/3 of severely mentally handicapped children. Facial ...earance is characteristic with brachycephaly, mid-face retrusion, small ...e with flattened nasal bridge, and upward sloping palpebral fissures ...ngoloid slant). There is relative macroglossia and delayed eruption of ...h. Major relevant associations are heart defects, atlanto-axial subluxa-..., anaemia, and an ↑ risk of leukaemia. Most Down's children and adults ...extremely friendly and cooperative.

...e syndrome is dysphagia and pain on chewing and turning the head ...ociated with an elongated styloid process.

...rs–Danlos syndrome A group of disorders characterized by hyperflex-...y of joints, ↑ bleeding and bruising, and hyperextensible skin. There ...ears to be an underlying molecular abnormality of collagen in this inher-... disorder. Bleeding is commoner in type IV, early onset periodontal ...ase in type VIII. Pulp stones may be seen in all types.

...syndrome (Lucie Frey, a Polish physician) is a condition in which ...atory sweating and flushing of skin occur. It follows trauma to skin

overlying a salivary gland and is thought to be due to post-trauma crossover of sympathetic and parasympathetic innervation to the gla and skin, respectively. Its frequency following superficial parotidecto ranges from 0–100% depending on which surgeon you are talking to, bu almost certainly present in all cases to some degree if you looked for caref enough (use starch–iodine test).

Gardener syndrome This comprises multiple osteomas (particularly of jaws and facial bones), multiple polyps of the large intestine, epiderm cysts, and fibromas of the skin. It shows autosomal dominant inheritan The discovery on clinical or X-ray examination of facial osteomas manda examination of the lower gastrointestinal tract, as these polyps have tendency to rapid malignant change. This is a highly 'worthwhile' syndrom

Goldenhar syndrome is a variant of hemifacial microsomia and consists microtia (small ears), macrostomia, agenesis of the mandibular ramus a condyle, vertebral abnormalities (e.g. hemivertebrae), and epibul dermoids. Also, cardiac, renal, or skeletal abnormalities can occur. Up 10% of patients may have mental handicap—in other words, 90% **do no**

Gorlin–Goltz syndrome (multiple basal cell naevi syndrome) see, p. 5 Consists of multiple BCCs (epitheliomas), multiple jaw cysts (odontoge keratocysts), vertebral and rib anomalies (usually bifid ribs), and calcifi tion of the falx cerebri. Frontal bossing, mandibular prognathism, hyp telorism, hydrocephalus, eye, and endocrine abnormalities have also be noted.

Graves' disease Autoantibodies to thyroid stimulating hormone (TS cause hyperthyroidism with ophthalmopathy; women 30–50 yrs are co monly affected; exophthalmos can be helped by craniofacial approach orbital decompression.

Heerfordt syndrome (uveoparotid fever) is sarcoidosis with associat lacrimal and salivary (especially parotid) swelling, uveitis, and few Sometimes there are associated neuropathies, e.g. facial palsy.

Hemifacial microsomia Prevalence: 1 in 5000 births. Bilateral in 20% cases. Congenital defect characterized by lack of hard and soft tissue affected side(s), usually in the region of the ramus and external (i.e. first and second branchial arches). Wide spectrum of ear and cran deformities found.

'Histiocytosis-X' Really three broad groups of diseases with the histolog feature of tissue infiltration by tumour-like aggregates of macropha (histiocytes) and eosinophils.
1 *Solitary eosinophilic granuloma* Mainly affects males < 20. Mandible a common site. Responds to local Rx.
2 *Hand–Schüller–Christian disease* Multifocal eosinophilic granuloma causing skull lesions, exophthalmos, and diabetes insipidus. Affects younger group. May respond to cytotoxic chemotherapy.
3 *Letterer–Siwe disease* Rapidly progressive, disseminated histiocytosis. Associated pancytopenia and multisystem disease; can be fatal.

Horner syndrome Consists of a constricted pupil (miosis), drooping ey (ptosis), unilateral loss of sweating (anhydrosis) on the face, and occasion sunken eye (enophthalmos). It is caused by interruption of sympathetic nerve fibres at the cervical ganglion 2° to, e.g., bronchogenic carcinoma, invading the ganglion or neck trauma. Scores high on the 'worthwhile' rating.

Hurler syndrome is a mucopolysaccharidosis causing growth failure and mental retardation. A large head, frontal bossing, hypertelorism, and coarse features give it its classical appearance. Multiple skeletal abnormalities (dysostosis multiplex), corneal clouding, and serum and urinary acid mucopolysaccharide abnormalities also occur.

Hypohydrotic ectodermal dysplasia hypodontia found in association with lack of hair, sweating, and saddle nose.

Klippel–Feil anomalad is the association of cervical vertebral fusion, short neck, and low-lying posterior hairline. A number of neurological anomalies have been noted, and unilateral renal agenesis is frequent. Cardiac anomalies sometimes occur.

Larsen syndrome is a mainly autosomal dominant condition, with a pre-diliction for females, consisting of cleft palate, flattened facies, multiple congenital dislocations, and deformities of the feet. Sufferers are usually of short stature. Larynx may be affected.

Lesch–Nyhan syndrome is a defect of purine metabolism causing mental retardation, spastic cerebral palsy, choreoathetosis, and aggressive self-mutilating behaviour (particularly involving the lips).

MAGIC syndrome stands for Mouth And Genital ulcers and Interstitial chondritis and is a variant of the Behçet syndrome group.

Marfan syndrome is an autosomal dominant condition characterized by tall, thin stature and arachnodactyly (long, thin, spider-like hands), dislocation of the lens, dissecting aneurysms of the thoracic aorta, aortic regurgitation, floppy mitral valve, and high arched palate. Joint laxity is also common. This condition is highly prevalent among top-class basketball and volleyball players, for obvious reasons.

Melkerson–Rosenthal syndrome Consists of facial paralysis, facial oedema, and fissured tongue. It is probably a variant of the group of conditions now known as orofacial granulomatosis.

Multiple endocrine neoplasia A group of conditions affecting the endocrine glands. MEN IIb is of particular relevance as it consists of multiple mucosal neuromas which have a characteristic histopathology, pheochromocytoma, medullary thyroid carcinoma, and a thin wasted appearance. Calcitonin levels are elevated if medullary thyroid carcinoma is present. Index of suspicion should be high in tall, thin, wasted-looking children and young adults presenting with lumps in the mouth. Biopsy is mandatory and histopathology is suggestive the thyroid must be adequately investigated. This is another 'worthwhile' syndrome.

Orofacial–digital syndrome is one of the many CLP syndromes, all of which are associated with hypodontia (laterals especially) and supernumeraries. This one has finger abnormalities as well.

Papillon–Lefevre syndrome is palmoplantar hyperkeratosis and juvenile periodontitis, which affects both 1° and 2° dentition. Normal dental

development occurs until the appearance of the hyperkeratosis of t
palms and soles, then simultaneously an aggressive gingivitis and periodo
titis begin. The mechanism is not well understood.

Patterson–Brown–Kelly syndrome (Plummer–Vinson syndrome) is the occu
rence of dysphagia, microcytic hypochromic anaemia, koilonychia (spoo
shaped nails), and angular cheilitis. The dysphagia is due to a post-crico
web, usually a membrane on the anterior oesophageal wall, which is pr
malignant. The koilonychia and angular cheilitis are 2° to the anaemia b
may be presenting symptoms. The main affected group are middle-ag
women, and correction of the anaemia may both relieve symptoms a
prevent malignant progression of the web.

Peutz–Jeghers syndrome is an autosomal dominant condition of melano
pigmentation of skin (especially peri-oral skin) and mucosa, and intestir
polyposis. These polyps, unlike those of the Gardener syndrome, ha
no particular propensity to malignant change, being hamartomatous, and a
found in the small intestine. They may, however, cause intussusception
other forms of gut obstruction. Ovarian tumours are sometimes associat
with the condition (10% woman with Peutz–Jeghers).

Progeria is probably a collagen abnormality. It causes dwarfism and pr
mature ageing. Characteristic facial appearance occurs due to a dispropo
tionately small face with mandibular retrognathia and a beak-like no:
creating an unforgettable appearance; death occurs in the mid-teens.

Ramsay Hunt syndrome is a lower motor neurone facial palsy, with vesic
on the same side in the pharynx, external auditory canal, and on the fac
It is thought to be due to herpes zoster of the geniculate ganglion.

Reiter syndrome Consists of arthritis, urethritis, and conjunctivitis. The
are frequently oral lesions, which resemble benign migratory glossitis
appearance but affect other parts of the mouth. The condition is probal
an unwanted effect of an immune response to a low-grade pathoge
however, some still believe it to be a sexually transmitted disease, althou
there is no hard evidence for this.

Robin sequence Named after Pierre Robin (and mistakenly called Pier
Robin syndrome at times). This is micrognathia, cleft palate, and glo
optosis. Huge number of associated anomalies. Catch-up growth occurs

Romberg syndrome (hemifacial atrophy) consists of progressive atrophy
the soft tissues of half the face, associated with contralateral Jacksoni
epilepsy and trigeminal neuralgia. Rarely, half the body may be affected
starts in the first decade and lasts ~3 yrs before it becomes quiescent.

Sicca syndrome (primary Sjögren syndrome) is xerostomia and kerat
conjunctivitis sicca, i.e. dry mouth and dry eyes. There is an ↑ risk of dev
oping parotid lymphoma with this condition. Interestingly, although Sic
syndrome has certain serological abnormalities in common with system
connective tissue disorders such as rheumatoid arthritis, it does not ha
any of the symptomatology (unlike Sjögren syndrome).

Sjögren syndrome (secondary Sjögren syndrome) In addition to dry ey
and dry mouth this has both the serology and symptomatology of an aut
immune condition, usually rheumatoid arthritis, but sometimes SI

temic sclerosis, or primary biliary cirrhosis. Actual swelling of the salivary nds is relatively uncommon and late-onset swelling of the parotids may ald the presence of a lymphoma.

vens–Johnson syndrome   A severe version of erythema multiforme, a cocutaneous condition that is probably autoimmune in nature and preciped particularly by drugs. Classical signs are the target lesions, concentric rings which especially affect the hands and feet. Stevens–Johnson synome is said to be present when the condition is particularly severe, and ssociated with fever and multiple mucosal involvement. Viral infections, herpes simplex, are the second commonest cause.

:kler syndrome   Perhaps the commonest *syndrome* associated with cleft ate (20%). Consists of flat mid-face, cleft palate, myopia, retinal detachnt, hearing loss (80%), and arthropathy. 30% of Robin sequence patients ve Stickler syndrome, ∴ examine eyes.

rge–Weber anomalad   is due to a hamartomatous angioma affecting upper part of the face, which may extend intracranially. There may be ociated convulsions, hemiplegia (on the contralateral side of the body), intellectual impairment. The risks of surgery are obvious.

acher–Collins syndrome (mandibulofacial dysostosis)   Basically involves ects in structures derived from the first branchial arch. It is inherited as autosomal dominant trait with variable expressivity, and consists of wnward-sloping (antimongoloid slant) palpebral fissures, hypoplastic lar complexes, mandibular retrognathia with a high gonial angle, deformed nas, hypoplastic air sinuses, colobomas in the outer third of the eye, middle and inner ear hypoplasia (and hence deafness). 30% have cleft ates and 25% have an unusual tongue-like projection of hair pointing vards the cheek. Most have *completely normal intellectual function*, ich may be missed because they are deaf and 'funny-looking kids' (how uld you like to be called a funny-looking dentist/doctor?). These people y well miss out on fulfilling their potential because of society's (and ne professionals') attitude to deformity. This syndrome is a prime indiion for corrective craniofacial surgery.

tter syndrome   is unilateral deafness, pain in the mandibular division of trigeminal nerve, ipsilateral immobility of the palate, and trismus, due invasion of the lateral wall of the nasopharynx by malignant tumour. rygopalatine fossa syndrome is a similar condition where the first and ond divisions of the trigeminal are affected.

Recklinghausen neurofibromatosis/syndrome   Multiple neurofibromas h skin pigmentation, skeletal abnormalities, CNS involvement, and a disposition to malignancy are the basics of this syndrome. It undergoes osomal dominant transmission and has a large and varied number of nifestations. Lesions of the face can be particularly disfiguring.

Useful information and addresses

Tooth notation

FDI

Permanent teeth

R	18 17 16 15 14 13 12 11	21 22 23 24 25 26 27 28	L
	48 47 46 45 44 43 42 41	31 32 33 34 35 36 37 38	

Deciduous teeth

R	55 54 53 52 51	61 62 63 64 65	L
	85 84 83 82 81	71 72 73 74 75	

Zsigmondy–Palmer, Chevron, or Set Square system

Permanent teeth

R	8 7 6 5 4 3 2 1	1 2 3 4 5 6 7 8	L
	8 7 6 5 4 3 2 1	1 2 3 4 5 6 7 8	

Deciduous teeth

R	e d c b a	a b c d e	L
	e d c b a	a b c d e	

Because of the difficulties of including the grid notation in written documents it is common practice to indicate the quadrant by abbreviating the arch and side. Thus the upper right second premolar is UR5 and likewise the lower left second deciduous molar is LLE.

European

Permanent teeth

R	8+7+6+5+4+3+2+1+	+1+2+3+4+5+6+7+8	L
	8−7−6−5−4−3−2−1−	−1−2−3−4−5−6−7−8	

Deciduous teeth

R	05+04+03+02+01+	+01+02+03+04+05	L
	05−04−03−02−01−	−01−02−03−04−05	

American

Permanent teeth

R	1 2 3 4 5 6 7 8	9 10 11 12 13 14 15 16	L
	32 31 30 29 28 27 26 25	24 23 22 21 20 19 18 17	

Deciduous teeth

R	A B C D E	F G H I J	L
	T S R Q P	O N M L K	

Some qualifications in Medicine and Dentistry

BA	Bachelor of Arts
BC/BCh/BS	Bachelor of Surgery
BChD/BDS	Bachelor of Dental Surgery
BM	Bachelor of Medicine
DDPH	Diploma in Dental Public Health
DDR	Diploma in Dental Radiology
DDS/DDSc	Doctor of Dental Surgery/Science
DGDP	Diploma in General Dental Practice
DOrth	Diploma in Orthodontics
DPhil	Doctor of Philosophy
DRD	Diploma in Restorative Dentistry
DSc	Doctor of Science
FDS	Fellowship in Dental Surgery
FFD	Fellow in Faculty of Dental Surgery
FFGDP	Diploma of Fellowship in General Dental Practic
FRCGP	Fellow of Royal College of General Practitioners
FRCP	Fellow of Royal College of Physicians
FRCS	Fellow of Royal College of Surgeons
LDS	Licentiate in Dental Surgery
MBBCh/MBChB	Bachelor of Medicine and Bachelor of Surgery
MCCD	Membership in Clinical Community Dentistry
MCDH	Master of Community Dental Health
MD	Doctor of Medicine
MDS	Master of Dental Surgery
MDentSci/MDSc	Master of Dental Science
MFD	Member of Faculty of Dentistry
MFDS	Member of the Faculty of Dental Surgery
MFGDP	Diploma of Membership of Faculty of General Dental Practitioners (UK)
MGDS	Diploma of Membership in General Dental Surge
MOrth	Membership in Orthodontics
MPhil	Master of Philosophy
MRCGP	Member of Royal College of General Practitione
MRCS	Member of Royal College of Surgeons
MSc	Master of Science
NVQ	National Vocational Qualification
PhD	Doctor of Philosophy

Bur numbering systems

Maximum diameter of bur head	ISO	UK		
		Round	Inverted cone	Flat fissu
0.6	006	$\frac{1}{2}$	$\frac{1}{2}$	
0.8	008	1	1	$\frac{1}{2}$
0.9	009			1
1.0	010	2	2	2
1.2	012	3	3	3
1.4	014	4	4	4
1.6	016	5	5	5
1.8	018	6	6	6
2.1	021	7	7	7
2.3	023	8	8	8
2.5	025	9	9	9
2.7	027	10	10	10
2.9	029	11		11
3.1	031	12		12

File sizes (for endodontic therapy)

Size	Tip diameter	ISO colour
08	0.08	grey
10	0.10	purple
15	0.15	white
20	0.20	yellow
25	0.25	red
30	0.30	blue
35	0.35	green
40	0.40	black
45	0.45	white
50	0.50	yellow
55	0.55	red
60	0.60	blue
70	0.70	green
80	0.80	black
90	0.90	white
100	1.00	yellow
110	1.10	red
120	1.20	blue
130	1.30	green
140	1.40	black

Wire gauges

Size on wire gauge	Diameter	
	Imperial (inches)	Metric (mm)
14	0.080	2.0
19	0.040	1.0
20	0.036	0.9
21	0.032	0.8
22	0.028	0.7
23	0.024	0.6
24	0.022	0.55
25	0.020	0.5
26	0.018	0.45
27	0.0164	0.4
28	0.0148	0.37
29	0.0136	0.35
30	0.0124	0.3

Passing exams

Preparation   First, there is unfortunately no substitute for the sheer har
work of revising, and to have a chance of being adequate this should sta
well before the exam. Beware of those who try to impress by saying the
have passed every exam, first time, having only started revising the nigh
before. These people are not super-intelligent (in fact, their behaviou
suggests the reverse) they have probably only been lucky ... to date!

Equally well, the human brain is not a computer and revising for hour
day in day out, could result in 'burn-out'. Each person needs to find the
own method, but a break of 5–10 min every hour and a complete hour c
after 3 hours' work, has succeeded for others.

It is important to be sure that you are revising the correct material 1
sufficient depth. One way of ensuring this is to go over past questions.
some are tackled under exam conditions, this also gives practice in exam
technique.

Immediate pre-exam period   If your nerve is strong enough it is prob
ably wise to stop working 2–3 days before the exams start and have a res
doing something that you enjoy. Most people baulk at this suggestion, bu
see the logic as of a marathon runner resting before an important race
Studying the night before is akin to an élite runner going out the nigh
before the Olympic marathon and running 26.2 miles just to make sure h
can cover the distance.

Written exams   It is important to know beforehand how many questior
you have to answer and $\therefore$ how long can be spent on each. Do not b
tempted to overrun. Spend a few minutes deciding which questions t
answer and in what order. It is better to tackle your best question secon
thus allowing the butterflies to settle. Read each question carefully, ar
periodically stop to check that you are answering the question set, not th
one you'd like to answer. A rough plan helps to produce a more logic
essay and provides an *aide-mémoire* in case of panic halfway throug
Write neatly.

Multiple choice exams   are beloved of examiners, but feared by candidate
If they involve –ve marking, a careful approach is required for success.
1 Do the necessary revision; it is impossible to waffle hopefully round th
   subject in a multiple choice exam.
2 Go through the paper, only answering those questions of which you
   are completely sure.
3 Count up the number you have answered and see if it is over the pass
   mark. If yes, stop there.
4 If you have not answered enough, go back through the paper, only
   answering those questions which you are nearly sure of. DO NOT loc
   at the questions you have previously answered, as usually your first
   instinct is right.
5 Stop there, as the next step is to guess—which is usually
   counter-productive.

Clinical exams   Turn up neatly dressed, armed with a clean white coa
Although some patients are regularly wheeled out for exams, many will b
almost as nervous about what is going to happen as you are. Many patien

can give helpful hints towards their diagnosis and management if asked the right questions. Some candidates spend the whole of their time with the patient, scribbling furiously, and do not leave themselves any time to think. Present the patient to the examiners in a logical fashion, i.e. starting with their name and age, not the radiographs. Check the medical history.

Objective structured clinical examinations (OSCEs) have been developed to evaluate the clinical competence of medical and dental students in both undergraduate and postgraduate curricula. This type of exam is so-called because they should be:

Objective—independent and competent examiners should have agreed what skills are being examined, with agreed marking scales.

Structured—have agreed criteria (in advance) for the correct answer for each element of the exam.

Clinical—to test clinical and practical competence, including communication and problem-solving skills.

Examination—this may include evaluation of written responses &/or observation by an examiner.

They usually comprise a series of stations, which each test a different clinical skill. A set time is allocated to each station. The clinical proficiencies tested may include taking a history from a 'patient' (increasingly actors are used rather than actual patients), and establishing a diagnosis and psychomotor skills. Students may be evaluated by an examiner, who observes and marks their responses and actions at a particular station.

GOOD LUCK!

Web-based learning

Definitions
Web-based learning is one type of distance education that ↓ the barriers of time and space to learning—'anytime, anywhere learning'. It is a component of the broader term 'e-learning', defined as: the use of electronic technology and media to deliver, support, and enhance teaching and learning. This encompasses the Internet, Intranet, and the World Wide Web.

In education, the Web is increasingly used both to support lectures (printed course materials) and as a means of delivering online learning programmes. These may be interactive, with online activities (such as self-assessments), animations, and simulations, which can be more enjoyable and meaningful to learners. Discussion forums via e-mail, video-conferencing, and live lectures (videostreaming) are all possible through the Web. Another advantage is that Web pages and a virtual learning environment may contain hyperlinks to other parts of the Web, thus enabling access to a vast amount of Web-based information.

Glossary
e-conferencing   Use of online presentations and discussion forums (in real time or stored as downloadable files on a website) so that participants need not travel.

Hyperlinks   Links in web pages that enable the user to access another web page (either on the same or a different site) with just one mouse click.

Internet   Global network of computers divided into subsets (e.g. the Web or e-mail systems). Computers are linked to the Internet via host computers, which link to other computers via dial-up (e.g. via a modem) and network connections

Internet service provider (ISP)   Links the home user to the Internet. The ISP maintains a network of personal computers that are permanently connected to the Internet.

Intranet   A network of computers that share information, usually within an organization. Access normally requires a password and is limited to a defined range of users, e.g. the NHS.

Managed learning environment   Provides an integrated function, with administrative tools such as student records, and links with other management information systems.

Search engines (such as Lycos, Google)   Can be used to find information.

Videostreaming   The process by which video images are able to be stored on and downloaded from the Web. This might be done in real time (such as a conference) or the images may be used asynchronously.

Virtual learning environment   A set of electronic teaching and learning tools. Principal components can map a curriculum, track student activity, and provide online student support and electronic communication

World Wide Web (WWW)   Use of the Internet to present various types of information. Websites or home pages may be accessed with the aid o a browser program (such as Netscape Communicator or Microsoft Internet Explorer). All such programmes use HTML (hypertext mark-up language).

Advantages

Information in different formats, i.e. audio, visual.
Provides a central and comprehensive way of delivering course materials.
Resources can be made available from any location and at any time.
Can widen access, e.g. to part-time, mature, or work-based students.
Can encourage more independent and active learning.
Can provide a useful source of supplementary materials to conventional programmes.

Disadvantages

Access to computers can be difficult, especially for postgraduates.
Learners find it frustrating if they cannot access graphics, images, and video-clips because of non-user-friendly software and limitations in the hardware.
It is difficult to write good material that maintains interest and motivation.
Personal passwords needed to access selected sites.
Information varies in quality and accuracy. Requires guidance, or use that is limited to accredited sites, e.g. official organizations or education establishments.
Potentially, extremely non-productive and time-wasting, depending on one's learning style.

Summary

At undergraduate level e-learning is becoming engrained in the curriculum. At postgraduate level it has great potential for continuing professional development (CPD), and for providing resources, online logbooks, and competency assessments. At present, however, it is limited by current software and variable access to hardware. Also, newer technologies are not necessarily better (or worse) for teaching or learning than older technologies, just different. Therefore, it is necessary to pick and choose to find what is right for you.

Dentistry and the World Wide Web

As anyone who has surfed the Web will know, it is a big world out there and new websites are constantly appearing; ∴ the following is at best a sampler of interesting sites. If you have time on your hands then type the subject that interests you into a search engine … and stand back. For a more academic approach seek the advice of the librarian in your local hospital, as they are often only too keen to help you find reputable sites and sources of information. Happy surfing!

Acryonyms: **www.nottingham.ac.uk/cpcme/edu/**
American Dental Association: **www.ada.org**
Bad Breath Research: **www.tau.ac.il/~melros/**
British Association of Dental Nurses: **www.badn.org.uk**
British Association of Dental Therapists: **www.badt.org.uk**
British Dental Association: **www.bda-dentistry.org.uk**
British Dental Health Foundation: **www.dentalhealth.org.uk**
British Dental Hygienists Association: **www.bdha.org.uk**
British Medical Association: **www.bma.org.uk**
British National Formulary: **www.bnf.org**
British Society for CAL in Dentistry: **www.derweb.co.uk/asp/contacts.asp**
British Society for Disability and Oral Health (BSDH): **www.bsdh.org.uk**
British Society of Paediatric Dentistry (BSPD): **www.bda.org/bspd**
Chief Dental Officer: **www.dh.gov.uk/cdo**
Chief Medical Officer: **www.dh.gov.uk/cmo**
Centre for Reviews and Dissemination: **www.york.ac.uk/inst/crd/**
Clinical Dental Technicians Association: **www.cdta.org.uk**
Clinical evidence: a compendium of research findings on clinical questions: **www.clinicalevidence.org**
Cochrane Collaboration: **www.cochrane.co.uk**
Committee of Postgraduate Dental Deans and Directors: **www.copdend.org.uk**
Conference of Postgraduate Medical Deans: **www.copmed.org.uk**
Confederation of Dental Employers (CODE): **www.derweb.co.uk/code**
Dentanet: **www.dentanet.org.uk**
Dental Practice Managers Association: **www.derweb.co.uk/bdpma**
Dental systematic reviews: **www.cochrane-oral.man.ac.uk/**
DERWeb (Dental Education resources on the web): **www.derweb.co.uk**
Department of Health: **www.dh.gov.uk**
Evidence-based courses, links, and guides: **www.shef.ac.uk/scharr/ir/scebm.html**
General Dental Council: **www.gdc-uk.org**
Kings Fund: **www.kingsfund.org.uk**
Institute of Healthcare Management: **www.ihm.org.uk**
National Counselling Service for Sick Doctors: **www.ncssd.org.uk**
National Electronic Library for Health (NeLH): **www.nelh.nhs.uk/**
National Institute for Clinical Excellence: **www.nice.org.uk**
Royal College of Surgeons of Edinburgh: **www.rcsed.ac.uk**
Royal College of Surgeons of England: **www.rcseng.ac.uk**
Royal College of Physicians and Surgeons of Glasgow: **www.rcpsglasg.ac.uk**

Scottish Intercollegiate Guidelines Network (SIGN): **www.sign.ac.uk**
TRIP database: **www.tripdatabase.com**
Voluntary Services Overseas: **www.vso.org.uk**

For when it all gets a bit stressful . . . try the following

www.bbc.co.uk/weather
www.bored.com
www.extremeironing.com
www.lastminute.com
www.lovelaughs.com
www.multimap.com
www.oofun.com
www.upmystreet.com

NB All these addresses were correct at the time of going to press.

Useful addresses

Barts and the London Dental School, Queen Mary's School of Medicine and Dentistry, Turner Street, London E1 2AD. Tel: 020 7882 5555.
Birmingham Dental School, St Chad's Queensway, Birmingham B4 6NN. Tel: 0121 236 8611.
Bristol Dental School, Lower Maudlin Street, Bristol BS1 2LY. Tel: 0117 923 0050.
British Dental Association, 64 Wimpole Street, London W1M 8AL. Tel: 020 7935 0875.
British Dental Health Foundation, Smile House, 2 East Union Street, Rugby CV22 6AJ. Tel: 0870 770 4000.
British Library, Boston Spa, Wetherby, N. Yorkshire LS23 7BQ. Tel: 0870 444 1500.
British Medical Association, BMA House, Tavistock Square, London WC18 9JT. Tel: 020 7387 4499.
Cardiff Dental School, Heath Park, Cardiff CF4 4XY. Tel: 01222 755944.
Cork Dental School, John Redmond Street, Wilton, Cork, Eire. Tel: 00 353 2154 5100.
Dental Defence Union, 230 Blackfriars Road, London SE1 8PJ. Tel: 020 7202 1500.
Dental Practice Board, Eastbourne, East Sussex BN20 8AD. Tel: 01323 433 550.
Dental Protection, 33 Cavendish Square, London W1G OPS. Tel: 020 7399 1400.
Dental Vocational Training Authority, Masters House, Temple Grove, Compton Place Road, Eastbourne BN20 8AD.
Department of Health, Chief Dental Officer, Richmond House, 79 Whitehall, London SW1A 2NL.
Dublin Dental School, Dublin University, Trinity College, Dublin 2, Eire. Tel: 00 353 1612 7200.
Dundee Dental School, Park Place, Dundee DD1 4HN. Tel: 01382 660111.
Edinburgh Dental Institute, 4th Floor, Lauriston Building, Lauriston Place, Edinburgh EH3 9YW. Tel: 0131 536 4970.
European Union of Dentists, 138 Chirsh Hill, Loughton, Essex. IG10 1LJ. Tel: 020 8508 4205.
Faculty of Dental Surgery, The Royal College of Surgeons of England, 35–43 Lincoln's Inn Fields, London WC1A 3PE. Tel: 020 7869 6810.
Faculty of General Dental Practitioners (UK), The Royal College of Surgeons of England, 35–43 Lincoln's Inn Fields, London WC2A 3PE. Tel: 020 7312 6671.
FDI World Dental Federation, 7 Carlisle Street, London W1V 5RG. Tel: 020 7935 7852.
General Dental Council, 37 Wimpole Street, London W1M 8DQ. Tel: 020 7887 3800.
General Dental Practitioners' Association, Victoria House, Victoria Road, Barnsley S70 2BB. Tel: 01226 299020.
Glasgow Dental School, 378 Sauchiehall Street, Glasgow G2 3JX. Tel: 0141 211 9600.

KT Dental Institute, Guy's Tower, Kings College London SE1 9RT. Tel: 020 7955 5000.

Institute of Dental Surgery, Eastman Dental Hospital, 256 Gray's Inn Road, London WC1X 8LD. Tel: 020 7915 1000.

Leeds Dental Institute, Dental and Medical Building, Clarendon Way, Leeds LS2 9LU. Tel: 0113 2440111.

Liverpool Dental School, Pembroke Place, PO Box 147, Liverpool L69 3BX. Tel: 0151 706 2000.

London School of Hygiene and Tropical Medicine, Keppel Street, London WC1E 7HT. Tel: 020 7636 8636.

Manchester Dental School, University Dental Hospital of Manchester, Bridgebridge Street, Manchester M15 6FH. Tel: 0161 276 1234.

Medical and Dental Defence Union of Scotland, 120 Blythswood Street, Glasgow G2 4EA. Tel: 0141 2215858.

Medical and Dental Retirement Advisory Service, Hartlands House, Primett Road, Stevenage SG1 3EE. Tel: 01438 742727.

National Advice Centre for Postgraduate Dental Education, The Royal College of Surgeons of England, 35–43 Lincoln's Inn Fields, London, WC2A 3PE. Tel: 0207 809 6804.

National Oral Health Promotion Group, 22 Leighton Close, Leamington Spa CV22 7BW. Tel: 01926 887 381.

National Radiological Protection Board, Cookridge, Leeds LS16 6RW. Tel: 0113 269 9643.

Newcastle Dental School, Framlington Place, Newcastle upon Tyne NE2 4BW. Tel: 0191 222 8347.

Postgraduate Medical & Dental Education, 33 Millman Street, London WC1N 3EJ. Tel: 020 7692 3184.

Queen's University of Belfast, School of Dentistry, Grosvenor Road, Belfast BT12 6BP. Tel: +44 01232 240503.

Royal College of Physicians and Surgeons of Glasgow, 234–242 St Vincent Street, Glasgow G2 5RJ. Tel: 0141 221 6072.

Royal College of Surgeons of England, 35–43 Lincoln's Inn Fields, London WC2A 3PE. Tel: 020 7405 3474.

Royal College of Surgeons of Edinburgh, Nicolson Street, Edinburgh EH8 9DW. Tel: 0131 527 1608.

Royal College of Surgeons of Ireland, 123 St. Stephen's Green, Dublin 2, Eire. Tel: 00 353 1402 2239.

Royal Society of Medicine, 1 Wimpole Street, London W1G 0AE. Tel: 020 7290 2900.

Scottish Dental Practice Board, Trinity Park House, South Trinity Road, Edinburgh EH2 1EL. Tel: 0131 552 6255.

Sheffield Dental School, Charles Clifford Dental Hospital, Wellesley Road, Sheffield S10 2SZ. Tel: 0114 271 7801.

The Fluoridation Society, Liverpool Dental School, Liverpool, L69 3BN. Tel: 0151 706 5216.

Women in Dentistry, 5 Sudbury Court Drive, Harrow, Middlesex HA1 3TZ. Tel: 020 8904 7933.

World Health Organization, Avenue Appia, CH-1211, Geneva 27, Switzerland. Tel: 022-91 3453.

Index